Cornwall Dermatology Research.

J. Krutmann   H. Hönigsmann   C. A. Elmets   P. R. Bergstresser (Eds.)

Dermatological Phototherapy and Photodiagnostic Methods

Springer
Berlin
Heidelberg
New York
Barcelona
Budapest
Hong Kong
London
Milano
Paris
Singapure
Tokyo

J. Krutmann   H. Hönigsmann
C. A. Elmets   P. R. Bergstresser (Eds.)

Dermatological Phototherapy and Photodiagnostic Methods

With 104 Figures, 50 in Color, and 71 Tables

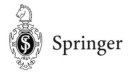 Springer

Prof. Dr. Jean Krutmann
Clinical and Experimental
Photodermatology
Heinrich-Heine-Universität
Moorenstraße 5
D-40225 Düsseldorf
Germany

Prof. Dr. Helmut Hönigsmann
Abt. für spezielle Dermatologie
und Umweltdermatosen
Universitäts-Hautklinik AKH
Währinger Gürtel 18 – 20
A-1090 Wien
Austria

Craig A. Elmets, M. D.
Department of Dermatology
University of Alabama at
Birmingham SDB 67
Birmingham, AL 35294-0007
USA

Paul R. Bergstresser, M.D.
Department of Dermatology
UT Southwestern Medical
Center
5323 Harry Hines Blvd.
Dallas, TX 75390-9069
USA

ISBN 3-540-67789-5 Springer-Verlag Berlin Heidelberg New York

Library of Congress Cataloging-in-Publication Data
Dermatological phototherapy and photodiagnostic methods / J. Krutmann ...
[et al.] eds. p. cm.
Includes bibliographical references and index.
  ISBN 3540677895 (alk. paper)
  1. Skin-Disease-Phototherapy. 2. Skin-Diseases-Photochemotherapy.
  I. Krutmann, Jean, 1959 –
  RL120.P48 D47 2001
  616.5'0631-dc21

Springer-Verlag Berlin Heidelberg New York
a member of Bertelsmann Springer Science + Business Media GmbH

© Springer-Verlag Berlin Heidelberg 2001
Printed in Germany

The use of general descriptive names, registered names, trademarks, etc. in this
publication does not imply, even in the absence of a specific statement, that such
names are exempt from the relevant protective laws and regulations and therefore free for general use.

Product Liability: The publisher cannot guarantee the accuracy of any information about dosage and application thereof contained in this book. In every individual case the user must check such information by consulting the relevant literature.

Cover design: design & production, Heidelberg
Typesetting: Mitterweger & Partner, Plankstadt
Printed on acid free paper   SPIN 10773859   22/3130   – 5 4 3 2 1 0 –

This book is dedicated to:
Carl and Claudia Krutmann,
Laurie, Joshua, Michael,
and David Elmets

Foreword

One form of what was called heliotherapy 2000 years ago consisted of ingestion of an infusion (boiled extract) derived from a weed growing in the Nile Delta, *Ammi majus* L., followed by exposure to the Egyptian sun for the treatment of vitiligo, a disorder that was a serious disfigurement in this population with brown and black skin colored population. This crude treatment was the very earliest form of what is now called PUVA photochemotherapy, a treatment for psoriasis, vitiligo, and 34 other diseases and that uses the same chemical, psoralen, derived from the same plant source, *Ammi majus* L., and followed by exposure to specially designed computerized UVA irradiators.

Phototherapy in the practice of dermatology was, in fact, not an efficacious and practical therapeutic option until as late as the mid-1970s, when lighting engineers, photophysicists, and dermatologists worked together to develop ultraviolet (UV) irradiators emitting high-intensity UVA. The UVA irradiators were designed to deliver uniform irradiation from fluorescent tubes lining a vertical cylinder in which the patient stands upright. The dose-delivery was computerized, and the doses were not designated in minutes but in joules (UVA) or in millijoules (UVB). The result was what has been termed photochemotherapy, which is defined as the use of chemicals that are "activated" by exposure of the molecules to radiant energy. The first example of photochemotherapy was the oral ingestion of a photoactive chemical, psoralen, followed by exposure to long-wave ultraviolet, UVA. The acronym PUVA was created and the modality represented the first use of light and drug together for a beneficial effect in humans.

The introduction of PUVA was the driving force in the mid-1970s that sparked a whole new series of discoveries during the next two decades, i.e., newly created high-intensity ultraviolet sources: UVA (320–400 nm) Sylvania of the USA and narrowband UVB (311–312 nm) Philips of Holland which has now replaced broadband UVB, as the first-line therapy for psoriasis, and more recently UVA-1 (340–400 nm). These new effective therapies have been a boon particularly for patients with generalized psoriasis providing efficacious ambulatory treatments but avoiding the systemic problems of methotrexate and cyclosporin.

The successful use of the new ultraviolet techniques for the treatment of disease was the "flywheel" for the development of a new sub-specialty called photomedicine, which encompasses all of the applications of the diagnosis and treatment of photo-induced disorders as well as the use of the new modalities such as photodynamic therapy for therapy of skin tumors and other diseases. There is now a Photomedicine Society and specialized journals of photodermatology.

We should be aware that the modern methods of phototherapy and photochemotherapy are part of a whole new discipline requiring special equipment and special knowledge of photophysics and photochemistry, and there are at present a limited number of phototherapy centers in the world. In a manner of speaking, present-day phototherapy is comparable to the use of X-radiation therapy in dermatology with special hardware, specific indications, the selection of patients, and the need for careful and precise dosimetry.

The practicing dermatologist needs to be educated to correctly use these sophisticated techniques, which have been evolved by large (over 5,000 patients using prospective randomized clinical trials in the United States and Europe), beginning in 1974. Alas, in the last two decades, although there was a new impetus for phototherapy, there has not been enough specialized training in phototherapy. Therefore, this updated practical manual is welcome. In this impressive volume, the indications and methodology of these various light sources are presented by an excellent international cadre of dermatologists experienced in the use of these various modalities.

It is fitting that one of the editors is from Vienna because the Dermatology Department of the Vienna General Hospital was the second in the world to use PUVA in 1975. This detailed and up-to-date practical monograph is a "must" for any group doing phototherapy or contemplating a phototherapy unit. It is also a handy instruction manual for training personnel (technicians and residents) in phototherapy.

Boston, USA, July 2000

Thomas B. Fitzpatrick, M.D. Ph.D.

Preface

During the past 25 years, phototherapy has greatly influenced treatment concepts in dermatology. Consequently, photomedicine has developed from empiricism into one of the most exciting fields in biomedical research. Studies on the effects of visible and ultraviolet radiation on skin have led to a fruitful collaboration between basic scientists and clinicians. Thus, phototherapy may be regarded as a prime example of applied skin biology.

UV radiation has been used for decades in the management of common skin diseases such as psoriasis and atopic dermatitis. More recently, the introduction of selective spectra in the UVB and UVA range such as narrowband UVB and UVA-1 phototherapy, as well as the inclusion of new indications, has much stimulated the interest in photodermatology. Visible light in combination with photosensitizers is currently in use for diagnosis and treatment of selected tumors. Extracorporeal photochemotherapy has proven to be effective beyond dermatology, in particular, in transplantation medicine.

Most phototherapeutic regimens have been developed empirically and without knowledge about the biological mechanisms involved. Recent progress in the understanding of basic photobiological principles has made phototherapy more effective and, even more importantly, safer at the same time.

The present handbook takes this dualism into account by presenting clinical information on the background of current knowledge of photobiological principles. Besides the detailed description of photo- and photochemotherapy for selected skin diseases, this volume contains standardized test protocols for photodermatoses and the diagnosis of skin tumors.

There exists a variety of phototherapeutic modalities, and clinicians can now select the therapy of choice. A specific disease can thus be treated with the regimen that fits best the particular situation of a given patient. Therefore, the major focus of this volume is on the use of different treatment modalities for a specific disease. The clinically oriented chapters are supplemented by practical guidelines for phototherapy that have proven successful over many years.

The leading experts have contributed to this project. Most of the authors are not only experienced clinical photodermatolo-

gists but also internationally renowned experts in basic photobiological research.

We are very grateful to all authors for their excellent contributions. We hope that this monograph will serve as a state-of-
the-art reference for "Dermatological Phototherapy and Photodiagnostic Methods" in daily practice, clinical settings, and
research.

Kitzbühel, Spring 2000

Jean Krutmann
Herbert Hönigsmann
Craig A. Elmets
Paul R. Bergstresser

Contents

III Special Phototherapeutic Modalities

IV Photoprotection in daily practice

V Photodiagnostic procedures in daily practice

VI Appendix

List of Contributors

Christoph Abels, M.D.
Klinik und Poliklinik für
Dermatologie, Universität
Regensburg,
Franz-Josef-Strauß-Allee 11,
93052 Regensburg,
Germany

Claudia Alge, M.D.
Abteilung für spezielle
Dermatologie und Umwelt-
dermatosen,
Universitäts-Hautklinik AKH,
Währinger Gürtel 18–20,
1090 Vienna,
Austria

Paul R. Bergstresser, M.D.
Department of Dermatology,
UT Southwestern Medical
Center,
5323 Harry Hines Blvd.,
Dallas, TX 75390–9069,
USA

Reinhard Breit, M.D.
Theodor-Körner-Strasse 6,
82049 Pullach,
Germany

Ponciano D. Cruz, Jr., M.D.
Department of Dermatology,
UT Southwestern Medical
Center, 5323 Harry Hines
Blvd., Dallas, TX
75390–9069,
USA

Craig Elmets, M.D.
Department of Dermatology,
University of Alabama
at Birmingham, SDB 67,
Birmingham,
AL 35294–0007, USA

Ludwig Endres, Ph.D.
Achheimstrasse 1a,
82319 Starnberg,
Germany

James Ferguson, M.D.
Photobiology Unit, Ninewells
Hospital,
Dundee, DD1 9S4, Scotland,
UK

Clemens Fritsch, M.D.
Hautklinik and Institut für
Physiologische Chemie I,
Heinrich-Heine-Universität
Düsseldorf,
Moorenstrasse 5, 40225
Düsseldorf, Germany

John Hawk, M.D.
Department of Environmental
Dermatology, St. Thomas
Hospital,
London SE1 7EH, UK

Peter Heald, M.D.
Department of Dermatology,
Yale University School of
Medicine,
333 Cedar Street, 501 LC1,
New Haven, CT 06520, USA

Erhard Hölzle, M.D.
Department of Dermatology
and Allergology,
City Hospital Oldenburg,
Dr.-Edenstrasse 10,
26133 Oldenburg,
Germany

Herbert Hönigsmann, M.D.
Abt. für spezielle Dermatolo-
gie und Umweltdermatosen,
Universitäts-Hautklinik AKH,
Währinger Gürtel 18 – 20,
1090 Vienna, Austria

Sigrid Karrer, M.D.
Klinik und Poliklinik
für Dermatologie,
Universität Regensburg,
Franz-Josef-Strauß-Allee 11,
93052 Regensburg,
Germany

Robert Knobler, M.D.
Department of Dermatology,
Division of Special and Envi-
ronmental Dermatology, Uni-
versity of Vienna Medical
School, Vienna General
Hospital – AKH,
Währinger Gürtel 18 – 20,
1090 Vienna,
Austria

Jean Krutmann, M.D.
Clinical and Experimental
Photodermatology,
Heinrich-Heine-University,
Moorenstrasse 5,
40225 Düsseldorf,
Germany

Michael Landthaler, M.D.
Universitäts-Hautklinik,
Franz-Josef-Strauß-Allee 11,
93053 Regensburg,
Germany

Kerstin Lang, M.D.
Universitäts-Hautklinik der
Heinrich-Heine-Universität,
Moorenstrasse 5,
40225 Düsseldorf,
Germany

Percy Lehmann, M.D.
Universitäts-Hautklinik der
Heinrich-Heine-Universität,
Moorenstrasse 5,
40225 Düsseldorf,
Germany

Henry W. Lim, M.D.
Department of Dermatology,
Henry Ford Hospital,
2799 W. Grand Blvd.,
Detroit, MI 48202 – 2689, USA

Renz Mang, M.D.
Clinical and Experimental
Photodermatology,
Heinrich-Heine-University,
Moorenstrasse 5,
40225 Düsseldorf,
Germany

Akimichi Morita, M.D., Ph.D.
Department of Dermatology,
Nagoya City University,
1-Kawasumi, Mizuho-cho,
Mizuho-ku,
Nagoya 467 – 8601, Japan

Warwick L. Morison, M.D.
10753 Falls Road,
Suite S – 355,
Lutherville, MD 21093,
USA

Norbert J. Neumann
Universitäts-Hautklinik der
Heinrich-Heine-Universität,
Moorenstrasse 5,
40225 Düsseldorf,
Germany

Wilfried H. G. Neuse, B.Sc.
Universitäts-Hautklinik,
Heinrich-Heine-Universität,
Moorenstrasse 5,
40225 Düsseldorf, Germany

Bernhard Ortel, M.D.
Wellmann 2,
50 Blossom Street,
Boston, MA 02114, USA

Amit Pandy, M.D.
Wellmann 2,
50 Blossom Street,
Boston, MA 02114, USA

Kristi J. Robson, M.D.
Department of Dermatology,
Henry Ford Health System,
Detroit, MI, USA

Anita Rütter, M.D.
Wilhelms-Universität
Münster,
Hautklinik,
Von-Esmarchstrasse 56,
48149 Münster, Germany

Thomas Ruzicka, M.D.
Heinrich-Heine-Universität
Düsseldorf,
Moorenstrasse 5,
40225 Düsseldorf, Germany

Klaus Werner Schulte, M.D.
Heinrich-Heine-Universität
Düsseldorf,
Moorenstrasse 5,
40225 Düsseldorf, Germany

Thomas Schwarz, M.D.
Hautklinik der Universität
Münster,
Von-Esmarchstrasse 56,
48149 Münster, Germany

Dr. med. Helger Stege, M.D.
Clinical and Experimental
Photodermatology,
Moorenstrasse 5,
40225 Düsseldorf, Germany

Rolf-Markus Szeimies, M.D.
Klinik und Poliklinik für
Dermatologie Regensburg,
Franz-Josef-Strauß-Allee 11,
93053 Regensburg, Germany

Adrian Tanew, M.D.
Universitätsklinik für Derma-
tologie, Abtlg. für Spezielle
Dermatologie und Umwelt-
dermatosen, Allgemeines
Krankenhaus der Stadt,
Währinger Gürtel 18 – 20,
1090 Vienna, Austria

Beatrix Volc-Platzer, M.D.
Division of Immunology,
Allergy and Infectious
Diseases, Department of
Dermatology,
University of Vienna Medical
School,
Währinger Gürtel 18 – 20,
1090 Vienna, Austria

Peter Wolf, M.D.
Universitätsklinik für Derma-
tologie und Venerologie,
Karl-Franzens-Universität,
Auerbruggerplatz 8,
8036 Graz, Austria

Anthony R. Young, Ph.D.
Photobiology Department,
St. John's Institute of Derma-
tology, Guy's King/St. Thomas
Hospital,
London SE1 7EH, UK

I Basic mechanisms in Photo(chemo)therapy

1 UV Radiation, Irradiation, Dosimetry

Ludwig Endres, Reinhard Breit

Contents

Concerning the Nature of Optical Radiation

The existence of invisible rays in sunlight was not known until the beginning of the nineteenth century. First in 1800, Friedrich Wilhelm Herschel was able to detect in the rainbow-colored solar spectrum, adjoining the red end, invisible rays that generated heat when they impinged on absorbent surfaces. Shortly thereafter, in 1801, Johann Wilhelm Ritter likewise discovered radiation at the other end of the visible spectrum as well, beyond the violet, which radiation was capable of initiating "intense chemical effects."

By reason of the detection processes and the geometric positions within the spectrum, it was accordingly an obvious idea to designate these two newly discovered radiation ranges as infrared (IR) and ultraviolet (UV) radiation respectively; in regard to the wavelengths, it would have been correct to refer to ultra-red and infraviolet.

But there were not yet any clear concepts concerning the nature of these types of radiation, their propagation, or, in particular, the manner in which light is able to generate effects. There were certainly various theories, the best known of these were the emanation theory of Isaac Newton, dating back to the year 1669, and the undulatory theory of Christiaan Huygens, dating back to 1677. Newton, in his theory, postulated that light consists of small particles, which, when they have been absorbed in material, were capable of generating the known effects. In contrast, Huygens took the view that light was a wave, which, just like a water wave, required a medium for its propagation. He named this medium the optical ether, which, in his opinion, was omnipresent, but was not detectable with the means available to him.

Each one of these theories was able to offer conclusive explanations for specified phenomena – Newton's for the radiation effects, Huygens' for the interference phenomena – but neither was capable of offering a total solution.

It is therefore understandable that these contradictory matters led to many discussions and attempts to set up a theory of light which was valid for all types of phenomena. However, for almost two centuries there were no further noteworthy findings in the state of knowledge on this matter.

The first decisive advance took place in 1871, when James Maxwell propounded an electromagnetic theory of light which inspired Heinrich Hertz to the experiments which, in 1888, led to the discovery of electrical oscillations. These results now furnished the proof that any electromagnetic radiation, thus including the complete optical radiation (light, UV and IR radiation), propagates in the manner of waves and that does not need any medium for this purpose. He found out, that all electromagnetic waves, independent from wavelength or frequency, propagate in the vacuum with the velocity of light, which was already known at that time. However, the attempts of to explain phenomena concerning the generation and absorption of these waves continued to be unsatisfactory.

The processes implemented in this connection were not established until the beginning of our century: In 1900, Max Planck published the radiation laws in which light is considered not as a steady process, but as a discontinuous sequence of small energy states, which are however not divisible any further. In 1902, Philipp Lenard discovered, in the course of investigations of the photoelectric effect, particular properties of light that led him to formulate an optical quantum hypothesis. And then in 1905, Albert Einstein was able to show that the experimental results of Lenard may be fully explained by the quantum theory of Planck.

Thus, beginning at this time, two theories, standing side by side with equal status, were necessary to provide a complete description of the behavior of electromagnetic waves; with regard to all questions concerned with the creation, absorption and effect of radiation, whether it be the visual process, the perception of heat, or the reactions to UV radiation, it was necessary to apply the laws of quantum theory, while the processes involved in the propagation of electromagnetic radiation and its behavior in optical systems could be described only by the wave theory.

Not until the second half of our century did new findings of quantum physics provide a connection between these two theories which, in a mathematical presentation, formed initial principles appertaining to a generally valid theory of radiation. Nevertheless, as so frequently occurs in modern physics, even when applying this model, all attempts at explanation go beyond the conceptual power of non-specialists for whom – although it is omnipresent – the manifestation of light continues, even nowadays, to be a mysterious process.

Characterization of Radiation

In spite of the very complicated interrelationships which, as briefly described above, underlie the various manifestations of electromagnetic rays, for the purpose of technical applications their behavior can be described with sufficient accuracy by just a few formulae. These concern on the one hand the features such as wavelength, frequency, photon energy, and spectral composition of a mixed radiation, while in the second main group statements are made which are concerned with the quantitative recording of the transferred radiation intensity and its spatial distribution.

Features of a Wave

Wavelength and Frequency

Electromagnetic radiation propagates in a undulatory form in which the shapes can differ to a wide degree. But mathematics can prove to us (Fourier analysis),

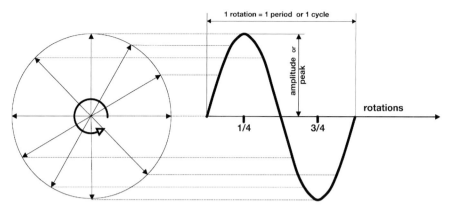

Fig. 1. Sinusoidal wave

that any shape can be reduced to a number of sinusoidal curves. So, for understanding the points treated in this chapter it is sufficient to consider only the properties of a simple sinusoidal wave.

In Figure 1 you can see how to create a sinusoidal wave. A rotating arrow describes a circle around a central point with its head. If transferring the several positions of the arrow head within a full turn to an axis divided in the rotation angles, you will perform a graph with a sinusoidal shape, exactly. Doing this way, the length of the arrow is corresponding to the maximum amplitude of the wave. The distance between the points at the beginning and the end of a full revolution is called one period or cycle of the wave.

If the arrow is rotating with a constant velocity, you can transfer the points of the arrow head to a time axis in the same manner. The higher the speed, the more cycles will be within a given time section (Fig. 2a).

At least, if you know the propagation velocity of a wave, you can transform the ordinate axis with a length segmentation (Fig. 2b).

With the numerical examples in Figure 2 we are now able to deduce the basic characterization of a sinusoidal wave.

Frequency means cycles per second (cps). In Figure 2a frequencies with 2, 4, and 8 cps have been plotted.

Wavelength is the length distance between the beginning and the end of a period. In Figure 2b wavelength with 0.5, 0.25 and 0.125 m have been plotted.

Propagation velocity is defined by the distance which covers an optional point P in a specified time. The dimension is m/s. In Figure 2 the propagation velocity of all three waves is 1 m/s.

From these quantities now it is possible to deduce the following correlations:

$$\text{frequency 1/s} = \frac{\text{propagation velocity m/s}}{\text{wavelength m}} \tag{1}$$

$$\text{wavelength m} = \frac{\text{propagation velocity m/s}}{\text{frequency 1/s}} \tag{2}$$

$$\text{propagation velocity m/s} = \text{wavelength m} \cdot \text{frequency 1/s} \tag{3}$$

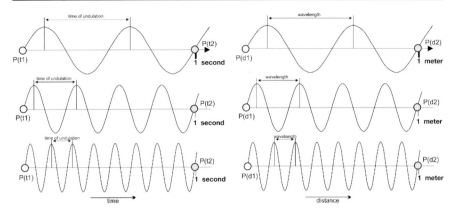

Fig. 2. Frequency and wavelength of a sinusoidal wave

This equations generally are valid for all types of electromagnetic waves, independent from frequency, wavelength, and intensity.

Optical radiation have shorter wavelength and higher frequencies as in the examples shown above. In order to avoid inconveniently large or small numbers, derived units are frequently used for the numerical characterization of electromagnetic waves. Thus, it is conventional to measure the wavelengths of light, UV, and IR radiation in the following units:

- Angstrom unit (AU) = 1×10^{-10} m
- Nanometer (nm = 1×10^{-9} m
- Micrometer (μ) = 1×10^{-6} m

To characterize frequencies it is common practice using the following units:

- Kilohertz (kHz)=$1 \times 10^{+3}$ cycles per second (cps or 1/s)
- Megahertz (MHz)=$1 \times 10^{+6}$ cps
- Gigahertz (GHz)=$1 \times 10^{+9}$ cps

Propagation Velocity

Any electromagnetic radiation energy propagates in the vacuum at the "velocity of light."

$$\text{Velocity of light } c = 299{,}792 \text{ km/s} \qquad (4)$$

The accentuation is on the word "vacuum." In all other cases, when the radiation enters a medium, the propagation velocity is reduced in accordance with the spectral refractive index n of the pertinent substance. For the velocities in different media see Table 1.

Normally these facts are without any influence for practice. But you can note: the propagation velocity in the earth's atmosphere differs so little from that in a vacuum that the difference in the vast majority of cases is negligible.

Formula 3, which states that the propagation velocity results from the product of frequency and wavelength, is valid too for radiation passing a medium. At a

Table 1. Velocity of light with a wavelength of 500 nm

Medium	Refractive index	Symbol	Velocity	Percentage of c
Vacuum	$n = 1$	c	= 299,792 km/s	
Air	$n = 1.0003$	c_{air}	= 299,690 km/s	→ 99.9 %
Water	$n = 1.33$	c_{water}	= 225,410 km/s	→ 75.2 %
Quartz glass	$n = 1.49$	$c_{qu.gl.}$	= 200,860 km/s	→ 67.0 %

reduced velocity, therefore, either the frequency or the wavelength must vary. Physics tells us that the frequency remains constant in all media and that the wavelength becomes shorter in proportion to the deduced velocity.

Hence, it would be more meaningful to characterize radiation by its frequency. Nevertheless, within the optical range, the characterization of the radiation by stating the wavelength in vacuum has become established, while within the range of the longer waves, the radio waves, stating the frequency is in most cases customary.

Photon Energy

Electromagnetic waves transport energy. The supporters of this energy are the photons. According to the Einstein relation, the energy E of a photon has a fixed relationship with the frequency v

$$E_{photon} = h \cdot v \text{ (with: } h = \text{Planck constant)}, \tag{5}$$

which, related to the wavelength in vacuum, may be written in numerical terms as follows:

$$E_{photon} = \frac{1.98 \cdot 10^{-19} \text{ watt} \cdot \text{seconds}}{\text{wavelength in nanometres}} \tag{6}$$

Another unit for the energy of radiation is the so-called electron-volt (eV). One eV corresponds to the acceleration that an electron experiences when it passes through the potential difference of 1 V in an electric field.

Since 1 watt second (W s)=1 joule (J)=0.624×10^{19} eV, it is also possible to write

$$E_{photon} = \frac{1240 \text{ electron-volts}}{\text{wavelength in nanometres}} \tag{7}$$

It is seen from this that the photon energy of electromagnetic radiation increases as the wavelength decreases; therefore: UV radiation has greater energy than visible light.

Classification of Electromagnetic Waves

The wavelengths of the electromagnetic spectrum cover the enormous range of roughly $10^{-16} - 10^7$ m. Accordingly, they subdivide into various divisions, which

Table 2. Overview of the electromagnetic spectrum

Designation	Wavelength	Frequency	Generation
Electric waves	$10^7 - 10^{-3}$ m	$10^1 - 10^{11}$ Hz	Oscillator circuits
Infrared radiation	$10^{-3} - 8 \times 10^{-7}$ m	$10^{11} - 4 \times 10^{14}$ Hz	Thermal radiators
Visible radiation	$8 \times 10^{-7} - 4 \times 10^{-7}$ m	$4 \times 10^{14} - 8 \times 10^{14}$ Hz	Thermal excitation, electron collision
UV radiation	$4 \times 10^{-7} - 10^{-7}$ m	$8 \times 10^{14} - 3 \times 10^{15}$ Hz	Electron collision
X-ray radiation	$5 \times 10^{-8} - 10^{-13}$ m	$6 \times 10^{15} - 3 \times 10^{21}$ Hz	Internal atomic electrons
Nuclear radiation	$10^{-13} - 10^{-16}$ m	$3 \times 10^{21} - 3 \times 10^{24}$ Hz	Nuclear reaction

Hertz (Hz) is the unofficial, but in the German language frequently used, designation for oscillations/second (s^{-1}).

are based, in terms of the most important distinctive feature, on the nature of the generation of the radiation. Table 2 shows a course classification on this basis.

Thus, within the regions of overlap, X-ray radiation can be generated both using X-ray tubes and also using the processes of generation of UV radiation, or electric waves can be generated using oscillator circuits and by thermal processes.

Conventionally, IR, visible, and UV radiation form the range of optical radiation. They are classified even more finely with regard to their chemical and physical effects:

Infrared Radiation

Long-wavelength infrared	IR-C (10 μ – 1 mm)
	Low-energy radiation, of little biological significance
Medium-wavelength infrared	IR-B (3 μ – 10 μ)
	The main emission range of heated glasses (light bulbs). This is not perceived as heat radiation by humans since it is already absorbed in the outermost layer of the skin. Remaining under intense IR-B radiation is perceived as unpleasant, since no counter-reaction to the regulation of the body temperature takes place.
Short-wavelength infrared	IR-A (800 – 3,000 nm)
	The main emission range of the thermal radiation of the sun. The radiation penetrates deeply into the skin and, within broad limits, is perceived as pleasant. The range 800 – 1400 nm is also designated as the therapeutic thermal octave.

Visible Radiation

The main distinctive feature of visible radiation is the color impression generated by the individual wavelength ranges in the human eye. The sensitivity of the eye to the different colors differs in magnitude. The eye is most sensitive to shades of green and least sensitive to violet and red colors. Since this sensitivity has quite essential significance with regard to the economy of light sources, a standard eye was determined on the basis of experimental investigations and its sensitivity progression was incorporated into the standardization as the spectral luminosity factor, or V (λ) curve.

In the psychological area as well, the wavelength and thus the color can be relevant. Bluish colors are intended to increase activity, while reddish color shades are intended to have a calming and relaxing effect.

Although the color impressions merge continuously into one another as the wavelength increases, it is nevertheless possible to stipulate approximate limits for the individual color ranges:
- Violet,   380–420 nm
- Blue,   421–495 nm
- Green,   496–566 nm
- Yellow,   567–589 nm
- Orange,   590–627 nm
- Red,   628–780 nm

Ultraviolet Radiation

Long-wavelength UV	UVA-1 (340–380 nm)
	A definite component of all natural and artificial, unfiltered light, and UV sources. This is not absorbed by unstained glasses. The lowest energy UV radiation. Having regard to its chemical effectiveness, it can be combined with the short wavelength, visible radiation (440 nm).
Long-wavelength UV	UVA-2 (315–340 nm)
	Transitional range between UVA and UVB in which the effects of both spectral ranges can be found.
Medium-wavelength UV	UVB (280–315 nm)
	The boundaries are defined in accordance with the erythema effect curve for human skin on the basis of the fundamental investigations by Karl Wilhelm Haußer and Wilhelm Vahle. Note: In the international literature, the boundaries are frequently defined differently: UVA-1: 340–400; UVA-2: 320–340; UVB: 280–320 nm.
Short-wavelength UV	UVC (100–280 nm)
	The shortest wavelength and thus highest energy part of UV radiation. In physical terms, UV extends to 15 nm and thus directly adjoins X-ray radiation.

Thus, the short wavelength boundary of UV radiation of the optical range was stipulated as 100 nm, in order to avoid conflicts with radiation protection regulations. Between 100 and 200 nm, oxygen and nitrogen absorb UV radiation. Thus, this range, which is also designated as vacuum-UV, cannot occur in air.

Spectral Composition of Radiation

Only in exceptional cases, e.g., in the case of lasers, does optical radiation consist of a single wavelength. Normally a mixture of many wavelengths having different intensities is emitted. The composition of specific radiation is the determining factor of the effects it can exert. Therefore, to evaluate the efficiency, it is necessary to know the portions of the power emitted in the various wavelength areas.

The representation of a wavelength-related composition of a mixture of radiation is designated as spectrum, or, listed in a numerical manner, as spectral power distribution (SPD).

Spectral power distributions can be realized with physical equipment only. Impinging radiation with different wavelength on our eye, we can perceive only one impression at one place of the retina. This impression primarily is dependent from the spectral distribution, but it allows no conclusions to the structure of the spectrum. Different spectra can cause identical impressions, which then are called metameric color stimuli.

Spectral Instruments

Investigations of such mixtures of optical radiation are performed with spectrometers or spectrographs. The principle construction is shown in Figure 3. Functionally you can subdivide these instruments in the components into the:
- Entrance area. The radiation to be measured is collected to the aperture of the spectrometer, which mostly is shaped as a slit.
- Imaging optics. Concave mirrors transform the divergent beam, coming from the entrance slit, to a parallel incidence. After passing the dispersing elements, they retransform them to a convergent bundle, focused in the exit plane of the spectrometer.
- Dispersing elements, either prisms or gratings. Prisms refract the radiation, depending on the wavelength, to different angles (see Fig. 4). Gratings reflect the radiation into different directions (optical diffraction). Generally, the following is true: The shorter the wavelength, the greater the change of direction. Blue is deflected more than red, and UV radiation more than visible. In the case of a prism, this basic principle may be represented in a simple manner. If a prism is held in sunlight and a piece of paper is placed behind the exit surface one can see the known colors of the rainbow appear on the paper (see Fig. 5). Accordingly, the rainbow is the spectrum of sunlight, but the eye

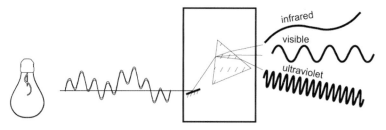

Fig. 3. Principle of the radiation path in a prism spectral instrument

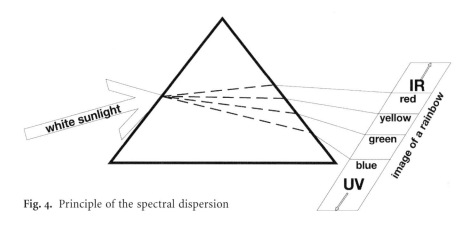

Fig. 4. Principle of the spectral dispersion

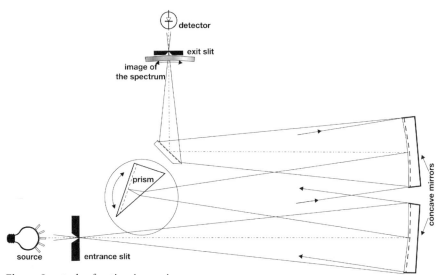

Fig. 5. Spectral refraction in a prism

cannot recognize the composition of the sunlight. The brain only perceives the impression "white".
- Exit area. It is defined by the imaginary plane on which the spectral dispersed radiation is focused. To record the intensities of it, three different procedures are in use:
  - Mounting a photographic detector. After exposure and development, a very fine structure of the spectrum appears. The blackening of the emulsion is typically for the spectral intensity at this point. A quantitative interpretation takes pains, because the blackening of the film is not linearly to the intensity.
  - Mounting a narrow (exit) slit with a single detector behind it. Revolving the dispersing element, in temporal sequences, the whole spectrum will penetrate the slit and can be recorded by steps. Disadvantages: A lot of time is necessary to carry out the measurements and a rotating prism necessitates a high precision of mechanical construction.
  - Mounting pixel detectors. In an array, the pixel detectors are closely packed on a disk. They are placed directly in the image of the spectrum so that each of these detectors is coordinated to a definite wavelength range. The exposure time with such an arrangement is within a tenth of a second, so evaluating the distribution with a computer, it is possible to perform spectral power distributions in a very short time.

The width of the exit slit and the dimensions of the detectors are the determining factors of spectral resolution. The narrower the slit, or the higher packed the detectors, the smaller is the selected range and the higher is the spectral resolution. It is primarily limited by the intensities of the signals, which become progressively weaker the smaller the wavelength area that has been seized. In practice, therefore, it is recommended to confine measurements to a resolution necessary for the respective application. Mostly it is sufficient to record in the visible range a value every 5 nm, while in the UV range, the spectrum must be recorded at least in 1 nm steps to guarantee a sufficiently precise allocation of the spectral radiation components.

Representation of Spectral Power Distributions

A spectral power distribution can be represented in the form of a table or as a diagram. At both, the intensity of the spectrally dispersed radiation is plotted against the wavelength (or frequency). The unit of the spectral radiation is to conform with the unit of the radiation entering the spectral equipment supplemented with the unit of the wavelength, which in the UV region usually is the nanometer. For example: for measuring irradiance (see Chap. 2, this volume) the unit is W/m^2. The quantity of the spectral unit then is $W/(m^2 nm)$.

Note: In some diagrams you will see the spectral unit W/m^3. This is mathematical playing, for you can combine m^2 and $nm = 10^{-9}$ m to 10^{-9} m^3.

In Figure 6 you can see the graphic possibilities of how to plot spectral power distributions. For this purpose, we have chosen a theoretical radiator, which emits in the wavelength range from 295 to 405 nm a power of 100 W and which has been measured in steps of ten to 10 nm.

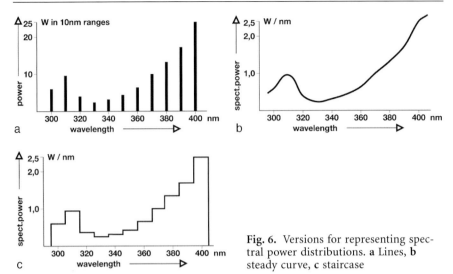

Fig. 6. Versions for representing spectral power distributions. a Lines, b steady curve, c staircase

In the first example (*a*) the intensities measured are plotted as lines drawn in the center of the wavelength range (the line at 300 nm encloses the range from 295 to 305 nm). The ordinate unit is W, supplemented with the index "in a range of 10 nm."

If we can be sure the measured spectrum is steady, we can connect the top of the lines to a continuous curve (*b*). The characterization of the ordinate now is spectral power with the unit W/nm. Note that the numerical values are 10 times lower than in Figure 6a.

If we intend to plot the spectrum by hand, it is more favorable to draw the distribution in the shape of a staircase (*c*).

In the example mentioned above, we see a so-called continuous spectrum, which is characterized by the fact that radiation is emitted in the total wavelength range. If we are measuring a continuum, the shape of the distribution stays nearly the same, independent from the spectral solution chosen. But especially, if we are measuring low-pressure discharge lamps we will find spectra in which emission is only on a few, definite wavelengths, while the neighborhood is free of any emission. In Figure 7 we show shapes of such a line spectrum, recorded with different spectral resolutions.

You can see that the lower the spectral resolution the broader becomes the shape of the line contour. Through evaluating the line intensity, you will find the same result, independent from the resolution. The deceptive shift from parts of the line intensity to adjoining wavelength can lead to errors if you calculate the efficiency of radiation. For this reason, we shall never specify a spectrum within smaller wavelength steps than the spectral resolution of the spectral instrument.

There are line spectra, continuous spectra, and spectra exhibiting both of these characteristics (see Fig. 8).

The spectra of sunlight and that of incandescent lamps are typical representatives of spectral radiation distributions which have no gaps, i.e., irrespective of

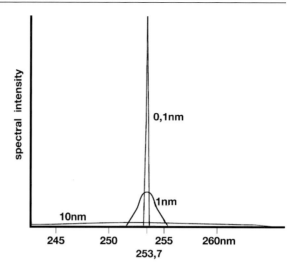

Fig. 7. Records of the line spectrum (mercury 253 nm) with spectral solutions of 10, 1, and 0.1 nm

how narrow the slit is chosen, radiation intensity can be detected at any wavelength setting. Such spectra are designated as continuous. These are typical of sources that generate their radiation through high temperatures.

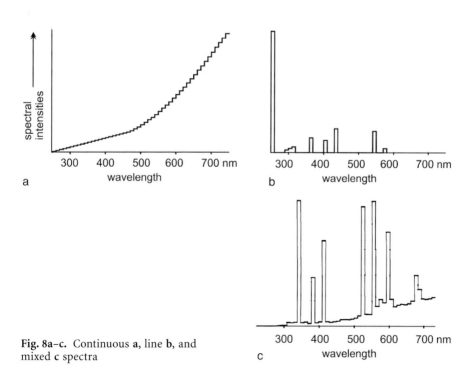

Fig. 8a–c. Continuous **a**, line **b**, and mixed **c** spectra

If, however, as in the case of sodium and mercury lamps, gases or vapors are excited to emit, then the result is a spectrum in which, at preferred wavelengths, radiation of very high intensity occurs, while in the neighboring areas, virtually no emission can be detected. Accordingly, such spectra are designated as line spectra.

From the majority of artificial radiation sources emerges a spectrum that represents a mixture of continuous distribution and line distribution. The reason for this is that modern light manufacturers have been making increasing use of several physical processes for radiation generation. For example, in the case of fluorescent lamps, the fundamental discharge of the mercury gives a line spectrum that is distributed over the UV and visible range. The visible lines make a contribution to the light directly, while the UV lines excite to fluorescence a mixture of fluorescent materials applied to the internal surface of the bulb. The spectrum of the fluorescent materials is approximately continuous and is superposed upon the line spectrum. This type of distribution is designated as a mixed spectrum.

The real quality of a spectrum is of great interest for physicists and chemists. From it they obtain fundamental information about the structure and the elements of a radiator. In the case of continuous radiators, the type of distribution gives an indication of the temperature of the radiator (see section "Bulb Materials" below); in the case of line and mixed spectra, the position of the lines and the form of the continuum give indications of the components excited to emission in a radiator (spectral analysis).

For a user whose primary interest is with the effectiveness of specific radiation, the presentation of a spectrum, such as a staircase, showing the intensity within definite wavelength ranges, is sufficient.

The spectral radiation distributions are of great importance for all investigations which are concerned with the arithmetic determination of effects of irradiation. To this end, there is a need not only for the emission spectrum of the radiation source but also for an action spectrum that shows how great the spectral sensitivity within the individual wavelength ranges is. Action spectra are known from many effects and have in some cases also been incorporated in standards. Examples of frequently employed action spectra are, within the visible range, the luminosity factor of the eye and the spectral value curves for color computation or, in the photobiological sector, the activity curves of erythema, pigmentation, or destruction of bacteria.

The effect of radiation is computed in that the intensity value of each wavelength is multiplied by the associated value of the spectral sensitivity curve and these arithmetic products are summated. The result is only one number, which is typical of the efficiency of the radiation mixture under investigation.

Quantitative Features of the Radiation

In addition to the spectral properties of radiation in application engineering, we also need quantities that enable us to make statements concerning the intensity and to describe the geometric conditions under which the radiation is present.

Table 3. Comparison of the most important radiant and luminous quantities and units

Quantity	Unit	Quantity	Unit
Radiant flux Φ_e	Watt (W)	Luminous flux Φ	Lumen (lm)
Radiant efficiency η_e	W/W	Luminous efficacy η_v	lm/W
Radiant energy Q_e	Joule (J)=W s	Quantity of light Q_v	lm s
Radiant intensity I_e	W/sr	Luminous intensity I_v	cd=lm/sr
Radiance L_e	W/m^2 sr	Luminance L	cd/m^2
Irradiance E_e	W/m^2	Illuminance E	lx=lm/m^2
Radiant exposure H_e	J/m^2	Light exposure H	lx s

From the vast amount of quantities that have in the past been proposed for these purposes, nowadays seven quantities have become established, which are internationally standardized and which are sufficient to solve all tasks occurring in practice (see Table 3).

Light is the best-known example of evaluated radiation. In this case, the radiation is evaluated by the spectral luminous efficiency of the human eye. By reason of their importance, in Table 3 luminous units have been added, which are correlated to the radiant units.

Statements on these quantities are also found in the majority of product specifications of radiation sources and irradiation systems so that the interpretation of these quantities permits an evidentially cogent comparison.

On the other hand, they are constructed in such a simple manner that, in the mode of writing related to the particular application, they require only the four basic types of computation in order to be understood.

The unit watt is the generally valid unit for any type of power. It applies not only to radiation but also to the electrical power take-up of a system or to the power of a car engine.

For these reason, in the case of all physical radiation measurements, it is absolutely necessary to make more detailed statements concerning the nature of the measured power. In the case of unevaluated radiation, the wavelength range must be stated, e.g., radiation of 300 – 400 nm or UVB radiation, and in the case of evaluation, by reference to an activity function, it is necessary to state the nature of the evaluation, e.g., radiant power of the erythema-effective radiation.

Comments to Radiant Quantities and Units

- Radiant power Φ_e is the total radiation emitted by a source. Whether the emission of radiation takes place uniformly into the entirety of space or only in preferred directions is of no importance in this connection.
- Radiant efficiency η_e is the ratio of the radiant flux of the emitted radiation to the power consumed by the source. It must be specified whether or not the power dissipated by an auxiliary, such as ballast, is included in the power consumed by the source.
- Radiant energy Q_e is the radiant power which is emitted during a specified time interval.

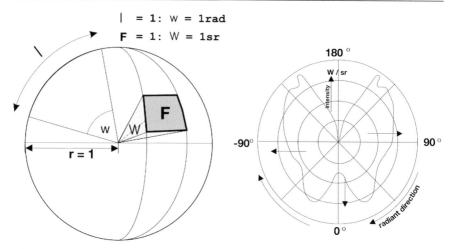

Fig. 9. Radian and steradian   Fig. 10. Spatial distribution

- Radiant intensity *I* is the radiant power which is emitted in a specified direction. The unit of the radiant intensity is W/sr (sr is the abbreviation for the solid angle unit, steradian. We assume that this term is not of common knowledge, so we will try to explain steradian in a few words).
  - A plane angle can be defined with degrees or with the length that an angle is cutting off from a circle (Fig. 9).
  - If this length equals the radius of the circle, you can say this angle equals 1 radian. This principle has been adopted in three-dimensional geometry to

    define a solid angle. If a cone or a pyramid is cutting off from a sphere an area equal to the square of the radius, you can say this solid angle has an amount of 1 sr. The shape of this area is of no importance. As the whole surface of a sphere is $4\pi \times r2$, it can be defined with 4π sr.
  - The radiant intensity is of significance especially in headlight engineering, since by this means the spatial intensity distribution can be characterized (see Fig. 10).
  - Radiance *L*. With neither with the definition of the radiant flux or the radiant intensity have statements been made about the size of the source. It is regarded as a mathematical point without any dimensions.
  - In the definition of radiance, information about the properties of the radiating part of a source is included. Radiance describes the radiant intensity emitted from a definite area. In photometry, radiance corresponds to luminance or brightness, which is responsible for the glare of a light source.
  - Figure 11 illustrates the correlation of intensity, radiation field, and radiance.
- Irradiance *E*. This characterizes the radiant power that is incident on a surface. In this connection, it is insignificant whether the radiation originates from one or more radiators and from which directions it is incident. Accord-

tive current/voltage curve. After ignition, which takes place automatically by means of a built-in ignition probe, a few minutes are required before the mercury has fully vaporized and a vapor pressure of a few kg/cm^2 has been built up. This pressure has two effects: first, the discharge is constricted in the center of the discharge vessel, so that a high radiation concentration, i.e., a high radiance, occurs there. Second, the center of the spectral emission is displaced as compared with the low-pressure discharge from the 254-nm line to the UVA line at 366 nm and the visible lines at 405, 546, and 578 nm. Thus, by reason of its simple construction and, compared with the incandescent lamp, its high light output, the high-pressure mercury lamp was one of the first discharge lamps to be used for illumination purposes. This type of lamp is relatively economical, has a long service life of many thousands of hours, and is accordingly still used even nowadays in the therapeutic treatment of psoriasis. Lamps are available on the market under the brand names HOK or HQA at the power levels 125 – 1,000 W.

A special design of the high-pressure mercury lamp is the above-mentioned Ultra-Vitalux radiator, in which the burner is built into a mushroom-shaped reflector. With a total power take-up of 300 W, it can be screwed into any normal lamp mounting and, by reason of this simple operation, is even nowadays still a widespread system for home therapy and for cosmetic applications.

High-pressure mercury lamps are manufactured at the power level of 125 W, also with a so-called black glass bulb which absorbs the visible lines and transmits only the UVA line at 366 nm. By reason of the fluorescence, which is thus made visible, the lamp is also used in diagnostics.

Mercury high-pressure lamps for illuminating purposes, as offered at times, are unfit for applications in the UV. They have an outer bulb, in some cases covered with phosphors, which allows UV radiation only in an insignificant quantity.

Summary of the Technical Attributes

– Wattage	125 – 1,000 W
– Lamp lengths	130 – 390 mm
– Efficacy UVA, -B, -C	Each 5 % (max)
– Supply voltage	125 – 230 V
– Operation	Using chokes. At a line voltage lower then 220 V a combination of transformer and choke is required.
– Brand designations	HOK, HQA, HQS, HQV radiators

Metal Vapor Halogen Lamps

These are likewise high pressure mercury lamps, to which metal halides are added. These radiators emit not only the Hg spectrum but also the typical spectrum of the metals that have been introduced, in most cases consisting of many lines. The admixing of various halides provides the lamp developer with the possibility of generating almost any desired spectrum. By means of iron, nickel, and cobalt halide additives, the spectral range between the UVA and -B lines is filled in to such extent that an almost continuous spectrum is formed between

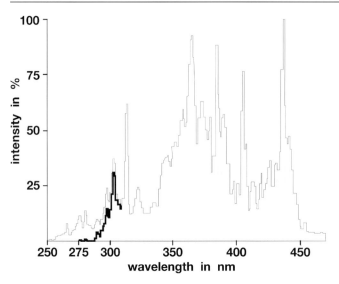

Fig. 16. Spectra of ULTRAMED metal halide UV radiator in UVA, -B, and -C design. Thick lines show the UVA and -B version

280 and 450 nm. A higher radiation output in the UV range is also associated with this improvement in the spectral progression. Accordingly, it has to a large extent displaced the pure mercury lamps.

These types of lamps mostly are supplied only as burners without an outer bulb. The small dimensions, the short discharge paths between 1 and 3 cm, and the associated high radiance make these lamps particularly suitable for incorporation in reflectors. Accordingly, their field of application resides principally in relatively large irradiation systems, with which high irradiances can be achieved, even at relatively large distance from the source.

When these lamps are used in therapy or as cosmetic radiators, because of the high radiation intensity of these lamps, in order to avoid undesired radiation effects, it is absolutely necessary to give consideration to appropriate filtering. Information on the subject should be requested from the manufacturers of the systems or radiators.

Properties

- Power levels   150 – 2,000 W
- Lamp lengths   50 – 200 mm
- Supply voltage   125 – 400 V
- Area of the fields of illumination   0.5 – 5 cm^2
- Operation   Possible only if using special control gears
- Ignition   Two versions are offered. Cold ignition: the lamp can be ignited only when cooled. Hot ignition: after being switched off, the lamp

can be ignited again immediately. Since in this case high frequency ignition voltages of several thousands of volts are used, appropriate screening for protection against leakage pulses is required.

– Brand designations   ULTRAMED, ULTRATECH, HMI, S MSR, HPA, and HPI lamps.

Short Arc Mercury Vapor Lamps (Maximum-Pressure Lamps)

These are almost point radiation sources, the radiance of which reach that of the sun in some UV ranges. This property makes them suitable as a radiation source in fluorescence microscopy and in fluorescence endoscopy. However, they are also successfully employed as irradiation monochromators, with which, for photobiological investigations, high irradiances can be generated with high spectral purity.

When the lamps have been warmed up, which requires a few minutes until the mercury has been fully vaporized, the spectrum of these lamps does indeed still show its radiation maxima in the region of the mercury lines, the contour

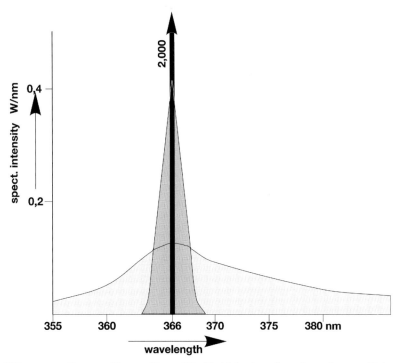

Fig. 17. UV mercury line at 366 nm of low- (*black*), high- (*gray*), and maximum- (*light gray*) pressure lamps

of which is, however, at the pressures of a few hundred N/cm^2 prevailing in the lamp, broadened to such an extent that it is possible to refer to an almost continuum-like progression. In this case, the tails of the lines overlap, so that within the entire range, in contrast to the low- and high-pressure lamps, in the case of which low-radiation regions occur between the lines, useful radiation is present at every wavelength (see Fig. 17).

At the lower power levels, the arc length, i.e., the length of the discharge path, is only fractions of a millimeter (the smallest field of illumination is only $0.25 - 0.25$ mm^2 in magnitude), but an arc length of 4 mm is not exceeded, even in the case of the larger types.

These lamps are ideal for the purpose of injecting high radiation intensities into light guides having small diameters. Incorporated in ellipsoidal mirrors, the total field of illumination of the lamp may be imaged on the entrance surface of a light guide on the scale 1:1 with only slightly attenuated intensity and may be transmitted with low loss if the aperture angles of the reflectors are suitable. Such combinations are already supplied in ready-assembled condition.

No special UV types are offered. But all types have sufficient energy in UVA and -B for UV applications.

Properties
- Power levels   50 – 1,750 W
- Lamp lengths   5 – 26 cm
- Area of the fields of irradiance   0.06 – 4 mm^2
- Electrical supply   Direct or alternating current, depending up-
                                           on the type
- Operation   Using special systems
- Brand designations   CS lamps, HBO lamps

Xenon Short Arc Lamps

Xenon short arc lamps are sources with high radiance and having a daylight-like spectrum in the visible range. In the industrial sector, they are mainly used in film projection and in solar simulation. In the scientific sector, they are used in photochemistry, in analytical measurements, and also in irradiation monochromators for photobiological investigations.

Just like the spectrum of the sun, the spectrum proceeds almost isoenergetically within the entire visible range; only within the range between 450 and 500 nm are there a few band-like peaks (Fig. 18). This reveals that the color temperatures of the xenon radiation and of the sun are almost identical (5,800 K).

In UV as well, the xenon discharge shows a purely continuous spectrum, the intensity of which, related to the visible range, is even greater than in the solar spectrum. The intensity declines slowly towards the shorter wavelengths and is limited only by the material of the bulb.

When using appropriately transitive quartzes, in the case of xenon lamps in the vacuum UV, radiation may still be detected as far as 170 nm.

The discharge vessel contains only the rare gas xenon and no other materials that must first vaporize when the lamp has been switched on. Accordingly, just

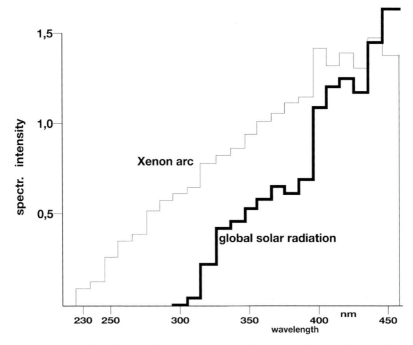

Fig. 18. Spectral power distribution of a Xenon short arc lamp and the global (sun+sky) solar radiation. Both distributions are referred to the same photometric value

like incandescent lamps, xenon lamps give full radiant power within a few seconds of ignition.

Further important properties of these lamps are the high constancy of the spectral radiation distribution and a slight decline of the radiant power over the entire surface life of the lamp. This and its high intensity make xenon short arc lamps a well-proven reference radiation source for the entire UV range. However, partly for reasons of cost but also because of the useful life maximum of 3,000 h, which is short for discharge lamps, they are used in irradiation therapy only in special cases.

In a similar design, there are krypton lamps which exhibit a marked radiation center at 220 nm.

Properties
- Power levels   75 – 10,000 W
- Lamp lengths   8 – 48 cm
- Area of the fields of illumination   0.25 – 40 mm^2
- Electrical supply   Direct current
- Operation   Using special systems
- Brand designations   XBO lamps, CSX lamps

Fluorescent Lamps

The primary radiation source in fluorescent lamps is a low-pressure mercury discharge. The line spectrum of this discharge has two strong lines in the UVC, at 185 and 254 nm, in which approximately 50 % of the energy emitted as radiation is contained. The remainder of the energy is distributed among the UVA and -B range (~20 %), the visible (~20 %) and weak lines in the IR.

To the internal surface of the bulb wall there are applied fluorescent substances in a thickness of 20–30 mm, which convert the short-wavelength UV lines into longer wavelength UV or visible radiation. Almost every UV quantum is converted into a photon with longer wavelength; the energy content of the photon is, however, in accordance with the Einstein relation, lower than that of the exciting radiation. Generalizing you can say, a maximum of 50 % of the radiation generated in the mercury discharge is available as fluorescence radiation. Nevertheless, fluorescent lamps are one of the most economical types of lamp.

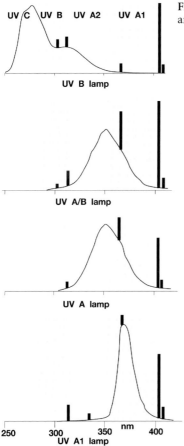

Fig. 19. Spectra of UVB, -AB, -A, and -A-1 fluorescent lamps

Fluorescent lamps are mainly used in illumination engineering. The UV radiation of these, so-called white lamps, starts with low intensity at about 300 nm, is dimensioned so that in no case will they exceed the currently stipulated limits for protection from radiation dangerous to health. By using appropriate bulb material, it is additionally ensured that in no case can the exciting UVC lines also penetrate to the outside.

For UV applications and for phototherapy, lamps are supplied with various spectra (see Fig. 19).

Lamps whose radiation center lies within UVA are used in photochemotherapy, in phototherapy, and, in large unit numbers, in solaria and sunbeds. In the case of these lamps, the emission maximum is between 350 and 370 nm; some types also have tails extending into the UVB, but all still have residual radiation in the violet and blue, and are therefore clearly distinguishable, even visually by their bluish light color, from white L-lamps.

Fluorescent lamps for UVA applications also exist with semi-laterally reflector layers. By this means, the lamps can be mounted closely side by side in irradiation systems and the irradiation intensity can be increased up to twofold as compared with systems having external reflectors.

Only an indication of the suitability of the individual types for specified practical applications may be taken from the graphical representations of the radiation spectra. As a result of the differing progressions of action curves, the center of action can be displaced markedly, so that only a spectral evaluation can give information on the active output.

In terms of the shape, a distinction is drawn between bar-shaped, ring-shaped, and U-shaped lamps. During recent years, compact lamps have been developed from the U-shaped L lamps, and these are approximately of the same size as incandescent lamps; because of their high light output and the longer service life, they are increasingly gaining acceptance in areas that were previously reserved for incandescent lamps. These compact fluorescent lamps are also manufactured for special UV applications, e.g., for treating psoriasis of the scalp.

Properties

– Power levels, compact lamps	7–18 W
– Power levels, tubes	40–100 W
– Lamp lengths, compact lamps	14–24 cm
– Lamp lengths, tubes	60–180 cm
– Supply voltage	125–230 V
– Operation	Using chokes and starters or using electronic adapter systems. All systems must be approved for the respective type of lamp.
– Brand designations	Light colors 78 and 79, EVERSUN SUPER, TL/10, 12, TL/09, CLEO

Influences That Can Change the Radiation of a Lamp

Lamp specifications include the lamp data for operating under normal conditions. But, depending on time, temperature, or mechanical, and electrical adjustments, variations of the lamp emission can result. Sometimes also, the bulb material will change without consequences in the visible range, but it is possible that by this constructive variation, the UV radiation will be changed.

Some of these influences you can ameliorate, for example, by prolongation of the irradiation time or by better cooling. With others, nothing can be done. The following section, therefore, shall provide some remarks about what kind of effects these influences can bear.

Bulb Materials and Their Influence on the UV Spectrum

Untreated bulb glass has a spectral transmission curve in the form of a cut-on filter, i.e., they hold back short wavelength radiation, start to transmit radiation in a wavelength range typical of the material, and then remain open to the short wavelength IR. Figure 20 shows, in this respect, a few typical examples.

Depending upon the composition of the glass, the cut-on may lie within the vacuum UV below 180 nm, but also only at the limit of the UVB, at 315 nm. In the UVA, from 340 nm, untreated bulb glasses and broad glass are always transmissive.

It is possible to characterize a cut-on filter by the three wavelengths which correspond to transmission values of 1 %, 50 %, and 90 %. In Table 6, these values are presented for frequently employed types of bulb glass.

Principally, the bulb material is selected for its processibility and its thermal and chemical resistance. Only where in these circumstances possibilities for selection still remain can the spectral transmissivity also be included in the deliberations. In many cases, however, the technological and optical requirements cannot be satisfied together, so that it is necessary to treat the glass.

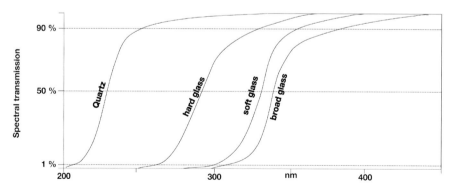

Fig. 20. Typical progression of the spectral transmission of bulb glasses in the UV

Table 6. Spectral transmission of some bulb glasses

Wavelengths (nm) for transmission value

Type of glass	1 %	50 %	90 %
Broad glass d = 2.5 mm	295	330	360
Broad glass d=5 mm	310	340	380
Soft glass/soda glass	290	330	350
Hard glass/silicate glass	260	290	340
Vycor glass	210	230	250
Quartz glass	175	190	240
Suprasil quartz	165	175	220

When assessing the spectral transmission values of bulb glasses, it is necessary to give consideration to the temperature dependence of this quantity. The customary list values only ever specify the values measured at room temperature, whereas the properties at operating temperature are of importance to the user. All bulb glasses have a tendency to displace their transmission cut-on in the long-wavelength direction as the temperature rises.

The magnitude of this displacement is dependent upon the material and can lie between 0.03 and 0.15 nm per 1 °C temperature rise. At temperatures of 800 °C, which occur in the case of halogen incandescent lamps and high-pressure burners, displacements of up to 100 nm are therefore possible.

The magnitude of the effects of the phenomenon of cut-on displacement in the event of a temperature rise may even be demonstrated without measuring equipment in the case of xenon lamps with quartz glass-Ultrasil bulbs. Xenon lamps have only a very short warm-up period, so that the full spectrum is emitted already when the lamp is switched on. According to Table 4, Ultrasil transmits to below 200 nm at room temperature, and, since xenon also radiates within this range, ozone-generating radiation must emerge directly after ignition. The fact that this is so is rapidly recognized by reference to the occurring typical "odor of ozone," which, however, disappears again after a brief period. (Note: Ozone is an odorless gas. The pungent odor originates from oxides of nitrogen, which are formed together with the ozone.) Since, however, the upper limit for the generation of ozone by radiation is approximately 210 nm, the transmissivity must have been displaced beyond this range by the heating.

However, this cut-on displacement is also significant with regard to the question of whether a lamp emits UVC or UVB; according to the brochure details in the case of the majority of bulb glasses, this would have to be the case. In fact, however, as is shown by the spectra of the lamps, the UV components are substantially smaller than would be expected on the basis of these curves.

Alteration of the Bulb Transmissivity by Thin Layers

By distinctive techniques, such as
– alteration of the glass wall thickness,
– staining within the mass,
– coloring the surface,
the transmission of the bulb material can be altered. These processes are mainly used in the visible range and, because of the temperature rise associated therewith, can be used only in the case of lamps that are not under an excessively high loading. By coating with thin, interfering layers, it is possible to alter the transmission properties of the bulbs in a variety of ways.

Since, in this case, the effect is not achieved by absorption, but by selective reflection, it does not bring about any direct rise in temperature of the bulbs and can therefore be used in the case of lamps under high loading, by reason of the high thermal stability of these layers as well. Cut-on replacements are possible, as is also the selection of specified spectral ranges.

Besides the possibility of altering the color of the light, there are at present two other areas of application for this process. In the first, a layer that reflects only in the IR is applied to incandescent lamp bulbs (IRC layers), by which the thermal radiation is retained within the bulb. This improves the radiation output of the lamps, since less electrical energy needs to be supplied for the same radiant power. The energy saving achieved thereby amounts to approximately 20 % at the present time.

In the second area of application, the layer reflects approximately the range of one wavelength octave and is transmissive for the adjacent ranges. Applied to reflectors, only radiation of the desired spectral range is then present in the main beam path, while the remaining radiation is transmitted or absorbed within the glass body. The preferred radiation range may lie within the UVA, within the visible or within the near IR (see Fig. 21).

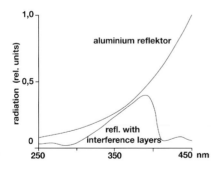

Fig. 21. Alteration of the lamp spectrum by selectively acting reflectors

Alteration of the Bulb Transmissivity by Doping

A further possibility for reducing the excessively high UV transmissivity of a bulb is the doping of the glass. Doping can take place as early as during manufacture, using small amounts of additives, in order thereby to increase the bonding strength of the oxygen ions, which is essential for transmissivity (Fig. 22).

This process is used in halogen incandescent lamps for general illumination, in order to avoid the undesired UVC radiation, as well as in projection lamps under high loading, in order thereby to avoid the risk of damage to materials due to high energy UV radiation.

Fig. 22. Effect of doping on the spectral transmissivity

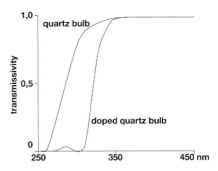

Influences of the Ambient Temperatures

The temperature of the ambient air for the various lamp types is of different significance. For all types in which the generation of the radiation occurs in small volumes, the environment of the bulb can reach temperatures of some hundred degrees. Therefore, in operating these kind of lamps, it has to be ensured that the temperatures do not exceed a level at which a lamp can be damaged. Possibly a socket can be loosened or the bulb can blow up. Both would lead to an immediate destruction of the lamps.

Applied to these dangers are all high-pressure discharge lamps and incandescent lamps with higher wattage, whilst the radiant flux of these types is largely independent from the ambient temperature.

With low-pressure discharge lamps (the most important exponents are fluorescent lamps) there is an evident interdependence of the radiant flux from the ambient temperature. The reason is to be found in the temperature dependence of the mercury vapor pressure.

At low temperatures an insufficient quantity of mercury vaporizes, so that too few charge carriers are present. As the temperature rises, there is an increase in the number of excitable mercury atoms and thus also in the luminous flux. However, if the temperature is increased still further beyond a specified value, the Hg atoms become so numerous that it is no longer possible for all of them to be excited. However, unexcited Hg atoms have the property that they absorb the UV mercury radiation (self-absorption), which is then no longer available to

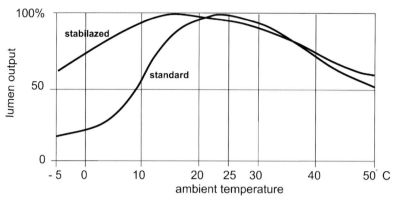

Fig. 23. Radiation emitted from standard, and temperature-stabilized fluorescent lamps as function of the ambient temperature

excite fluorescent material. The radiation maximum of a standard lamp is at an ambient temperature of 25 °C.

By means of design measures, the maximum of the luminous flux may be displaced between 15 (see Fig. 23) and 35 °C, so that, for operation externally, lamps are available which are optimized for 15 °C, while lamps having an emission maximum of 35 °C can be employed in enclosed-room lighting systems.

The vapor pressure can be influenced by physical methods, e.g., enlargement of the bulb surface by twisting or by means of additional convexities on the lamp, or with chemical methods, whereby amalgams are added to the lamp, which appears according to the current findings to be the more promising route. In this process designated as the amalgam technique, a lower vapor pressure becomes established at the same temperature, so that the maximum luminous flux appears only at higher temperatures. This would be nothing new, but, as a result of combinations with several amalgams and corresponding design adaptations, as is shown in Figure 22, the temperature progression can also be broadened and thus it is possible to manufacture lamps that can be employed more universally than before.

At the moment it is not possible to produce fluorescent lamps at which the maximum emission is higher than 35 °C. Although, in equipment in which a great number of lamps have been installed in a compact manner (for example in solaria), the temperature increases considerably more than 35 °C. To yield an optimal irradiation in these applications, a correct forced cooling is necessarily.

Influences of Time

After starting a lamp, it takes some time to reach its full emission. This burning-in time differs to a wide degree with the lamp types and is additionally dependent on electrical and environmental conditions. For this reason the burning-in times noted in Table 7 provide only rough estimates.

Table 7. Burning-in times and average rated life of some lamp types

Lamp type	Burning-in time	Lamp life
GLS incandescent lamps	5 s	1.000 h
Halogen lamps low voltage		
$T_f = 3000$ K	20 s	3.000 h
$T_f = 3200$ K	15 s	200 h
$T_f = 3500$ K	10 s	25 h
High-voltage	20 s	1.500 – 3.000 h
Infrared-coated	15 s	3.000 h
Fluorescent lamps		
Standard	5 min	10.000 h
With amalgam	15 min	10.000 h
Electrodeless	5 min	60.000 h
With UV phosphors	5 min	300 – 1.000 h
Mercury low-pressure HNS	10 min	6.000 h
Mercury high-pressure HQL	15 min	15.000 h
Metal halide lamps HQI, HMI	15 min	6.000 – 8.000 h
Xenon lamps XBO	10 s	400 – 1.200 h
ULTRA-VITALUX	5 min	1.000 h
ULTRAMED	3 min	500 h

Also, there is interest is the total time a lamp operates before it becomes useless, or is considered to be so according to specified criteria. To determine this life or average life of lamps, there are different methods. Unfortunately, most of the lamp manufacturers give no information about the methods on which their data have been based. For a better comparison, therefore, in Table 5 only the data of one manufacturer (OSRAM – SYLVANIA) have been used. This way, only the lamps and not the methods are compared.

For some lamp types the switching cycles have a great influence on the lamp life. For example, a metal halide lamp, burning for 8 h, reaches a lamp life of 6,000 h. With a switching cycle of 1 h, it decreases to 1,200 h. On the other hand, incandescent lamps can be switched on and off often without any influence on the lamp lives.

Further Influences

Operating with lamps inserted in luminaires there are many other influences that can alter the properties of the radiation and the life of a lamp.

If you have the choice, think to the following:

– The operating voltage shall not differ more than 5 % from the nominal value. At some types, even a low voltage is able to shorten the lamp life.
– Ballast's must have been constructed for the supply frequency.
– Refer electronic ballast.
– Use only burning position which are allowed. Pick up the position with the highest output.

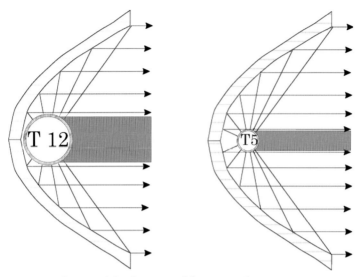

Fig. 24. Influence of the diameter of fluorescent lamps

- Fluorescent lamps with thinner diameter give a higher radiance and a higher
  yield of radiant intensity in the reflectors, more radiant intensity, and better
  luminaire efficiency (see Fig. 24).

Daylight

Sunlight and its adjacent spectral regions, UV and IR, are the basic requirement
for life on Earth. Knowingly or unknowingly, we are always exposed to their
influence, and their therapeutic action has been known to man since time
immemorial. However, daylight has nowadays been to a large extent displaced
as a therapeutic agent since, by way of replacement, artificial radiation sources
are available that are ready for use at any time and whose intensities and spectra
can be adapted to the respective treatment function. Nevertheless, daylight is
also included in the compilation of the UV radiation sources used in the medical sector, principally for the purpose of enabling a comparison between the
properties of artificial light and natural radiation. Particular attention should be
paid to the spectral alterations of sunlight in the course of the daily and seasonal
cycles.

Spectrum of the Extraterrestrial Radiation Outside of the Atmosphere

The totality of the optical radiation proceeds from the photosphere of the sun,
i.e., the outermost layer of the sun, which has a thickness of about 300 km. In
the superjacent chromosphere with the gaseous phases of the corona that are
situated there, a selective attenuation of the radiation takes place by absorption,

while the self-radiation of the corona, although at a temperature of 1 million degrees, makes only a slight contribution to the total emission spectrum of the sun because of its small optical density.

In terms of its spectral radiation distribution, solar radiation does not behave as a black body. Only in partial regions is it possible to assign a temperature to the progression, applying the Planck laws. Within the visible and the near UV, the distribution corresponds to a black body radiation of 5,700 K. However, in the shorter wavelength section, the intensity then increases more strongly than is to be expected because of this temperature. Within the range of the short wavelength UVC, the progression of the spectral distribution then no longer corresponds to a black body temperature of 4,700 K.

Terrestrial Solar Radiation

The alterations of the solar spectrum on passing through the atmosphere arise on account of scattering at air molecules and suspended substances (aerosols) and on account of absorption in atmospheric gases and vapors. In the case of the UV range, the absorption of ozone within the wavelength range below 300 nm and a strong spectral dependence of the scattering behavior are of importance in this connection. As a result of the latter, the short-wavelength components of the direct solar radiation decrease all the more strongly, the longer is their path through the atmosphere. In contrast, the scattered component, discernible in the visible as blue-sky radiation, increases as the sun gets lower, since in those circumstances it has to penetrate greater air masses.

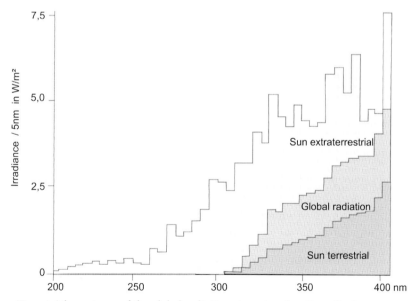

Fig. 25. Terrestrial spectrum of the global radiation at a solar elevation of 45°

Table 8. Solar illuminance and irradiance based on the sun's altitude in degrees [°]

Altitude of sun	Illuminance E			Irradiance E_e (W/m²)		Comparison to sun's altitude at 90° (%)		
(°)	(klx)	Total	UVB	UVA	Total	Visible	UVB	UVA
90	120	1.150	2.48	43.7	100	100	100	100
60	105	980	1.84	36.3	88	85	74	83
45	80	720	1.18	28.0	67	63	48	64
30	55	510	0.54	17.7	46	44	22	40
15	25	230	0.10	7.7	21	20	4	18

Table 9. Sky and direct sun radiation based on the sun's altitude [°]

Altitude of sun	Visible					UVB	UVA		
(°)	Sun W/m²	Sky W/m²	Sun/sky %	Sun W/m²	Sky W/m²	Sun/sky %	Sun W/m²	Sky W/m²	Sun/sky %
90	510	90	570	0.87	1.61	54	26.2	17.5	150
60	450	97	460	0.55	1.29	43	20.0	16.3	120
45	345	86	400	0.24	0.94	26	12.6	15.4	85
30	200	78	260	0.06	0.49	12	6.2	11.5	55
15	70	50	140	0.01	0.09	10	0.8	7.1	13

Figure 25 shows within the UV range these spectral influences of the atmosphere, by comparing for a solar elevation of 45° the extraterrestrial solar radiation with the global radiation and terrestrial radiation of the sun. Global radiation is the sum of sunlight and sky light. Tables 8 and 9 show how differently individual spectral ranges behave at the various solar elevations and how, in this case, the relationships between direct solar radiation and indirect sky radiation distribute.

All portions of the UV radiation are strongly dependent on the sun's elevation. The lower the sun altitude, the less is the radiation in the UV areas.

Dosimetry

A dose within the range of optical radiation, in terms of standards also referred to as irradiation H, is – in contrast to nuclear medicine and chemistry, in which it relates to a volume – the product of an irradiance E on a plane and the irradiation time.

Dosimetry is an attempt to determine the effects of the optical radiation with metrological methods. The term "attempt" has been picked up, because, especially in the field of biology, the reactions are of such a complex nature (as is evident in other chapters of this volume) that an exact calculation with simple mathematical proceedings is impossible. You can only approximate values characterizing the typical UV effects of a source. On the other side, beginning with the development of modern artificial lamps in the early 1930s, people looked for a procedure to compare the UV properties of a source. For this purpose, activity related functions have been introduced to test the suitability of a source for destined tasks.

To day, these procedures have been included in the international recommendations of the CIE (Commission Internationale de l'Eclairage) or in the German standard DIN 5031 Part 10. Some of them have also become components of further publications, for example in the Federal Health Gazette, the American Food and Drug Administration reports, or the proceedings of the International Electrotechnical Committee (IEC). In the USA, specified irradiation systems must already be officially approved with respect to possible risk to health due to UV radiation, and it is foreseeable that similar regulations are also to be expected in Europe.

To calculate an activity-related dose, the following quantities have to be known:
- Spectral distribution of the irradiance $E_{e\lambda}$ with a sufficient fine resolution
- Spectral dependence $s_x(\lambda)$ of the activity related function x
- Irradiation time t

Mathematically, then, we arrive at the definition of irradiation with the following formula:

$$H_x = \left(\int E_{e\lambda} \cdot S_x(\lambda) \cdot d\lambda \right) \cdot t \tag{12}$$

Usually H_x is calculated by summarizing of finite wavelength ranges with $\Delta\lambda=5$ resp. 1 nm:

$$H_x = \left(\Sigma\ E_e(\lambda) \cdot S_x(\lambda) \cdot \Delta\lambda \right) \cdot t \tag{13}$$

Activity Spectra

The activities that can be generated by optical radiation have spectral centers with a high effectiveness and one or more regions in which – with differing sensitivity – activity can still be detected. This spectral dependence is designated as the spectral action curve or as the activity spectrum of the pertinent reaction.

The progression of these activity functions, which may be of a physical, chemical or – as fits our theme – photobiological nature have been determined by experimental investigations. Accordingly, it is also understandable that relatively great ranges of scatter have occurred as a result of differences in the individual sensitivities, as well as owing to differing experimental conditions, in the spectral progressions. Therefore, for standardization purposes, often several of these results have been averaged or have been simplified. Figure 26 shows the size of such modifications withthe example of the action curve of erythema.

For binding statements concerning the activities of optical radiation, reference should accordingly always be made only to standardized activity spectra. In Fig. 27 some of these action curves have been pictured.

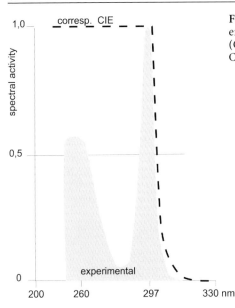

Fig. 26. Spectral activity functions of erythema experimentally determined (Coblentz) and erythema corresponding CIE recommendations

Photobiological activities are in many cases initiated only within a small wavelength range and accordingly have, in many instances, very steep gradients in their progression.

But, activity curves should not be confused with spectral absorption diagrams, which are frequently relied upon as evidence of effectiveness. According to the Grothus-Draper law, only absorbed radiation can initiate a reaction, whilst the converse conclusion, that any absorbed radiation quantum also makes a contribution to a specified activity, is not permissible.

Photobiological activities can occur not only in UV but also in visible radiation. For examples are mentioned the activity curve of the brightness perception of the eye on which all optical engineering and thus all measuring systems of illumination engineering are based, perceiving colors, or the growth of plants.

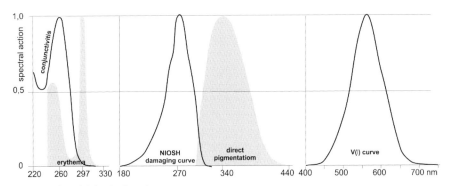

Fig. 27. Photobiological action curves

Computation of Activity-Related Quantities

Starting quantities for the determination of activity-related quantities are the spectral radiation distribution of an irradiation system and the action spectrum of the activity to be investigated, standardized to the value 1 for the maximum. These two prescribed quantities are used to determine a so-called fold integral, which signifies, in non-infinitesimal notation, that the radiation intensity in small wavelength ranges is multiplied by the spectrally associated sensitivity, and these individual values are then summated to form the total quantity.

In Figure 28 and Table 10, the computation process is explained by reference to a numerical example; in order to keep the numerical quantity within bounds, only the most intensive lines of the UVB spectrum of a mercury lamp were selected as a radiation source.

In Figure 28 you will find:
– The action curve of erythema in 50-nm steps, as published in the tables of standards
– The action curve of erythema interpolated to 1-nm steps
– Irradiance of the UV B lines of a mercury low-pressure lamp

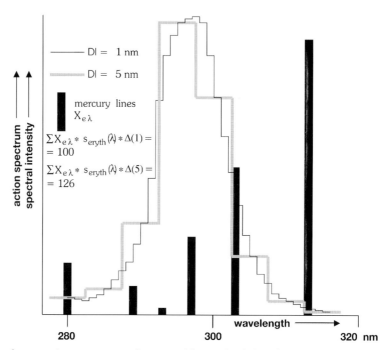

Fig. 28. Erythema action curve according to Coblentz, divided in five 1-nm steps, demonstrating the differing coordination to the lines of a mercury low-pressure lamp

Table 10. Weighted irradiance of erythema activities

1	2	3		5 (column 2×3)	6 (column 2×4)
Line	Irradiance E_e	Spectral activity of erythema $s_{eryth}(\lambda)$ 5-nm steps	Erythema-weighted irradiance E_{eryth} 1-nm steps	$s_{eryth}(\lambda) \times E_e$ mW_{eryth}/m^2	$s_{eryth}(\lambda) \times E_e$ mW_{eryth}/m^2
nm	mW/m^2				
280	300	0.06	0.06	18	18
289	160	0.31	0.18	50	29
292	40	0.99	0.87	40	35
296	450	0.99	1.00	450	450
302	960	0.19	0.37	182	355
313	1.560	0.01	0.03	16	47
Total	3.470			756	934

In Table 10 you will find:
- Column 1: wavelength of the line centers
- Column 2: line intensities
- Column 3: erythema activities in 5-nm steps [s(λ) 5]
- Column 4: erythema activities in 1-nm steps [s(λ) 1]
- Column 5: line intensities multiplied with [s(λ) 5]
- Column 6: line intensities multiplied with [s(λ) 1]

Columns 2, 5, and 6 have been summarized to the total intensities in the UVB range.
    Already this simple example shows three important findings:
- Unweighted radiation differs widely from the weighted intensities (compare column 2 with columns 5 and 6). The amount of these differences is dependent form the distributions of the spectra. So we cannot draw conclusions from the UVA or UVB content to the weighted activities. Comparing the activities of different spectra only on the base of wavelength ranges may lead to strong discrepancies.
- Different resolutions of the spectral distributions, as well from the source as from the action curve, may also lead to discrepancies. In our example, you can find a difference of 25 %, changing the resolution from 5 to 1 nm.
- At action curves with steep gradients, mostly only a small area is decisive for the activity. In our example, the intensity of the line at 296 nm is 13 % of the total UV B radiation but about 50 % weighted with the erythema action curve.

These statements also are also valid in continuance or mixed spectra, where several hundred individual procedures may be required. In earlier times, this was a laborious procedure, but nowadays, in the age of electronic data processing, it is an automatic sequence. Thus, the weighted radiation quantities of the most important photobiological activities are available for all radiators and may be requested from the manufacturers, where they have not already been incorporated in the product specifications.

In most cases, the operator of UV irradiation systems is not aware of those absolute values of the spectral irradiance distribution that are incident on the object surface, and in a normal case it is also not possible for him to carry out these costly measurements himself. Since, however, these values are a prerequisite for the determination of activity-related quantities, the following auxiliary process is recommended for the purpose of determining the respective radiation values by simple measurements on one's own. To do this, it is necessary to request from the manufacturer, if it has not been supplied, a system-specific spectral distribution of the UV and of the visible range in which the ordinate values are standardized so that the optical evaluation gives an illuminance of 1,000 lx. It is even better, because this saves computation work if the desired activity-related quantity is given directly, such as related to 1,000 lx. In the first case, the ordinate must be designated in $mW/m^2/1,000$ lx, and in the second case the following must be stated: active quantity/1,000 lx.

The measuring instrument employed is a commercially available illuminance meter, with which the illuminance is determined at the place to be irradiated.

The measured illuminance is then divided by 1,000 lx and the output values are multiplied by this quotient. Thus, where 500 lx are measured, the values should be halved; in the case of 4,000 lx, fourfold higher values should be inserted.

This process has the advantage of a progressive control, in which the decline in radiation due to aging and contamination is also recorded and, where appropriate, can be corrected. Differing changes in the visible and in the UV have a disadvantageous effect on the accuracy of measurement, since in all instances reference is made only to the visible. According to experience, errors of up to a maximum of 15 % may occur as a result of this; this should be negligible in the vast majority of cases.

Determination of a Dose

In physical notation, it can be written

$$\text{Dose } H = \text{irradiance } E_{actin.} \times \text{irradiation time } t \qquad (14)$$

with the units $W/m^2 \times s$ or J/m^2.

This definition is valid for all quantities that the several components may have. But evaluating a dose with respect to an effect caused by it, you must specify the range in which a true relationship between cause (irradiation, irradiance time) and effect is met. Within this range the following conditions must be complied with:

– The Bunsen-Roscoe law must be valid.

   This law states that it has to be immaterial whether one and the same dose is generated with a high irradiance during a brief period or with a low irradiance during a long period. A dose of 1,000 units can be generated both

by an irradiance of 1,000 during the time 1 and with the irradiance 1 during the time of 1,000.
- Additivity of the activity.
  In the case of an integral irradiation, radiation of differing wavelengths participate in the generation of the activity. It has to be ensured that all spectral ranges generate effects which can be brought into register with one another, and that, depending upon their intensity, these individual effects may be linearly added to form the total activity. If the activities of λ_1 and λ_2 are equal and 1, than the activity of both, influencing at the same time must be 2.
- Proportionality of the radiation activity.
  The individual activity of one spectral range may be distinguished from another only by a proportionality factor. In the event of a weighted radiation, this factor is predetermined by the value of the activity curve at the pertinent wavelength. Consequently, the radiation of any selectable wavelength of an intensity 1 and a spectral weighting of 1 must generate the same activity as the radiation of another wavelength having the intensity 5 and a spectral weighting of 0.2.

In the case of photobiological processes, with its complicated processes which form the basis of a reaction, these conditions only approximately can be performed. Three examples shall verify this contention.

It is known that, in the case of UV erythema below a determined irradiance level, no reddening of the skin can be achieved even with arbitrarily long irradiation times, since the reaction products are more rapidly broken down than generated. In the case of erythema, this limit is undershot if it is necessary to irradiate for more than 1 h to achieve the initial reaction.

The starting point of all manifestations of the erythema is not located at zero. Only if a defined actinic irradiation is exceeded does an erythema appear after a latency time on the skin (see Fig. 29).

As long ago as 1934, Haußer and Vahle had established that the gradient of the skin reddening curve was highly wavelength-dependent (Fig. 30). On this basis, the gradation becomes flatter the shorter the wavelength of the radiation. The result of this is that, in order to increase the level of reddening from 1 to 2 at a wavelength of 250 nm, it is necessary once again additionally to administer 1.5 doses while, to achieve this result using radiation of wavelength 300 nm, only 10 % of the dose with which stage 1 was achieved is necessary.

Further you have to regard the skin type you are testing, and the fact that sensitizers in the blood, generated by nutrients or medicaments, are able to increase the effectiveness of specified wavelengths, and in some cases even to broaden the entire activity spectrum. Known examples of this are furocoumarin or psoralen.

Threshold Dose

The expression "threshold dose" is used in the case of activities that require a minimum irradiation before the initial appearance of a reaction, which, in the case of skin investigations, is in most cases determined visually. In medicine,

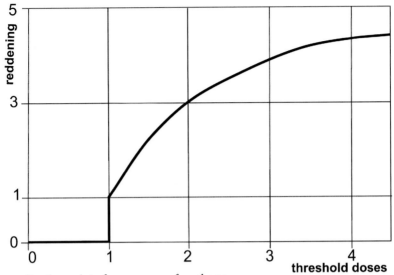

Fig. 29. Starting point of appearance of erythema

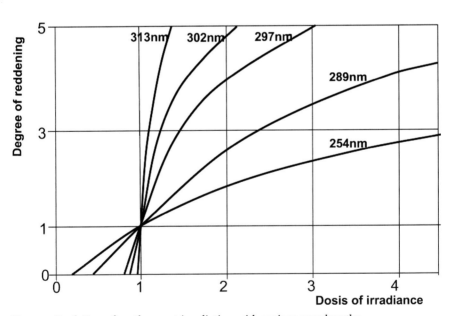

Fig. 30. Gradation of erythema at irradiation with various wavelengths

these are principally UV erythema, the various types of skin pigmentation and conjunctivitis and keratitis of the eye. If the reactions to the radiation do not appear until after a time delay, the time interval between irradiation and assessment is also relevant in determining the threshold dose.

Conclusion

Although the experimental conditions and the evaluation process for the determination of the threshold values are nowadays to a large extent standardized or at least agreed, it must nevertheless be stated that, in the case of all photobiological processes, a precomputation of the activity generated by the irradiation is loaded with an uncertainty which is about an order of magnitude greater than the uncertainty of the physical bases of computation. Even in the case of careful procedures, a not negligible uncertainty of measurement and reproduction must be expected in the determination of the threshold doses. Therefore, is the purpose of an evaluation an other then a general specification of a radiant source you have to control the calculations by experiments.

In some instances, the literature contains indications to the effect that a specified number of erythema threshold doses would be necessary before an average sunburn appears. What is meant by this is that the product – irradiated for this special case – of irradiance and time is the specified multiple of the erythema threshold dose. Since, however, there are also differing gradation curve progressions for differing wavelengths, it is no longer possible to describe the dose required for the activity which has occurred as a multiple of the erythema threshold dose in this simple way. The proportionality of the radiation activity would first have to be assessed for each individual wavelength. Thus, in this special case concerning the attainment of an average sunburn, a change in irradiance cannot be compensated by a computational adaptation of the irradiation time in accordance with the Bunsen-Roscoe law. The following formulation is correct in these cases: with an erythema-active irradiance of W/m² and an irradiation time of y seconds, an average sunburn has been observed z h after termination of the irradiation. However, such statements make sense only in circumstances in which the situation involves a frequently occurring irradiance level, e.g., under the midday sun; however, this is then to be specified.

If, however, such details concerning the radiation range which has been irradiated are not available for the purposes of the assessment of an observed sunburn, then data concerning the irradiation time which was necessary for the skin reaction that occurred can only be formulated experimentally. In these circumstances, the prerequisites for the application of the formula for the determination of the irradiation H are no longer satisfied in respect of the skin reactions which go beyond the erythema threshold reaction.

References

1. Bartels J (1960) Geophysics. Fischer, Frankfurt
2. Endres L (1989) Radiators. In: Erb W (Editor) Introduction to spectroradiometry. Springer, Berlin Heidelberg New York
3. Gerlach W (1960) Physics. Fischer, Frankfurt
4. Lompe A (1969) Technical-scientific proceedings of the Osram company, vol 10. Springer, Berlin Heidelberg New York
5. Meyer AEH, Seitz EO (1949) Ultraviolet rays. De Gruyter, Berlin
6. Schulze R (1970) Radiation climate of the earth. Steinkopf, Darmstadt
7. Anonymous (1987) Pocket book of lamp engineering. Osram, Berlin
8. Westphal WH (1990) Physics. Springer, Berlin Heidelberg New York
9. Anonymous (1993) Technical information – principles of optical radiation. Philips Light, Hamburg
10. Anonymous (1998) Light program '98/99. Osram, Munich
11. Anonymous (1987) International lighting vocabulary. International commission on illumination publication no 17.4
12. DIN 5031 part 10 (draft) German standard

2 Mechanisms of Photo(chemo)therapy

Jean Krutmann, Akimichi Morita, Craig A. Elmets

Contents

Introduction

Ultraviolet (UV) radiation has been used for decades with great success and at a constantly increasing rate in the management of skin diseases and has thereby become an essential part of modern dermatological therapy [28]. Its success as a therapeutic agent has stimulated studies about the mechanisms by which UVB and UVA phototherapy work. The knowledge obtained from this work is an indispensable prerequisite for making treatment decisions on a rational rather than empirical basis. Modern dermatological phototherapy has just begun to profit from this knowledge, and it is very likely that this development will continue and provide dermatologists with improved phototherapeutic modalities and regimens for established and new indications. This chapter aims to provide an overview about current concepts of the mode of action of dermatological phototherapy. Special emphasis will be given to studies that have identified previously unrecognized immunosuppressive/anti-inflammatory principles of photo(chemo)therapy.

Historical Concepts

The prototypic skin disease showing a favorable response to UVB phototherapy is psoriasis. This inflammatory dermatosis is characterized by keratinocyte hyperproliferation. Initially it was thought that UVB phototherapy worked through antiproliferative effects resulting from UVB-induced DNA damage [1, 2]. The number of skin diseases responding to UVB and UVA phototherapy, however, extends far beyond psoriasis. Most UV-responsive diseases are not characterized by hyperproliferative processes, but are immunologic in nature [51]. The capacity of UV radiation to affect the skin immune system was first recognized in the early 1970s in numerous studies (reviewed in [16, 23]). It is therefore now generally believed that UVB, UVA, and psoralen plus UVA (PUVA) therapy exert a variety of immunomodulatory effects on human skin, and that this is of critical importance for the therapeutic efficacy of UV phototherapy.

Therapeutic Photoimmunology

It should be noted that most of the immunomodulatory effects that have been described thus far are not specific for a single modality. At least under in vitro conditions, UVB, UVA, and PUVA radiation may have very similar or even identical immunosuppressive consequences. The actual therapeutic relevance of these effects, however, is determined by the physical properties of the type of UV radiation employed [3]. Ultraviolet B radiation mainly affects epidermal keratinocytes and Langerhans' cells, whereas UVA radiation can penetrate more deeply into the dermis and thereby also affect dermal fibroblasts, dermal dendritic cells, endothelial cells, and skin-infiltrating inflammatory cells such as T lymphocytes, mast cells, and granulocytes (Fig. 1). Many of these effects have been identified by using animal models or through in vitro studies employing cultured human skin cells. It is beyond the scope of this chapter to give a comprehensive review of photoimmunology. The reader is referred to a recent monograph for a more extensive discussion of immunological effects of ultraviolet radiation [23]. The emphasis will instead be on work in the field of human photoimmunology describing immunomodulatory effects of phototherapeutic relevance. In particular, recent studies employing in situ techniques in order to analyze immunomodulatory/anti-inflammatory effects that occur in the skin of patients while they undergo photo(chemo)therapy will be discussed in greater detail.

In general, photoimmunological effects of therapeutic relevance fall into three major categories:
1. effects on production of soluble mediators,
2. modulation of the expression of cell-surface-associated molecules and
3. the induction of apoptosis in pathogenetically relevant cells.

Effects on Soluble Mediators

The beneficial effects induced by photo(chemo)therapy are thought to result from the induction of mediators with anti-inflammatory, immunosuppressive, or both properties. There is also evidence that phototherapeutic modalities suppress the production of proinflammatory cytokines. In addition, beneficial effects observed after UVA-1 phototherapy in scleroderma patients have been attributed to the production of cytokines, which upregulate matrix metallopro-

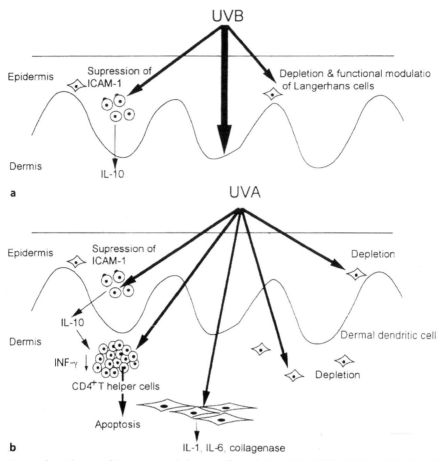

Fig. 1a, b. Scheme of immunomodulatory effects induced by UVB- [A] or UVA(1)-[B] photo(chemo)therapy. *ICAM-1*, intercellular adhesion molecule-1; *IFN-γ*, interferon-γ; *IL-10*, interleukin-10

teinase expression in human skin. The capacity to modulate the production of soluble, immunomodulatory mediators has been demonstrated in extenso for UVB and more recently also for UVA and UVA-1 radiation [32, 36]. In contrast, little is currently known about the effects of PUVA on the release of cytokines, neuropeptides, and prostanoids.

Induction of Anti-inflammatory/Immunosuppressive Factors

Therapeutic effects induced by UVB or UVA radiation can be attributed, at least in part, to the induction of mediators with anti-inflammatory or immunosuppressive properties. In vitro studies employing cultured human keratinocytes have demonstrated that UVB, and to some extent also UVA radiation, are capable of inducing the production of cytokines, neuropeptides, and prostanoids with such properties. For example, a keratinocyte-derived cytokine of particular therapeutic relevance is interleukin (IL)-10, which is functionally defined by its capacity to suppress the production of interferon (IFN)-γ by T lymphocytes of the T helper-1-like subtype. There has been some debate about the capacity of human keratinocytes to secrete IL-10, but recent in vitro and in vivo studies have unambiguously demonstrated that UVB and, in particular UVA-1 radiation, have the capacity to increase significantly IL-10 mRNA and protein expression in cultured normal human keratinocytes, and IL-10 protein expression is increased in epidermal keratinocytes following in vivo UV irradiation of human skin [10, 11]. Successful phototherapy (UVA-1 or UVA/UVB) of atopic dermatitis is associated with downregulation of IFN-γ expression in atopic eczema [9] and this effect may, at least in part, be explained by phototherapy-induced expression of IL-10 and subsequent paracrine suppression of IFN-γ production.

Another example of a UVB- and UVA-1-inducible soluble factor that is increasingly produced by irradiated keratinocytes and which exerts anti-inflammatory/ immunosuppressive effects is the neuropeptide alpha-melanocyte-stimulating hormone (alpha-MSH). In vitro exposure of human keratinocytes to UVB or UVA-1 radiation increases the synthesis of proopiomelanocorticotropin-derived peptides including alpha-MSH [32]. Alpha-MSH has a variety of anti-inflammatory (e.g., inhibition of IL-1 or tumor necrosis factor (TNF)-α-mediated inflammation) and immunosuppressive effects (e.g., inhibition of cell-mediated immune responses). It has therefore been proposed that UV radiation-induced production of alpha-MSH constitutes a UV-inducible, anti-inflammatory agent.

A third example is UVB and UVA radiation-induced production of prostaglandins in epidermal keratinocytes [8]. Prostaglandin (PG)E_2 is a potent immunosuppressant that affects the expression of costimulatory molecules on the surface of antigen-presenting cells and thereby prevents the activation of selected T-cell subsets (especially Th_1-like cells) [12]. Very recent studies indicate that in addition to keratinocytes, UV-irradiated epidermal Langerhans' cells may constitute an important cellular source for immunosuppressive prostanoids. Ultraviolet B and, in particular UVA-1 irradiation of human dendritic cells, markedly induced cyclooxygenase activity and caused the production and release of significant amounts of PGE_2 and thromboxane (J. Krutmann et al., unpublished observation).

Regulation of Proteolytic Enzymes by UV-Inducible Cytokines

Ultraviolet radiation-inducible soluble factors also include cytokines such as IL-1 or IL-6, which exert proinflammatory, and thus therapeutically unfavorable, effects. It is of interest, however, that successful UVA-1 phototherapy of patients with localized scleroderma was associated with an up to 20-fold induction of matrix metalloproteinase (MMP)-1 expression in sclerotic skin lesions that had improved under phototherapy [47]. In these patients, skin sclerosis is due to increased collagen production and deposition. Phototherapy-induced softening and dissapearance of sclerotic skin lesions may thus result from induction of the MMP-1 protease. Similar to UVB radiation, UVA-1 radiation might induce MMP-1 expression directly, but in vitro studies employing human dermal fibroblasts indicate that UVA-1 radiation-induced MMP-1 expression is in part caused by an autocrine mechanism involving the UVA-1-inducible cytokines IL-1 and IL-6 [52]. At least for the treatment of sclerotic skin lesions, induction of these proinflammatory cytokines by high-dose UVA-1 phototherapy may thus be beneficial rather than detrimental.

Effects on Cell Surface Receptors

There is increasing evidence that UVB and UVA radiation as well as PUVA treatment can directly affect the expression and function of cell surface receptors including adhesion molecules, cytokine, and growth factor receptors.

Modulation of Adhesion Molecule Expression

A hallmark of UV- or PUVA-responsive skin diseases such as psoriasis, atopic dermatitis, and cutaneous T-cell lymphoma is an increased expression of the adhesion molecule intercellular adhesion molecule-1 (ICAM-1) on the surface of epidermal keratinocytes [31]. The ICAM-1 molecule is functionally defined by its capacity to serve as a counter-receptor for the lymphocyte function associated antigen-1 (LFA-1), which is present on the surface of leukocytes. There is strong in vitro and in vivo evidence that ICAM-1/LFA-1 mediated cell-cell adhesion is an important prerequisite for the generation and maintenance of a variety of inflammatory and immune reactions in the skin [21, 25–28]. In healthy human skin, keratinocytes express little or no ICAM-1 on their surface. This is in sharp contrast to inflamed skin, in which keratinocyte ICAM-1 expression is markedly upregulated. Stimulation of keratinocytes by proinflammatory cytokines including IFN-γ, TNF-β, and TNF-α is responsible for this upregulation [31]. It has therefore been of particular phototherapeutic interest to learn that cytokine-induced ICAM-1 expression may be efficiently inhibited by irradiation of cultured keratinocytes with sublethal doses of UVB or UVA radiation [18, 40]. This anti-inflammatory property of UV radiation is also observed in vivo [44, 49]. Exposure of human skin to suberythemal doses of UVB radiation was sufficient to effectively suppress upregulation of keratinocyte ICAM-1 expression, which was induced through i.c. injection of rh-IFN-γ. In vitro and in vivo inhibition of ICAM-1 expression was observed only if UVB irradiation preceded cytokine stimulation. In additional studies it has been demonstrated that the UVB radiation-induced suppression of ICAM-1 induction was transient in nature, because 24 h after UVB radiation exposure significant induction of keratinocyte ICAM-1 expression was observed [20, 40]. If UVB irradiation was repeated 24 h after the first exposure, reinduction of ICAM-1 suppression was achieved, indicating that a maximal anti-inflammatory effect required repetitive exposure to UVB phototherapy.

The gene regulatory mechanisms responsible for this anti-inflammatory effect are poorly understood. Inhibition of cytokine-induced ICAM-1 expression does not depend on the nature of the ICAM-1 inducing cytokine [20]. It is therefore unlikely that UVB radiation interferes with intracellular signal transduction induced by a specific cytokine, but it may very well be that UVB radiation induces a mechanism that in a more general way prevents transcription of inducible genes. The latter possibility is supported by a series of recent observations indicating that UVB radiation also suppresses the upregulation of other cytokine-inducible genes including HLA-class II molecules and IL-7 [15].

The successful treatment of psoriasis with PUVA is associated with a marked reduction in keratinocyte ICAM-1 expression in lesional skin [31]. It should be noted, however, that there is currently no convincing evidence that PUVA, similar to UVB or UVA radiation, is capable of directly modulating cytokine-induced or constitutive keratinocyte ICAM-1 expression. PUVA therapy-induced downregulation of keratinocyte ICAM-1 expression may therefore best be explained by an indirect mechanism, e.g., the reduction of cytokine-producing, skin-infiltrating inflammatory cells, which could also result in reduced ICAM-1 expression.

In addition to keratinocytes, UVB radiation has been found to significantly suppress adhesion molecule expression in antigen-presenting cells such as monocytes or epidermal Langerhans' cells [19, 45]. These downregulatory effects appear to be relatively specific, and they mainly affect the ICAM-1 molecule and members of the B7 family. UVB radiation-induced inhibition of adhesion molecule expression is of functional relevance because the resulting alteration of the costimulatory repertoire of antigen-presenting cells appears to cause anergy in effector Th_1 cells and preferential activation of regulatory Th_2 cells.

Targeting of Cytokine and Growth Factor Receptors

Keratinocyte-derived IL-1-α is one of the key cytokines in the initiation of cutaneous inflammation. The regulation of keratinocyte IL-1 receptor expression, therefore, has a major impact on the course of inflammatory reactions in the skin. Human keratinocytes express two different receptor molecules for IL-1: the IL-1 receptor type I (IL-1RI) and the IL-1 receptor type II (IL-1RII). These molecules differ markedly from a functional point of view. IL-1RI serves as a signaling receptor, whereas IL-1RII does not mediate IL-1 induced signals. However, by virtue of its capacity to bind IL-1, IL-1RII functions as a decoy receptor limiting or suppressing IL-1-mediated tissue responses. It has, therefore, been of phototherapeutic interest to learn that UVB radiation regulates IL-1RI and IL-1RII expression differentially in human keratinocytes [13]. Expression of IL-1RII is rapidly and dramatically induced after UVB radiation, whereas IL-1RI expression decreases at the same time (though at a later point it gradually increases). It has therefore been proposed that UVB radiation may limit excessive responses to IL-1 stimulation of keratinocytes under inflammatory conditions by two complementary mechanisms:

1. increased expression of the decoy receptor IL-1RII and
2. decreased expression of the signaling molecule IL-1RI.

Downregulation of the signaling receptor by UVB radiation is not specific for IL-1α, but may also be observed for other cytokines including TNFα. Accordingly, in vitro exposure of human keratinocytes to sublethal doses of UVB radiation initially decreased mRNA and protein expression of the 55-kDa TNF receptor, which was subsequently followed by TNF receptor re-expression, eventually exceeding baseline levels [50]. Moreover, at time points of decreased TNF receptor expression, TNF responsiveness of UVB-irradiated keratinocytes was significantly reduced. UVB radiation did not affect the release of soluble TNF receptors from human keratinocytes. In a similar manner, UVB or UVA-1 radiation also failed to modulate the production of soluble ICAM-1 molecules produced by human keratinocytes [22].

In addition to cytokines, growth factor receptors such as the epidermal growth factor (EGF) receptor appear to be important target molecules for UV radiation as well as PUVA treatment. Modulation of EGF receptor expression and function is thought to be of central importance within the signal transduction cascade relevant for UV radiation-induced gene expression. These studies were mainly directed at analyzing the so-called "stress response" in mammalian cells, and the UV radiation doses used were of little therapeutic relevance. This is in contrast, however, to studies assessing the effects of PUVA treatment on EGF receptor function. In murine as well as human cells, PUVA radiation inhibits binding of EGF to its receptors [30]. Since EGF is a growth factor for keratinocytes, it has been proposed that PUVA-induced inhibition of EGF binding might contribute to the beneficial effects induced by PUVA therapy in psoriasis, a skin disease characterized by keratinocyte hyperproliferation.

Induction of Apoptosis in Skin-Infiltrating Cells

T cells have an increased susceptibility towards UV radiation-induced apoptosis compared to other cell populations such as monocytes or keratinocytes. Morita et al. were the first to demonstrate that induction of apoptosis in skin-infiltrating T cells is the basic mechanism in UVA phototherapy of atopic dermatitis [37]. Atopic dermatitis may be viewed as a T-cell-mediated skin disease in which activation of T-helper cells by inhalant allergens (or atopens) leads to T-cell cytokine production and the subsequent development of eczema. This process involves an early initiation phase that is dominated by the expression of Th_2-like cytokines, which is then switched into a second, later phase [14]. The latter is characterized by the predominance of the Th_1-like cytokine IFN-γ, which is responsible for the development and maintenance of clinically apparent eczema. Successful phototherapy of atopic dermatitis with UVA-1 radiation is associated with a marked reduction in the number of skin-infiltrating T cells and subsequent downregulation of IFN-γ expression in lesional atopic skin [9]. By employing a double labeling technique to identify $CD4^+$, apoptotic T cells, Morita et al. demonstrated that UVA-1 phototherapy induced apoptosis in T-helper cells present in the dermal compartment of atopic eczema. After only a few (1–3) exposures of patients to single doses of 130 J/cm^2 UVA-1, $CD4^+$, apoptotic T cells were present in lesional atopic skin [37]. Continuation of UVA-1 phototherapy lead to a gradual increase in the number of apoptotic T-helper cells and a subsequent reduction of the inflammatory infiltrate and improvement of clinical symptoms.

Induction of T-cell apoptosis is not specific for UVA phototherapy [6, 17, 33, 55]. Successful UVB phototherapy of psoriatic patients induced a reduction in the number of skin-infiltrating T cells, which was followed by a normalization of keratinocyte morphology. In vitro UVB irradiation induced T-cell apoptosis, suggesting that the reduction of the inflammatory infiltrate resulted from UVB radiation-induced T-cell apoptosis [17]. This hypothesis has recently been proven by the demonstration of apoptotic T cells in lesional psoriatic skin of patients undergoing UVB phototherapy [41]. Induction of T-cell apoptosis was observed regardless of whether broadband UVB or 311-nm UVB phototherapy was employed. It should be noted, however, that because of its physical properties, a much greater level of 311-nm UVB radiation penetrates into human dermis, and therefore apoptosis occurs in both epidermal and dermal T cells. This difference may at least partially explain the clinical observation that 311-nm UVB phototherapy is superior to broadband UVB phototherapy for the treatment of psoriasis [42].

Induction of T-cell apoptosis is also thought to be a key mechanism for PUVA therapy. Evidence for the appearance of apoptotic T cells under PUVA therapy has thus far been provided for peripheral blood T cells in patients with Sézary syndrome undergoing extracorporeal photopheresis [55]. Interestingly, the induction of apoptotic cells is not an immunologically null-event, but most likely it has immunosuppressive consequences. Phagocytosis of apoptotic cells has profound effects on mediator production by macrophages [54]. After phagocytosis of apoptotic T cells, macrophage production of the anti-inflammatory/immunosuppressive cytokine IL-10 is increased, whereas the production of proinflammatory cytokines such as TNF-α, IL-1, and IL-12 is downregulated [4, 54]. Further studies have demonstrated that inhibition of the production of proinflammatory cytokines is mediated through the autocrine production of TGF-β [34]. In addition, there is increased production of selected chemokines, in particular Mip-1-α and Mip-2. These studies provide a rationale to explain how extracorporeal photopheresis, through the induction of apoptosis in only a small percentage of circulating T cells, exerts immunosuppressive effects, as evidenced by the successful use of this modality in transplantation immunology.

The mechanisms by which UVA-1 and UVB radiation induce T-cell apoptosis differ markedly. In general, UVA-1 radiation can cause preprogrammed cell death (early apoptosis), which is protein synthesis independent, as well as programmed cell death (late apoptosis), which requires de novo protein synthesis [5]. In contrast, UVB irradiation (and also PUVA treatment) exclusively induces late apoptosis [6]. By employing atopen-specific human T-helper cells that have been cloned from lesional skin of atopic dermatitis patients, Morita et al. have demonstrated that UVA-1 radiation is able to cause both early and late apoptosis and that UVA1-R-induced singlet oxygen generation is the initiating event leading to T-cell apoptosis [37]. Singlet oxygen production induced the expression of Fas-ligand molecules on the surface of UVA-1-irradiated T cells. Subsequent binding of Fas ligand to Fas on the same or neighboring T cells was then shown to be responsible for T-cell apoptosis (Fig. 2). The key role of singlet oxygen in eliciting early apoptosis in human T cells has recently been corroborated in an

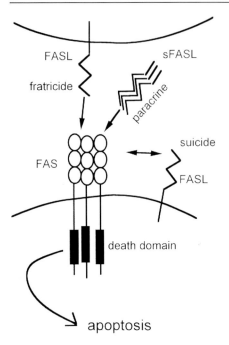

Fig. 2. Scheme of potential mechanisms by which T-cell apoptosis may be induced. *sFASL*, soluble Fas ligand

independent study employing Jurkat cells. Ultraviolet A-1 radiation/singlet oxygen has been postulated to act on mitochondria and induce Jurkat-cell apoptosis by opening the megachannel and by decreasing the mitochondrial membrane potential [6]. The capacity to induce early apoptosis in mammalian cells seems to be highly specific for UVA-1 radiation and singlet oxygen, respectively. From a photo-therapeutic point of view, this qualitative difference suggests that UVA-1 photo-therapy is superior to UVB or PUVA therapy for skin diseases in which induction of apoptosis in pathogenetically relevant cells is of critical importance. This assumption is supported by the observation that UVA-1 radiation, but not PUVA, is capable of inducing apoptosis in skin-infiltrating mast cells of patients with urti-caria pigmentosa (Fig. 3). As a consequence, UVA-1 phototherapy, but not PUVA was associated with mast cell depletion from skin and longer lasting remission periods in these patients [46, 48]. The unique properties of UVA-1 radiation have also stimulated interest in its therapeutic use for patients with cutaneous T-cell lymphoma [43]. In vitro studies indicate that malignant T cells are exquisitely sen-sitive to UVA-1 radiation-induced apoptosis, and UVA-1 phototherapy might thus prove to be at least equivalent, if not superior to PUVA for this indication [38].

Photobiological Aspects of Photo(chemo)therapy

Several immunomodulatory effects of phototherapeutic relevance, e.g., the induction of IL-10 or the suppression of ICAM-1 induction, may be achieved by both UVB and UVA-1 irradiation. The photobiological mechanisms responsible for these immunomodulatory effects, however, have been found to greatly differ depending on the type of UV radiation used [24].

Similar to antiproliferative effects, immunomodulation induced by UVB radiation appears to result from UVB radiation-induced generation of DNA photoproducts, in particular thymine dimers. UVB radiation-induced suppression of IFN-γ-stimulated keratinocyte ICAM-1 expression was associated with the formation of significant numbers of thymine dimers in UVB-irradiated human skin [49]. Topical application of a DNA repair enzyme encapsulated into liposomes not only decreased the number of thymine dimer positive keratinocytes in irradiated skin by about 40–50%, but it completely prevented UVB radiation-induced inhibition of ICAM-1. Essentially identical results were obtained from in vitro studies, in which the role of thymine dimer formation for UVB radiation-induced IL-10 expression in cultured murine keratinocytes was assessed [39]. Exposure of murine keratinocytes (PAM212 cells) to increasing doses of UVB radiation dose-dependently increased both thymine dimer formation and IL-10 protein expression, and treatment of irradiated cells with exogenously supplied DNA repair enzymes was sufficient to partially reduce the number of thymine dimers and at the same time to completely suppress UVB radiation-induced IL-10 protein synthesis. The precise reason for the discrepancy between the partial reversal in thymine dimers and the total prevention of immunomodulatory effects such as IL-10 synthesis or inhibition of ICAM-1 induction is currently unknown. It has been postulated that gene-specific repair mechanisms may explain this phenomenon. Thus, formation of thymine dimers appears to be of central importance for UVB radiation-induced therapeutic effects. It should be noted, however, that UVB radiation might also have cell membrane effects independent of DNA damage [29].

In contrast to UVB radiation, UVA-(1) radiation-induced immunomodulatory effects are thought to be based on oxidative mechanisms [22]. The generation of singlet oxygen plays a prominent role. This conclusion is based on the following three observations: UVA radiation-induced gene-regulatory events such as the regulation of ICAM-1 or collagenase I expression can be

1. inhibited by singlet oxygen quenchers,
2. enhanced through strategies that result in an increase in the half life of singlet oxygen, and
3. mimicked by stimulation of unirradiated cells with singlet oxygen generating systems [7, 53].

Of central importance to the understanding of these mechanisms is the recent finding that both UVA radiation- and singlet oxygen-induced gene expression are mediated through activation of transcription factor AP2, and that UVA radiation-induced gene expression is controlled through the balance between AP2 and its alternative splice product AP2B [7]. Singlet oxygen, however, is not only an important mediator for UVA radiation-induced gene regulatory events, but also plays a key role in UVA radiation-induced apoptosis in human T-helper cells [37].

In contrast to UVB or UVA radiation-induced immunomodulation, the photobiological base for PUVA-induced immunosuppressive effects has not yet been characterized.

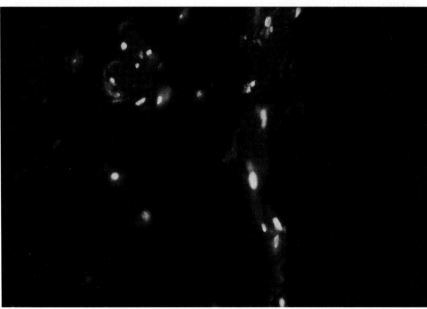

Fig. 3. Apoptotic mast cells in lesional skin of a patient with urticaria pigmentosa before (**A**) and after (**B**) UVA-1 phototherapy (3×130 J/cm^2). Mast cells were stained with an anti-mast-cell tryptase antibody in red, and apoptotic cells were detected by the transferase mediated d-UTP nick end-labeling (TUNEL) method in green. Apoptotic mast cells thus stain orange

Perspectives

There is compelling evidence that the efficacy of photo(chemo)therapy may not simply be attributed to antiproliferative effects, but most likely involves immunomodulatory consequences, some of which have been outlined above. It should be noted, however, that the majority of photoimmunological studies have been conducted either in vitro or in animal models, whereas only recently have in situ techniques been employed in order to monitor immunological changes induced in the skin of patients undergoing UV phototherapy. These studies have already contributed to our knowledge about the mode of action of UVA and UVB phototherapy, e.g., by identifying apoptosis as a key mechanism in phototherapy of T-cell-mediated skin diseases. This progress should prompt further interest in studies in this area of clinical research, which might best be described as "therapeutic photoimmunology".

References

1. Bevilaqua PM, Edelson RL, Gasparro FP (1991) High performance liquid chromatography analysis of 8-methoxypsoralen monoadducts and crosslinks in lymphocytes and keratinocytes. J Invest Dermatol 97:151–155
2. Epstein JH (1968) UVL-induced stimulation of DNA synthesis in hairless mouse epidermis. J Invest Dermatol 52:445–448
3. Everett M, Yeargers E, Sayre R, Olson R (1966) Penetration of epidermis by ultraviolet rays. Photochem Photobiol 5:533–542
4. Fadok VA, Bratton DL, Konowal A, Freed PW, Wstcott JY, Henson PM (1998) Macrophages that have ingested apoptotic cells in vitro inhibit proinflammatory cytokine production through autocrine/paracrine mechanisms involving TGF-ß, PGE2, and PAF. J Clin Invest 101:890–896
5. Godar DE (1996) Preprogrammed and programmed cell death mechanisms of apoptosis: UV-induced immediate and delayed apoptosis. Photochem Photobiol 63:825–830
6. Godar DE (1999) UVA 1 radiation mediates singlet-oxygen and superoxide-anion production which trigger two different final apoptotic pathways: the S and P site of mitochondria. J Invest Dermatol 112:3–12
7. Grether-Beck S, Olaizola-Horn S, Schmitt H, Grewe M, Jahnke A, Johnson JP, Briviba K, Sies H, Krutmann J (1996) Activation of transcription factor AP-2 mediates UVA radiation- and singlet oxygen-induced expression of the human intercellular adhesion molecule-1 gene. Proc Natl Acad Sci USA 93:14586–14591
8. Grewe M, Trefzer U, Ballhorn A, Gyufko K, Henninger HP, Krutmann J (1993) Analysis of the mechanism of ultraviolet B radiation induced prostaglandin E2 synthesis by human epidermoid carcinoma cells. J Invest Dermatol 101:528–531
9. Grewe M, Gyufko K, Schöpf E, Krutmann J (1994) Lesional expression of interferon-γ in atopic eczema. Lancet 343:25–26
10. Grewe M, Gyufko K, Krutmann J (1995) Interleukin-10 production by cultured human keratinocytes: regulation by ultraviolet B and ultraviolet A1 radiation. J Invest Dermatol 104:3–6
11. Grewe M, Duvic M, Aragane Y, Schwarz T, Ullrich SE, Krutmann J (1996) Lack of induction of IL-10 expression in human keratinocytes. Reply. J Invest Dermatol 106:1330–1331
12. Grewe M, Klammer M, Stege H, Krutmann J (1996) Involvement of direct and indirect mechanisms in ultraviolet B radiation (UVBR)-induced inhibition of ICAM-1 expression in human antigen presenting cells. Abstract. J Invest Dermatol 106:933

13. Grewe M, Gyufko K, Budnik A, Berneburg M, Ruzicka T, Krutmann J (1996) Interleukin-1 receptors type I and type II are differentially regulated in human keratinocytes by ultraviolet B radiation. J Invest Dermatol 107:865–871

14. Grewe M, Bruijnzeel-Koomen CAFM, Schöpf E, Thepen T, Langeveld-Wildschuh AG, Ruzicka T, Krutmann J (1998) A role for Th1 and Th2 cells in the immunopathogenesis of atopic dermatitis. Immunol Today 19:359–361

15. Khan IU, Boehm KD, Elmets CA (1993) Modulation of IFNγ-induced HLA-DR expression on the human keratinocyte cell line SCC-13 by ultraviolet radiation. Photochem Photobiol 57:103–106

16. Kripke ML (1981) Immunologic mechanisms in UV radiation carcinogenesis. Adv Cancer Res 34:69–106

17. Krueger JG, Wolfe JT, Nabeja RT, Vallat VP, Gilleaudeau P, Heftler NS, Austin LM, Gottlieb AB (1995) Successful ultraviolet B treatment of psoriasis is accompanied by a reversal of keratinocyte pathology and by selective depletion of intraepidermal T cells. J Exp Med 182:2057–2068

18. Krutmann J, Koeck A, Schauer E, Parlow F, Moeller A, Kapp A, Foerster E, Schoepf E, Luger TA (1990) Tumor necrosis factor β and ultraviolet radiation are potent regulators of human keratinocyte ICAM-1 expression. J Invest Dermatol 95:127–131

19. Krutmann J, Khan IU, Wallis RS, Zhang F, Koehler KA, Rich EA, Ellner JJ, Elmets CA (1990) The cell membrane is a major locus for ultraviolet-B-induced alterations in accessory cells. J Clin Invest 85:1529–1536

20. Krutmann J, Czech W, Parlow F, Trefzer U, Kapp A, Schoepf E, Luger TA (1992) Ultraviolet radiation effects on human keratinocyte ICAM-1 expression: UV-induced inhibition of cytokine induced ICAM-1 mRNA expression is transient, differentially restored for IFN-γ versus TNFα, and followed by ICAM-1 induction via a TNFα-like pathway. J Invest Dermatol 98:923–928

21. Krutmann J, Czech W, Diepgen T, Niedner R, Kapp A, Schöpf E (1992) High-dose UVA1 therapy in the treatment of patients with atopic dermatitis. J Am Acad Dermatol 26:225–230

22. Krutmann J (1994) Regulatory interactions between epidermal cell adhesion molecules and cytokines. In: Luger TA, Schwarz T (eds) Epidermal growth factors and cytokines. Dekker, New York, pp 415–432

23. Krutmann J, Elmets CA (eds)(1995) Photoimmunology. Blackwell Science, Oxford

24. Krutmann J, Grewe M (1995) Involvement of cytokines, DNA damage, and reactive oxygen species in ultraviolet radiation-induced modulation of intercellular adhesion molecule-1 expression. J Invest Dermatol 105:67S–70S

25. Krutmann J (1996) Phototherapy for atopic dermatitis. Dermatol Therapy 1:24–31

26. Krutmann J (1997) High-dose UVA-1 therapy for inflammatory skin diseases. Dermatol Ther 4:123–128

27. Krutmann J, Diepgen TL, Luger TA, Grabbe S, Meffert H, Sönnichsen N, Czech W, Kapp A, Stege H, Grewe M, Schöpf E (1998) High-dose UVA1 therapy for atopic dermatitis: results of a multicenter trial. J Am Acad Dermatol 38:589–593

28. Krutmann J (1999) Therapeutic photomedicine: phototherapy. In: Freedberg IM, Eisen AB, Wolff K, Austen KF, Goldsmith LA, Katz SI, Fitzpatrick TB (eds) Fitzpatrick's dermatology in general medicine, 5th edn. McGraw-Hill, New York, pp 2870–2879

29. Kulms D, Pöppelmann B, Yarosh D, Luger TA, Krutmann J, Schwarz T (1999) Nuclear and cell membrane effects contribute independently to the induction of apoptosis in human cells exposed to UVB radiation. Proc Natl Acad Sci USA 96:7974–7979

30. Laskin JD, Lee E, Yurkow EJ, Laskin DL, Gallo MA (1985) A possible mechanism of psoralen phototoxicity not involving direct interaction with DNA. Proc Natl Acad Sci USA 82:6158–6162

31. Lisby S, Ralfkier E, Rothlein R, Veijsgard GL (1989) Intercellular adhesion molecule-1 (ICAM-1) expression correlated to inflammation. Br J Dermatol 120:479–484

32. Luger TA, Schwarz T (1995) Effects of UV light on cytokines and neuroendocrine hormones. In: Krutmann J, Elmets CA (eds) Photoimmunology. Blackwell Science, Oxford, pp 55–76

33. Marks DI, Fox RM (1991) Mechanism of photochemotherapy induced apoptotic cell death in lymphoid cells. Biochem Cell Biol 69:754–760

34. McDonald PP, Fadok VA, Bratton D, Henson PM (1999) Transcriptional and translational regulation of inflammatory mediator production by endogenous TGF-β in macrophages that have ingested apoptotic cells. J Immunol 163:6164–6172

35. Morison WL (1993) Photochemotherapy. In: Lim HW, Soter NA (eds) Clinical photomedicine. Dekker, New York, pp 327–346

36. Morita A, Grewe M, Ahrens C, Grether-Beck S, Ruzicka T, Krutmann J (1997a) Ultraviolet A1 radiation effects on cytokine expression in human epidermoid carcinoma cells. Photochem Photobiol 65:630–635

37. Morita A, Werfel T, Stege H, Ahrens C, Karmann K, Grewe M, Grether-Beck S, Ruzicka T, Kapp A, Klotz O, Sies H, Krutmann J (1997b) Evidence that singlet oxygen-induced human T-helper cell apoptosis is the basic mechanism of ultraviolet-A radiation phototherapy. J Exp Med 186:1763–1768

38. Morita A, Yamauchi Y, Yasuda Y, Tsuji T, Krutmann J (2000) Malignant T-cells are exquisitely sensitive to ultraviolet A-1 (UVA-1) radiation-induced apoptosis. J Invest Dermatol (in press)

39. Nishigori C, Yarosh DB, Ullrich SE, Vink AA, Bucana CD, Roza L, Kripke ML (1996) Evidence that DNA damage triggers interleukin 10 cytokine production in UV-irradiated murine keratinocytes. Proc Natl Acad Sci USA 93:10354–10359

40. Norris DA, Lyons B, Middleton MH, Yohn JY, Kashihara-Sawami M (1990) Ultraviolet radiation can either suppress or induce expression of intercellular adhesion molecule-1 (ICAM-1) on the surface of cultured human keratinocytes. J Invest Dermatol 95:132–138

41. Ozawa M, Ferenci K, Kikuchi T, Cardinale I, Austin LM, Coven TR, Burack LH, Krueger JG (1999) 312-nanometer ultraviolet B light (narrow band UVB) induces apoptosis of T cells within psoriatic lesions. J Exp Med 189:711–718

42. Picot E, Meunier L, Picot-Deheze ML, Peyron JL, Meynadier J (1992) Treatment of psoriasis with a 311 nm UVB lamp. Br J Dermatol 127:509–512

43. Plettenberg H, Stege H, Megahed M, Ruzicka T, Hosokawa Y, Tsuji T, Morita A, Krutmann J (1999) Ultraviolet A1 (340–400 nm) phototherapy for cutaneous T-cell lymphoma. J Am Acad Dermatol 41:47–50

44. Roza L, Stege H, Krutmann J (1996) Role of UV-induced DNA damage in phototherapy. In: Hönigsmann H, Jori G, Young AR (eds) The fundamental bases of phototherapy. OEMF spa, Milano, pp 145–152

45. Simon JC, Krutmann J, Elmets CA, Bergstresser PR, Cruz D (1992) Ultraviolet B irradiated antigen presenting cells display altered accessory signaling for T cell activation: relevance to immune responses initiated in the skin. J Invest Dermatol 98:66S–69S

46. Stege H, Schöpf E, Ruzicka T, Krutmann J (1996) High-dose-UVA1 for urticaria pigmentosa. Lancet 347:64

47. Stege H, Berneburg M, Humke S, Klammer M, Grewe M, Grether-Beck S, Dierks K, Goerz G, Ruzicka T, Krutmann J (1997) High-dose ultraviolet A1 (UVA1) radiation therapy for localized scleroderma. J Am Acad Dermatol 36:938–943

48. Stege H, Budde M, Kürten V, Ruzicka T, Krutmann J (1999) Induction of apoptosis in skin-infiltrating mast cells by high-dose ultraviolet A-1 radiation phototherapy in patients with urticaria pigmentosa. J Invest Dermatol 114:791

49. Stege H, Roza L, Vink AA, Grewe M, Ruzicka T, Grether-Beck S, Krutmann J (2000) Enzyme plus light therapy to repair DNA damage in ultraviolet-B-irradiated human skin. Proc Natl Acad Sci USA 97:1790–1795

50. Trefzer U, Brockhaus M, Lötscher H, Parlow F, Budnik A, Grewe M, Christoph H, Kapp A, Schöpf E, Luger TA, Krutmann J (1993) The human 55-kd tumor necrosis factor receptor is regulated in human keratinocytes by TNFα and by ultraviolet B radiation. J Clin Invest 92:462–470
51. Volc-Platzer B, Hönigsmann H (1995) Photoimmunology of PUVA and UVB therapy. In: Krutmann J, Elmets CA (eds) Photoimmunology. Blackwell Science, Oxford, pp 265–273
52. Wlascheck M, Heinen G, Poswig A, Schwarz A, Krieg T, Scharfetter-Kochanek K (1994) UVA-induced autocrine stimulation of fibroblasts derived collagenase/MMP-1 by interrelated loops of interkeukin-1 and interleukin-6. Photochem Photobiol 59:550–556
53. Wlascheck M, Briviba K, Stricklin GP, Sies H, Scharfetter-Kochanek K (1995) Singlet oxygen may mediate the ultraviolet A-induced synthesis of interstitial collagenase. J Invest Dermatol 104:194–198
54. Voll RE, Herrmann M, Roth EA, Stach C, Kalden JR, Girkontaite I (1997) Immunosuppressive effects of apoptotic cells. Nature 390:330
55. Yoo EK, Rook AH, Elenitas R, Gasparro FP, Vowels BR (1996) Apoptosis induction by ultraviolet light A and photochemotherapy in cutaneous T-cell lymphoma: Relevance to mechanism of therapeutic action. J Invest Dermatol 107:235–242

II Photo(chemo)therapy in daily practice

3 Photo(chemo)therapy for Psoriasis

Herbert Hönigsmann, Adrian Tanew, Thomas Ruzicka, Warwick L. Morison

Contents

This chapter reviews the current practice of phototherapy with ultraviolet (UV) radiation and of psoralen photochemotherapy (PUVA) in the treatment of psoriasis. Both treatment modalities are well-established in today's armamentarium of dermatological therapy. Continued clinical research has helped to improve treatment protocols. Simultaneously, the understanding of mechanisms underlying the biological responses to UV exposure and psoralen photosensitization has much increased. Therefore, we are well prepared to minimize the potential long-term side effects such as skin carcinogenesis by optimizing therapeutic strategies. Phototherapeutic regimens use repeated, controlled UV exposures to alter cutaneous biology, which in this context aims at inducing remission of skin disease. In this chapter we will discuss the use of UVB radiation without sensitizer as well as psoralen photosensitization (PUVA). Although UVB has been used for a longer time than PUVA, the latter has been evaluated and validated in a more detailed and coordinated fashion.

Phototherapy

Historical Aspects

Phototherapy of psoriasis with artificial light sources has a tradition going back more than 70 years, and, if heliotherapy is considered, centuries. Early in the twentieth century, psoriasis phototherapy was performed with carbon arc lamps similar to the lamps developed by Finsen for the treatment of lupus vulgaris. Later, medium-pressure mercury arc lamps, which were more practical and had a higher output of ultraviolet (UV) radiation, replaced carbon arc lamps. In 1925, Goeckerman, at the Mayo Clinic, introduced a combination of topical crude coal tar and subsequent UV irradiation for the treatment of psoriasis. This treatment became a standard therapy for psoriasis for half a century, particularly in the USA. More recently, it was shown in the 1970s that broadband UVB radiation alone, if given in doses that produce a faint erythematous reaction, can clear certain clinical forms of psoriasis, particularly seborrheic and guttate types. A major step forward was the introduction in 1984 of a newly designed lamp emitting a narrow band at 312 nm. This lamp proved to yield better results than broad-spectrum UVB lamps. This treatment currently appears to represent the most effective phototherapy for psoriasis.

Heliotherapy

The beneficial effects of sunlight on psoriasis have been well-recognized since ancient times, and heliotherapy for psoriasis enjoyed special attention in the early twentieth century. More recently, heliotherapy, also called climatotherapy, has been successfully used at the Dead Sea. This area has an unusually high ratio of UVA to UVB radiation because of its location 400 m below sea level and the vapor in the atmosphere [1]. The treatment is believed to be cost-effective and pleasant. However, it seems that relapses occur quite early, probably because treatment is discontinued abruptly after clearing and no maintenance therapy schedule follows, as is usual for UV phototherapy with artificial UV.

Principles and Mechanisms of Phototherapy

Phototherapy for psoriasis traditionally refers to the use of artificial broadband UVB irradiations delivered by fluorescent lamps. It is the use of ultraviolet irradiations for therapeutic purposes without the addition of exogenous photosensitizers. The radiation is absorbed by endogenous chromophores. The photochemical reactions of these absorbing biomolecules result in alterations of skin biology and thus lead to the treatment effect.

The best-characterized chromophore for UVB is nuclear DNA. Absorption of UV by nucleotides leads to DNA photoproduct formation, mainly pyrimidine dimers [2]. Despite the quantitative predominance of the dimers, the pyrimidine (6–4) pyrimidone photoproduct may be biologically more significant [3].

Many biological consequences of UV radiation have been linked to specific DNA photoproducts [4, 5]. Much is known on how DNA photoproducts interfere with cell cycle progression and induce growth arrest for cell-fate decision [6].

UVB exposure is known to cause a reduction of DNA synthesis [7, 8]. Therefore, it can be used to suppress the accelerated DNA synthesis in psoriatic epidermal cells. A more detailed explanation of how UVB and UVB-induced DNA damage interfere with cell division has been developed. The tumor suppressor gene product p53 was shown to be upregulated after UVB exposure. It is involved in control of the cell cycle via regulation of the WAF 1/CIP 1 gene [9]. This mechanism may be relevant for the reversal of the shortened cell cycle in keratinocytes of psoriatic epidermis. The UVB-induced alteration of cell cycle control mechanisms is also important for apoptosis, which is seen in skin after UVB exposure ("sunburn cells"), and the control of skin carcinogenesis [10].

Besides the effect on cell cycle, UV radiation induces prostaglandin release and alters cytokine expression and secretion [11, 12]. Interleukins 6 and 10 seem to play important roles for systemic symptoms of UV phototoxicity (sunburn) and immunosuppression [13–16]. All these mechanisms may be equally important for therapeutic effectiveness and side effects. Also, UV-induced cellular molecular effects that are independent of nuclear DNA damage have been demonstrated. These involve membrane receptors and molecular signaling pathways that regulate transcriptional activity [17, 18]. Thus, gene expression may also be altered independently of DNA damage. The existence of such molecular regulatory mechanisms indicates additional or parallel molecular pathways but does not help to identify the actual cellular targets and effector mechanisms of phototherapy. One important aspect of the mechanisms of phototherapy is the effect on cutaneous immune response by UVB. Recently, UV-induced systemic immunosuppression has also been linked to the formation of pyrimidine dimers [19]. UV radiation suppresses contact allergy, delayed type hypersensitivity, and immunosurveillance against UV-induced non-melanoma skin carcinoma in mice. Langerhans' cells are very sensitive to UVB, which alters their antigen-presenting function. Keratinocytes secrete soluble mediators such as interleukin-1 and -6, prostaglandin E2, tumor necrosis factor alpha, and several others under the influence of UV radiation. This may alter the cutaneous immune response by direct effects on T lymphocytes or via their influence on the function of epidermal Langerhans' cells [20].

The interplay of the various photobiological pathways is far from being completely understood. In psoriasis, both epidermal keratinocytes and cutaneous lymphocytes may be targeted by UVB. Immune suppression, alteration of cytokine expression, as well as cell-cycle arrest may contribute to the suppression of disease activity in psoriatic lesions.

Action Spectrum and Radiation Sources

The term action spectrum defines the relative effectiveness of a particular wavelength for a specific radiation-induced process. In phototherapy this process denotes the therapeutic effect. The action spectrum for erythema induction is well defined, and therapeutic efficacy in psoriasis therapy usually parallels erythema formation. However, excessive erythema can be a limiting factor in phototherapy. Therefore an optimal relationship between antipsoriatic and erythemogenic activity appears desirable.

When comparing therapeutic spectra, Fisher noted an improved antipsoriatic efficacy of wavelengths around 313 nm [21]. Parrish and Jaenicke [22] reported an action spectrum for antipsoriatic activity demonstrating that wavelengths shorter than 296 nm were almost ineffective for treating psoriasis even when multiple minimal erythema doses (MEDs) were used for individual exposures. In contrast, the 304- and 313-nm bands were optimally effective even with suberythemogenic doses. This action spectrum is well matched by standard therapeutic UVB fluorescent lamps, which emit wavelengths between 295 and 350 nm with a peak at 305 nm. In the UVA range, erythemogenic doses are also therapeutically relevant, but require fluences more than 1,000 times higher than needed for UVB phototherapy and are therefore not practical. The addition of UVA does not enhance the therapeutic efficacy of UVB [23].

New lamps have been designed to meet the therapeutic action spectra better than conventional sources. One regimen using metal halide lamps with increased emission between 295 and 330 nm has been described as selective ultraviolet phototherapy (SUP) [24]. SUP is more efficient than broadband phototherapy but does not compare with PUVA [25]. The more recent development of 312 nm narrowband UVB (a narrow fluorescent band at 311–313 nm emitted by the Philips TL-01 lamp) was introduced to optimally meet the requirements for antipsoriatic activity [26].

Phototherapy Regimens

Prior to phototherapy, the individual UV sensitivity of the patient should be evaluated. This is done by exposing small areas (e.g., 1-cm-diameter circles) of the lower back to an incremental series of UVB irradiations. Increases are made by steps of 10 mJ/cm^2 or geometrically by multiplying with $\sqrt{2}$. The lowest fluence that leads to well-circumscribed pink erythema is called minimal erythema dose (MED). Recently, the use of the minimal detectable erythema reaction has been proposed as a more reliable threshold value [27].

The initial therapeutic UVB dose lies at 75–100% of the MED. Treatments are given 2–5 times weekly. As peak UVB erythema appears before 24 h after exposure, increments may be done at each successive treatment. The rate of increase depends on treatment frequency, the effect of the preceding therapeutic exposure, and of treatment. The objective of the dose increments is to maintain a minimally perceptible erythema as a clinical indicator of optimal dosimetry. For example, with thrice weekly treatments, increases of 40% are given if no erythema was induced, and 20% with slight erythema. If erythema is mild but persistent, no increment is made. With daily exposure, these rates are no more than 30%, 15%, and 0%, respectively. With more intensive or painful erythema, irradiations are withheld until symptoms subside. Treatments are given until total remission is reached or no further improvement can be obtained with continued phototherapy.

Phototherapy of Psoriasis

Primarily psoriatics with eruptive and seborrheic forms of psoriasis respond rapidly with broadband UVB. The results with chronic plaque-type psoriasis, however, are not so favorable. Although broadband UVB phototherapy can be very effective, it is second to PUVA both with clearing efficiency and remission times [28]. Besides the regimens outlined above, other regimens may be used. Some schedules use skin type-dependent starting doses and fixed increments regardless of skin reaction. The patient's head, if free of psoriasis, may be covered with UV-opaque material during exposures, in order to minimize unnecessary aggravation of environmental photodamage. Sometimes, the patient's extremities are given higher dose increments than the trunk.

Upon clearing treatment is either discontinued or the patients are subjected to maintenance therapy. It is generally felt that maintenance therapy keeps patients clear of disease. However, maintenance philosophy varies around the world; moreover, the efficacy and requirements of maintenance are controversial. In Europe, many dermatologists now avoid maintenance therapy, while in America some continue treatment for years after clearing.

A few problems exist with maintenance UVB therapy. Treatment becomes time-consuming and interferes with the patient's quality of life. As more maintenance treatments are given, cumulative UVB doses rapidly increase, thus risking premature aging and photocarcinogenesis. More multicenter trials are necessary to quantify the long-term risks and answer questions about the role of maintenance therapy.

Maintenance therapy is instituted in a fairly standard way. Generally, once clear, patients decrease the frequency of UVB treatments while maintaining the last dose given at the time of clearing.

The use of adjunctive agents and combination therapies is directed at an improved efficacy and a reduction of the cumulative UVB burden in order to reduce the incidence of long-term side effects. The efficacy of phototherapy may be enhanced by applying hydrophobic vehicles preceding exposure, so that the altered optical properties of psoriatic scales increase the effective UV dose to the psoriatic lesion [29]. UVB may be combined with topical tars [30] (Goeckerman regimen) or anthralin applications [31] (Ingram regimen). The combination with topical steroids is discouraged because it may result in reduced remission times [32]. Systemic drugs such as retinoids increase efficacy, particularly in patients with chronic and hyperkeratotic plaque-type psoriasis [33, 34]. Also, retinoids may possibly reduce the carcinogenic potential of UVB phototherapy.

The use of narrowband (312 nm) phototherapy is superior to conventional broadband UVB with respect to both clearing and remission times [26, 35, 36]. This is due to an improved adjustment of the lamp's emission to the therapeutic spectral requirements. In Europe, narrowband UVB has replaced conventional phototherapy in many areas. In the USA, the Philips TL-01 lamp has only recently come into usage, partly due to minor technical incompatibilities. From our own studies and other reports, we consider narrowband phototherapy nearly as effective as PUVA [37, 38]. Narrowband UVB has also been successfully used in a variety of combination therapies, such as with retinoids (RePUVA)

[39], anthralin [31, 40], and calcipotriol [41]. The antipsoriatic efficacy of sub-erythemogenic narrowband UVB irradiations indicates a potential for further developments and improvements.

Side Effects

The short-term side effects consist of erythema ("sunburn"), dry skin with pruritus, occasional phototoxic blisters, and an increased frequency of recurrent herpes simplex eruptions. Moderate painful erythema resulting from overexposure is treated with topical corticosteroids. Systemic nonsteroidal anti-inflammatory agents and corticosteroids have also proven useful for severe cases. Subacute effects such as pruritus and dry skin respond well to intensified lubrication with bland emollients after lukewarm baths.

Long-term side effects include photoaging and carcinogenesis. UVB is a known carcinogen, although its carcinogenic potential seems to be less than that of PUVA [42]. Stern and Laird [43] in their 16-center study failed to show a relationship between UVB phototherapy and nonmelanoma skin cancer. However, they strongly caution that future studies may reveal an increased risk of nonmelanoma skin cancer with UVB phototherapy.

Photochemotherapy with Psoralens

Psoralen photochemotherapy (PUVA) is the combined use of psoralens (P) and long-wave UV radiation (UVA). The drug-and-radiation combination results in a therapeutic effect that is not achieved by the single component alone. Remission of skin disease is induced by repeated controlled phototoxic reactions [44].

Historical Aspects

Topical exposure to extracts, seeds, and parts of plants (e.g., Ammi majus, Psoralea corylifolia) that contain natural psoralens and subsequent irradiation with sunlight as a remedy for what was then called leukoderma (vitiligo) has been used for thousands of years by the ancient Egyptian and Indian healers. In Western countries, early results of vitiligo treatment with exposure to sunlight or UV radiation were reported in the beginning of the 20th century. Encouraging results with topical and oral psoralens were initially reported by El Mofty and Lerner et al. [45, 46].

In 1974 it was shown that the combination of orally administered 8-methoxypsoralen (8-MOP) and subsequent exposure to artificial UVA was a highly effective treatment for psoriasis. This new therapeutic concept was termed photochemotherapy and is known acronymously as PUVA (psoralen and UVA radiation) [47]. The development of oral PUVA therapy was made possible because of the introduction of a new high-intensity UVA radiation source. It was first used to treat psoriatic patients at the department of dermatology,

Harvard University in Boston. In a parallel study, the excellent efficacy was confirmed by studies on a large patient cohort in Vienna, Austria [48]. Within a few years, the beneficial effects of PUVA were confirmed worldwide.

However, prior to the development of the high-intensity UVA source, it had already been shown that topically applied psoralens plus exposures to low-intensity UVA (black-light) could clear psoriatic lesions [49, 50].

The effectiveness of oral photochemotherapy has been widely documented and has profoundly influenced dermatological therapy in general because it provided treatment for a variety of different skin disorders besides psoriasis [51].

Principles and Mechanisms

PUVA is performed by the administration of a fixed dose of a certain psoralen preparation at a constant interval before UVA exposure. These parameters are kept unaltered in order to make psoralen plasma levels as reproducible as possible. Initial dose finding (phototoxicity testing) and dose adjustments are done by varying the UVA fluence.

Remission of psoriasis is induced by repeated, controlled phototoxic reactions. These reactions occur only when psoralens are activated by UVA radiation. Absorption of photons is confined to the skin according to the penetration characteristics of UVA. PUVA-induced phototoxic reactions manifest as delayed sunburn-like erythema and inflammation that, with an overdose, can progress to blister formation and even superficial skin necrosis. Therefore, UVA dosimetry is most critical for safe and efficient PUVA therapy [47, 48].

For maximum safety and also effectiveness of photochemotherapy, the following criteria have to be observed:
1. familiarity with the photobiological principles, the clinical reaction, and the course of the phototoxic reaction;
2. knowledge about UVA dosimetry and kinetics of psoralens;
3. exact definition and fluence rate of the UVA source;
4. determination of the individual photosensitivity of the patient after psoralen ingestion.

Psoralens are linear furocoumarins which were originally derived from plant compounds that were active in repigmenting vitiligo if combined with sun exposure [52]. For current clinical applications, 8-methoxypsoralen (8-MOP, methoxsalen) is most commonly prescribed, but 5-methoxypsoralen (5-MOP, bergapten) is also used where available. The synthetic linear furocoumarin, 4,5',8-trimethylpsoralen (TMP) is utilized for bathwater-delivered PUVA mainly in Scandinavia. These psoralens are all bifunctional, which means they have two photoactivatable double bonds. Currently, 8-MOP and 5-MOP are available as oral preparations that either contain crystals, micronized crystals, or solubilized psoralens in a gel matrix. The liquid preparation induces earlier, higher, and more reproducible peak plasma levels than the crystalline preparations. Oral psoralens are metabolized in the liver and excreted with the urine within 12 to

24 h. Due to a considerable first-pass effect, small alterations of the psoralen dose may alter plasma levels considerably. This may be the major source of the high intra- and inter-individual variability of plasma levels [53–55]. It is important for the best possible reproducibility that as many parameters as possible are kept constant, such as type and quantity of food eaten before or ingested with the drug and time of the day.

Psoralens are only reactive when activated by UV radiation and the activity is confined to those layers of skin that are reached by UVA. The radiation penetrates epidermis and papillary dermis and reaches also the superficial vascular plexus. Electronically excited psoralens may undergo photochemical reactions that modify biomolecules and thus alter skin biology.

The photochemical interaction with nuclear DNA seems biologically highly relevant and has been investigated thoroughly [56]. Bifunctional psoralens react with DNA in three steps. First, the psoralen intercalates into the DNA double strand, a process which occurs in the absence of UV radiation. Upon irradiation, either reactive double bond may form a cyclobutane adduct with a pyrimidine base. These are called 3,4 monoadducts (MAs) or 4',5'MA depending on which double bond of the psoralen is involved. Only the 4',5'MA can form a psoralen-DNA crosslink after absorbing a second photon. Under clinical conditions, MAs are the more prominent adducts, but the relationship between the different psoralen-DNA photoproducts depends on both the type of psoralen and irradiation wavelengths [57]. Although most is known about psoralen-DNA photoproducts, other photochemical reactions of 8-MOP may contribute to the therapeutic effect [58]. Excited psoralens can react with molecular oxygen, which results in the formation of reactive oxygen species such as singlet oxygen. Reactive oxygen species cause cell membrane damage by lipid peroxidation and may activate the cyclooxygenase and arachidonic acid metabolic pathways [59].

DNA-psoralen crosslinks inhibit DNA replication and cause cell-cycle arrest. The involved cellular molecular pathways have been elucidated, which has improved our understanding of the operative mechanisms. Psoralen photosensitization leads to an alteration of cytokine and cytokine receptor expression as well as cytokine secretion [60]. PUVA can revert the pathologically altered pattern of keratinocyte differentiation markers and reduce the number of proliferating epidermal cells. Infiltrating lymphocytes are strongly suppressed by PUVA, with variable effects on different T-cell subsets [61]. It has also been demonstrated that PUVA is far more potent in inducing apoptosis in lymphocytes than in keratinocytes at a similar level of the antiproliferative activity in both cell types [62]. This shows that PUVA readily induces apoptotic cell death in lymphocytes. This specific response pattern may explain the high efficacy in cutaneous T-cell lymphoma (CTCL) as well as in inflammatory skin diseases. Although these findings have improved our knowledge of pathways and mechanisms in psoralen photosensitization, the interactions and relative contributions to the clearing of a specific disease are not understood.

Action Spectrum

The action spectrum for 8-MOP-induced delayed erythema was originally believed to peak at 365 nm. More-recent studies have shown maximal activity in the 330-nm range [63, 64]. As with phototherapy, therapeutic relevance of the erythema action spectrum has been only evaluated in psoriasis. The data are harder to collect because of the relatively high intraindividual variability of psoralen levels in plasma and skin. At present, however, it seems that the antipsoriatic activity parallels the erythema action spectrum for 8-MOP [65, 66]. A spectrum has been obtained that matches the 8-MOP DNA crosslinking action spectrum in human skin in vivo [67]. This may indicate therapeutic relevance of psoralen-DNA crosslinks in the treatment of psoriasis.

The psoralen action spectrum is well covered by the conventional therapeutic UVA fluorescent tubes. Metal halide lamps, which are used for unsensitized UVA phototherapy, emit a broad spectrum that is filtered in the UVB and UVC range. These are also suitable for photochemotherapy, although they are relatively less efficient because of a spectral shift to longer wavelengths. But the high output of UVA greatly reduces treatment times [68].

PUVA Regimens

The initial clinical studies on the use of psoralens in psoriasis were performed with topical application of 8-MOP [49, 50]. Topical psoralen plus UVA irradiation is effective in clearing psoriasis but has several disadvantages. The phototoxic erythema reaction is unpredictable and may result in vesiculation. UVA dosimetry guidelines are therefore difficult to establish. Quite commonly cosmetically unacceptable hyperpigmentations are induced; if numerous lesions are present, the application of psoralens is laborious and time-consuming. Moreover, if psoriasis is still in an active phase new lesions may develop in previously non-affected, untreated areas. In our own experience, topical PUVA may be indicated in addition to oral PUVA in selected cases of recalcitrant plaques, and particularly in palmoplantar psoriasis. On the other hand, bath-PUVA therapy, which employs whole-body immersion in TMP or 8-MOP baths followed by total-body exposure to UVA, yields quite satisfactory results. Especially for patients with a strong ability for tanning, bath-PUVA (see below) may be a useful alternative treatment.

PUVA for Psoriasis

Practically all forms of psoriasis respond to PUVA, although the management of erythrodermic or generalized pustular psoriasis is more difficult than that of more common forms [69]. Two therapeutic concepts of PUVA treatment for psoriasis were developed simultaneously. Both have been shown to be highly efficient and have therefore remained in use. Owing to their origins, they are usually referred to as the American and the European regimens. Table 1 shows

Table 1. Protocols and therapeutic results of the European PUVA Study (EPS) and the U.S. 16-Center-Trial (UST)

	EPS	UST
Starting dose	1 MPD	Skin type dependent
Treatments per week	4	2–3
UVA dose increments	Individualized	Fixed
Clearing rate	88.8 %	88 %
Exposures	20	25
Time to clearing	5.7 weeks	12.7 weeks
Cumulative UVA dose	96 J/cm^2	245 J/cm^2

the characteristics of these two methods of administering oral 8-MOP PUVA [70, 71]. Our routine treatment includes oral administration of 0.6–0.8 mg/kg 8-MOP-liquid or 1.2 mg/kg 5-MOP-liquid 1 h and 2 h before UVA exposure, respectively. For plaque-type psoriasis, 4 treatments per week, with an intermission on Wednesdays, are performed until clearing is achieved. Maintenance therapy is recommended in the European regimen. It consists of 4 weeks of twice-weekly treatments at the last UVA dose used for clearing, followed by four once-weekly exposures. According to the recommendation of the British Photodermatology Group, maintenance treatment should be considered only if relapses are rapid following clearance [72]. To clarify the impact of maintenance therapy more studies are required.

New regimens or modifications of the existing protocols have been introduced to increase efficacy and reduce side effects of PUVA. One major accomplishment was the availability of 5-MOP, which gives a much lower incidence of gastrointestinal side effects, even at a dose of up to 1.8 mg/kg. After oral administration, 5-MOP is clinically less phototoxic than 8-MOP and therefore safer with regard to side effects related to overdosing of UVA [73].

One aggressive PUVA schedule optimizes UVA irradiations by repeated phototoxic threshold determination during the course of the therapy. Treatments are given twice weekly, 72 h apart. This procedure aims at an optimized dosimetry and thus increases efficacy and reduces total UVA fluences [74–76]. Most recently, the combination of dihydroxyacetone-induced UVA protection of uninvolved skin with PUVA has resulted in an improved clearing of psoriasis [77].

PUVA treatment of limited areas of affected skin may be performed by using topical delivery of psoralen solutions. 8-MOP is being used as a 0.15 % solution painted on the lesions 20 min before exposure. Topical application of TMP by bath water has been popular in Scandinavia for many years [78], but only recently has it attracted worldwide interest. Bathwater delivery of 8-MOP helps to avoid gastrointestinal and ocular side effects because there is no systemic photosensitization. Skin psoralen levels are more reproducible and photosensitivity is less persistent than after oral administration. The higher incidence of unwanted phototoxicity can be easily prevented by a lower starting dose (30–50 % of the MPD) and a more cautious dosimetry in the initial treatment phase [79]. 8-MOP is used at concentrations between 0.5 and 5.0 mg 8-MOP per liter of bath water. Baths are taken for 15–20 min and then the patient's skin is gently patted dry. The UVA exposure should ensue immediately, as photosensitivity decreases rather rapidly. TMP is more phototoxic after topical application and is used at lower concentrations (0.125–0.5 mg/l) than 8-MOP.

In a continuing quest for new psoralens with reduced side effects, researchers have synthesized the angular furocoumarin 4,6,4'-trimethylangelicin and the monofunctional 7-methylpyridopsoralen. Both compounds demonstrated promising photobiological parameters and antipsoriatic activity after topical application [80, 81]. Currently, these furocoumarins are not commercially available.

Combination Treatments

As with phototherapy, PUVA can be combined with other treatments to improve efficacy and reduce possible side effects [82]. Topical adjuvant therapies with corticosteroid, anthralin, and tar preparations have been tried with some success, and more recently the combination with calcipotriol yielded good results. However, topical therapy does not find all patients' acceptance since it is considered a step backward to conventional treatment.

A combination of PUVA and methotrexate can reduce the duration of treatment, number of exposures, and total UVA dose and is effective also in clearing patients unresponsive with PUVA or UVB alone [83].

Cyclosporine A plus PUVA therapy and RePUVA cleared widespread plaque-type psoriasis in a comparable time. However, RePUVA was significantly superior regarding the cumulative UVA dose required for clearance and the incidence of severe and early relapses [84]. Particularly in view of possible long-term side effects (immune suppression, skin carcinogenesis), the combination of PUVA plus cyclosporine A cannot be recommended [85, 86].

The combination of PUVA with systemic retinoids is one of the most potent therapeutic regimens for psoriasis [87, 88]. The therapeutic efficacy of PUVA therapy is dramatically increased when combined with daily oral retinoid (etretinate, acitretin, isotretinoin; 1 mg per kg body weight) administration 5–10 days before the initiation of PUVA, and this combination is continued throughout the clearing phase treatment [87–90]. This combined regimen, called RePUVA, was reported to reduce the number of exposures by one third and the total cumulative UVA dose by more than one half. RePUVA was shown to clear also "poor PUVA responders" who could not be brought into complete remission by PUVA alone [87, 91].

The mechanism of the synergistic action of retinoids and PUVA is unknown but it may be due to the accelerated desquamation of the psoriatic plaques that optimizes the optical properties of the skin and to the reduction of the inflammatory infiltrate. As an additional beneficial effect, etretinate and other retinoids may theoretically protect against long-term carcinogenic effects of PUVA by reducing the number of exposures and by its potential anti-cancer effect. Short-term side effects of retinoids are completely reversible at discontinuation and long-term toxicity is not a concern because the administration is limited to the clearing phase. The potential teratogenicity of retinoids represents a serious concern. In Europe etretinate has been replaced by its active metabolite acitretin (Neotigason) because it was believed that its elimination half-life were strikingly shorter than that of etretinate while being as effective as etretinate-PUVA [91, 92]. Meanwhile there is evidence that acitretin is, in part, metabolized into etretinate that again accumulates in the body [93, 94]. Therefore, this substance does not represent an advantage over etretinate. For women of childbearing age, the use of isotretinoin can be considered, because contraception is necessary for only 2 months after discontinuation of therapy as opposed to etretinate and acitretin, which require two years of contraception.

Phototherapy and PUVA in HIV-Infected Patients

Skin disease is common in HIV-infected individuals [95]. Psoriasis and other phototherapy-responsive dermatoses such as CTCL and vitiligo may be encountered in HIV patients [96, 97].

In 1985 the first patient with AIDS and psoriasis was reported [98]. The relationship between the two diseases is now well documented in the literature. However, it is still unknown if psoriasis is more frequent among HIV-infected individuals than in the general population. The two diseases have a paradoxical relationship because HIV results in immunosuppression, and psoriasis usually resolves with immunosuppressive treatments [99]. HIV's effect on the immune system may trigger the exacerbation or onset of psoriasis. HIV infects and depletes $CD4^+$ helper T cells and epidermal Langerhans' cells [100, 101]. The virus infects but does not necessarily kill the cells. It is able to alter the cell's gene expression patterns and cause abnormalities in the growth or function of the cell [100]. It is known that HIV causes dysregulation of both cellular and humoral immunity, disturbing the delicate balance of cytokines. This disruption of cytokine pattern is currently believed to trigger psoriasis [102]. Occasionally, the psoriasis of patients with very low CD4 counts spontaneously resolves, possibly because of the AIDS patient's inability to produce the cytokines needed for epidermal hyperproliferation. Such a phenomenon is seen in other terminally ill patients as well.

Psoriasis in HIV-infected individuals usually resists treatment with standard therapies such as topical steroids. Often UVB phototherapy or PUVA has to be employed to help these patients. Controversy existed over the safety of such treatments. Firstly, UVB and PUVA – both able to induce systemic immune suppression – may modify the immune status of the patient in a way that would lead to a worsening of the HIV disease status [103]. Secondly, it has been shown that UV radiation as well as psoralen photosensitization may activate the HIV promoter, which could boost viral gene transcription and eventually virus production [104]. In addition, the virus-induced immune suppression may support an accelerated development of skin carcinomas in UVB or PUVA-treated patients [105]. The therapies did not result in any worsening of HIV disease or increased complication rates [106]. If UVB phototherapy fails, PUVA may be the treatment of choice. In addition, with PUVA, the systemic treatment of psoriasis did not lead to a progression of HIV disease or an increase in side effects [107, 108]. It was concluded from these studies that UVB phototherapy and PUVA may be safe for HIV-positive psoriatics. Theoretical modeling of the UVB- and PUVA-induced HIV promoter activation in human skin actually indicated that UVB is more likely than PUVA to activate viral transcription in vivo [109]. The initial clinical studies are encouraging in their lack of accelerating HIV disease progression. Data from long-term observations are currently awaited. Therefore, it is not possible at the present time to generally advocate the use of PUVA or UVB phototherapy in (HIV-)immunosuppressed individuals, but major hazards appear unlikely. The available data and theoretical considerations indicate that UVB is more likely to be a hazard than PUVA in the treatment of an HIV-infected population [109, 110].

Long-term studies are needed to evaluate further the risk/benefit ratio of UVB phototherapy and PUVA in HIV-infected patients.

Side Effects and Long-Term Hazards

The short-term side effects of UVB and PUVA overdosing are quite similar and consist of redness, swelling, and occasionally blister formation as can be seen with excessive sunburns. The major difference lies in the time frame: while UVB-induced erythema peaks before 24 h, the maximal PUVA reaction is not reached before 72 h. A generalized pruritus or tingling sensation may herald phototoxic side effects and should be taken as a warning sign. With large skin areas affected, systemic symptoms of excess phototoxicity such as fever and general malaise may occur due to massive cytokine release. Besides an adjustment of dosimetry, additional measures depend on extent and degree of phototoxicity. Cool compresses, non-steroidal anti-inflammatory drugs, topical and even systemic corticosteroids may be required to alleviate the symptoms. PUVA-induced skin pain unrelated to actual phototoxic burns occurs rarely but may necessitate discontinuation of treatment. In the initial phase of PUVA using 5-MOP, an asymptomatic and transient maculopapular eruption unrelated to excess phototoxicity has been seen in a small number of patients [73]. Photoonycholysis and subungual hemorrhages are delayed signs of acute phototoxicity to the nail bed.

Besides the phototoxic episodes, psoralens can induce systemic side effects in the absence of light. Most notorious is nausea and vomiting induced by oral 8-MOP. The effect is more common with liquid formulations of 8-MOP. The grossly reduced incidence of these side effects with oral 5-MOP is the major reason for increased usage of this compound.

Eye protection is mandatory during UVA exposure and UVA-opaque glasses are required for ambient exposure until the evening of the treatment day. With these precautions, ocular side effects should not occur. Accidental ocular UVB overexposure may induce photokeratitis due to its absorption in conjunctiva and cornea. UVA penetrates into the ocular lens and is cataractogenic by itself with high fluences. With systemic psoralen sensitization, psoralen-protein photoproducts may be formed. The higher permeability of the ocular lens at a younger age resulted in the relative contraindication of oral PUVA in children younger than 12 years. Despite the experimental data, which indicated a risk of premature cataract formation, clinical evaluation shows no increase in lens opacities even in patients who neglected careful eye protection [111, 112]. These patients, however, suffer from other ocular side effects such as conjunctival alteration [112].

The long-term side effects of UVB and PUVA generally resemble those known as dermatoheliosis, which is the overall damage to skin by prolonged solar exposure with high cumulative fluences. These changes are usually confined to permanently sun-exposed areas such as the face, neck, and forearms. High cumulative doses of whole body UVB or PUVA exposures result in similar changes characterized by pigmentary changes, xerosis, loss of elasticity, wrinkle formation, and actinic keratoses. Additionally, PUVA may induce hypertrichosis and profuse formation of dark lentigines, termed PUVA lentiginosis [70].

The major concern with prolonged and repeated phototherapeutic regimens is the induction or promotion of skin cancers (for review see [113]). Solar radiation plays a role in the induction of both melanoma and non-melanoma skin carcinomas. Therefore, from the very beginning PUVA patients were carefully monitored for the development of precursors and malignant skin tumors. Almost all data were obtained from psoriatics since they are the largest group of patients receiving PUVA.

The risk is related to DNA damage, but PUVA-induced downregulation of immune responses could play an additional role. In PUVA patients, the risk of squamous cell carcinoma, but not of basal cell carcinoma, is significantly increased in comparison with matched controls, and the magnitude of the increase appears to be dose-dependent [114–117]. However, there is uncertainty about the contribution of PUVA to these observations; many of the reported patients had previous exposure to excessive sunlight and to treatments of known carcinogenicity, including arsenic, UVB, and antimetabolite therapy such as methotrexate [115, 118]. Male genitalia appeared to be particularly susceptible to carcinogenic stimuli of PUVA in patients previously treated with tar and UVB [119], but the risk seemed not to increase if only PUVA was used [120].

Carcinogenicity of 5-MOP-UVA therapy in PUVA-treated patients is unknown, but 5-MOP has shown a similar activity than 8-MOP via in vitro photomutagenicity studies and photocarcinogenicity studies in mice [121].

Only a few anecdotal cases of malignant melanoma have been observed in long-term PUVA treated psoriatics [122], and no increased risk of melanoma was found in all large-scale studies reported so far. However, recently, Stern et al. [123] reported 11 melanomas in 9 patients from the cohort of 1,380 patients enrolled in the PUVA Follow-up Study (16-Center Study). The authors concluded that about 15 years after the first treatment the risk increases, particularly in patients with more than 250 treatments. Only four melanomas were observed between 1975 and 1990, and this number equaled the expected incidence (relative risk, 1.1). In the same cohort, seven melanomas were detected from 1991 to 1996 (relative risk, 5.4). This increased incidence is alarming, especially considering the long latency period, which suggests that more cases are to be expected in the future. Also, the risk seemed to persist after discontinuation of PUVA. Since there are no data available on dosimetry, it is unclear whether melanomas are associated with a certain cumulative UVA dose or with episodes of phototoxic burns. Moreover, no information is given on other cocarcinogenic factors, on the clinical type of melanoma and, most importantly, on the patients' history (dysplastic nevi, family history of melanoma). One of the nine patients had three melanomas. If he had familial melanoma or dysplastic nevus syndrome and would be excluded from the cohort, there would be no significant increase in risk. Besides this lack of important information, this report has to be taken seriously and emphasizes that the guidelines for PUVA treatment must be rigidly observed. Patients with long-term PUVA must receive life-long monitoring [124].

In any case, to possibly reduce the risks, the cumulative doses must be kept low and therefore UVA sparing aggressive regimens without prolonged maintenance therapy may be safer than continuous non-aggressive regimens [125] and may possibly modify the time course of PUVA carcinogenesis [113].

Based on a study with 944 Swedish and Finnish patients [126] and on previous animal experiments [127], bath-PUVA with TMP seems to bear no relevant risk of carcinogenesis. In addition, no association between cutaneous cancer and 8-MOP bath PUVA was found in 158 psoriatic patients [128]. These data on the long-term safety of bath-PUVA are encouraging, but no premature conclusions should be drawn.

It is important to compare the risks of PUVA with UVB phototherapy for psoriasis. Animal studies show that UVB is carcinogenic, but model studies indicate that the observed risk of squamous cell carcinoma is much higher with PUVA than the calculated risk with UVB [129, 130]. There is a recent trend towards the use of narrow-band UVB (Philips TL-01). The carcinogenic risk of this source in comparison with PUVA is not known, and it will be crucial to monitor its long-term effects in psoriatics.

The management of severe psoriatics requires long-term planning. Informed and competent physicians with relevant experience may reach this goal with a careful patient selection and the use of individualized regimens and combination treatments. For disabling psoriasis, the choice of treatment lies not between risk and safety but among alternative options, such as methotrexate, cyclosporine A, or retinoids and UVB, no one of which can be considered absolutely safe. The risk/benefit ratio still seems very favorable for PUVA [131], and so far no single therapy, except perhaps narrowband UVB, has been accepted as equally safe and efficient.

References

1. Abels DJ, Kattan-Byron J (1985) Psoriasis treatment at the Dead Sea: a natural selective ultraviolet phototherapy. J Am Acad Dermatol 12:639–643
2. Cadet J, Anselmino C, Douki T, Voituriez L (1992) Photochemistry of nucleic acids in cells. J Photochem Photobiol B Biol 15:277–298
3. Petit Frere C, Clingen PH, Arlett CF, Green MH (1996) Inhibition of RNA and DNA synthesis in UV-irradiated normal human fibroblasts is correlated with pyrimidine (6–4) pyrimidone photoproduct formation. Mutat Res 354:87–94

4. Ronai ZA, Lambert ME, Weinstein IB (1992) Inducible cellular responses to ultraviolet light irradiation and other mediators of DNA damage in mammalian cells. Cell Biol Toxicol 6:105–126
5. Moan J, Peak MJ (1989) Effects of UV radiation of cells. J Photochem Photobiol B Biol 4:21–34
6. Liu M, Pellingo JC (1995) UV-B/A irradiation of mouse keratinocytes results in p53-mediated WAF-1/CIP-1 expression. Oncogene 10:1955–1960
7. Kramer DM, Pathak MA, Kornhauser A, Wisekmann (1974) Effects of ultraviolet radiation on biosynthesis of DNA in guinea pig skin. J Invest Dermatol 62:388–393
8. Epstein WL, Fukuyama K, Epstein JH (1969) Early effects of ultraviolet light on DNA synthesis in human skin in vivo. Arch Dermatol 100:84–89
9. Liu M, Pellingo JC (1995) UV-B/A irradiation of mouse keratinocytes results in p53-mediated WAF1/CIP1 expression. Oncogene 10:1955–1960
10. Brash DE, Rudolph JA, Simon JA, Lim A, McKenna GJ, Baden HP, Halperin AJ, Ponten J (1991) A role for sunlight in skin cancer: UV-induced p53 mutations in squamous cell carcinoma. Proc Natl Acad Sci USA 88:10124–10128.
11. Hruza LL, Pentland AP (1993) Mechanisms of UV-induced inflammation. J Invest Dermatol 100:35S–41S
12. Greaves MW (1986) Ultraviolet erythema: causes and consequences. In: Hönigsmann H, Stingl G (eds) Therapeutic photomedicine. Karger, Basel, pp 18–24 (Current problems in dermatology, vol 15)
13. Schwarz T, Luger TA (1989) Effect of UV irradiation on epidermal cell cytokine production. J Photochem Photobiol B Biol 4:1–13
14. Beissert S, Hosoi J, Grabbe S, Asahina A, Granstein RD (1995) IL-10 inhibits tumor antigen presentation by epidermal antigen-presenting cells. J Immunol 154:1280–1286
15. Urbanski A, Schwarz T, Neuner P, Krutmann J, Kirnbauer R, Köck A, Luger TA (1990) Ultraviolet light induces increased circulating interleukin-6 in humans. J Invest Dermatol 94:808–811
16. Ullrich SE (1995) Modulation of immunity by ultraviolet radiation: key effects on antigen presentation. J Invest Dermatol 105:30S–36S
17. Warmuth I, Harth Y, Matsui MS, Wang N, DeLeo VA (1994) Ultraviolet radiation induces phosphorylation of the epidermal growth factor receptor. Cancer Res 54:374–376
18. Devary Y, Rosette C, DiDonato JA, Karin N (1993) NF-kB activation by ultraviolet light not dependent on a nuclear signal. Science 261:1442–1445
19. Kripke ML, Cox PA, Alas LG, Yarosh DB (1992) Pyrimidine dimers in DNA initiate systemic immunosuppression in UVB-irradiated mice. Proc Natl Acad Sci USA 89:7516–7520
20. Cruz PD (1992) Photoimmunology. In: DeLeo VA (ed) Photosensitivity. Igaku-Shoin, New York, pp 25–32
21. Fisher T (1976) UV-light treatment of psoriasis. Acta Derm Venereol 56:473–479
22. Parrish JA, Jaenicke KF (1981) Action spectrum for phototherapy of psoriasis. J Invest Dermatol 76:359–362
23. Diette KM, Momtaz K, Stern RS, Arndt KA, Parrish JA (1984) Role of ultraviolet A in phototherapy for psoriasis. J Am Acad Dermatol 11:441–447
24. Schröpl F (1977) Zum heutigen Stand der technischen Entwicklung der selektiven Phototherapie. Dtsch Dermatol 25:499–504
25. Hönigsmann H, Fritsch P, Jaschke E (1977) UV-Therapie der Psoriasis. Halbseitenvergleich zwischen oraler Photochemotherapie (PUVA) und selektiver UV-Phototherapie (SUP). Z Hautkr 52:1078–1082
26. Van Weelden H, De La Faille HB, Young E, Van der Leun IC (1988) A new development in UVB phototherapy of psoriasis. Br J Dermatol 119:11–19
27. Quinn AG, Diffey BL, Craig PS, Farr PM et al (1994) Definition of the minimal erythema dose used for diagnostic phototesting (abstract). Br J Dermatol 131:56

28. Hönigsmann H, Calzavara-Pinton PG, Ortel B (1994) Phototherapy and photoche-motherapy. In: Dubertret L (ed) Psoriasis. ISED, Brescia, pp 135–150
29. Lebwohl M, Martinez J, Weber P, De Luca R (1995) Effects of topical preparations on the erythemogenicity of UVB: implications for psoriasis phototherapy. J Am Acad Dermatol 32:469–471
30. Tanenbaum L, Parrish JA, Pathak MA, Anderson RR, Fitzpatrick TB (1975) Tar pho-toxicity and phototherapy for psoriasis. Arch Dermatol 111:467–470
31. Storbeck K, Hölzle E, Schurer N, Lehmann P, Plewig G (1993) Narrow-band UVB (311 nm) versus conventional broad-band UVB with and without dithranol in pho-totherapy for psoriasis. J Am Acad Dermatol 28:227–231
32. Meola T Jr Soter NA, Lim HW (1991) Are topical corticosteroids useful adjunctive therapy for the treatment of psoriasis with ultraviolet radiation? A review of the lit-erature. Arch Dermatol 127:1708–1713
33. Steigleder GK, Orfanos CE, Pullmann H (1979) Retinoid-SUP-Therapie der Psoria-sis. Z Hautkr 54:19–23
34. Iest J, Boer J (1989) Combined treatment of psoriasis with acitretin and UVB photo-therapy compared with acitretin alone and UVB alone. Br J Dermatol 120:665–670
35. Green C, Ferguson J, Lakshmipathi T, Johnson BE (1988) 311 nm UVB phototherapy-an effective treatment for psoriasis. Br J Dermatol 119:691–696
36. Picot E, Meunier L, Picot-Debeze MC, Peyron JL, Meynadier J (1992) Treatment of psoriasis with a 311-nm UVB lamp. Br J Dermatol 127:509–512
37. Van Weelden H, Baart de la Faille H, Young E, Van der Leun JC (1990) Comparison of narrow-band UV-B phototherapy and PUVA photochemotherapy in the treat-ment of psoriasis. Acta Derm Venereol 70:212–215
38. Tanew A, Radakovic-Fijan S, Schemper M, Hönigsmann H (1999) Paired compari-son study on narrow-band (TL-01) UVB phototherapy versus photochemotherapy (PUVA) in the treatment of chronic plaque type psoriasis. Arch Dermatol 135:519–524
39. Green C, Lakshmipathi T, Johnson BE, Ferguson J (1992) A comparison of the effi-cacy and relapse rates of narrowband UVB (TL-01) monotherapy vs. etretinate (re-TL-01) vs. etretinate-PUVA (re-PUVA) in the treatment of psoriasis patients. Br J Dermatol 127:5–9
40. Karvonen J, Kokkonen EL, Ruotsalainen E (1989) 311 nm UVB lamps in the treat-ment of psoriasis with the Ingram regimen. Acta Derm Venereol 69:82–85
41. Kerscher M, Volkenandt M, Plewig G, Lehmann P (1993) Combination phototherapy of psoriasis with calcipotriol and narrow-band UVB. Lancet 342:9
42. Studniberg HM, Weller P (1993) PUVA, UVB, psoriasis, and nonmelanoma skin cancer. J Am Acad Dermatol 29:1013–1022
43. Stern RS, Laird N (1994) The carcinogenic risk of treatments for severe psoriasis. Cancer 73:2759–2764
44. Hönigsmann H, Szeimies RF, Knobler R et al (1999) Photochemotherapy and photo-dynamic therapy. In: Freedberg IM, Eisen AZ, Wolff K, Austen KF, Goldsmith LA, Katz SI (eds) Fitzpatrick's dermatology in general medicine, 5th edn. McGraw-Hill, New York, pp 2880–2900
45. El Mofty AM (1948) A preliminary report on the treatment of leukoderma with Ammi majus Linn. J R Egypt Med Assoc 31:651–655
46. Lerner AB, Denton CR, Fitzpatrick TB (1953) Clinical and experimental studies with 8-methoxypsoralen in vitiligo. J Invest Dermatol 20:299–314
47. Parrish JA, Fitzpatrick TB, Tanenbaum L, Pathak MA (1974) Photochemotherapy of psoriasis with oral methoxsalen and long wave ultraviolet light. N Engl J Med 291:1207–1211
48. Wolff K, Hönigsmann H, Gschnait F, Konrad K (1975) Photochemotherapie bei Pso-riasis. Klinische Erfahrungen bei 152 Patienten. Dtsch Med Wochenschr 100:2471–2477

49. Mortazawi SAM (1972) Meladinine mit UVA bei Vitiligo, Psoriasis, Parapsoriasis und Akne vulgaris. Dermatol Wochenschr 158:908–911
50. Walter JF, Voorhees JJ (1973) Psoriasis improved by psoralen plus light. Acta Derm Venereol 53:469–472
51. Honig B, Morison WL, Karp D (1994) Photochemotherapy beyond psoriasis. J Am Acad Dermatol 31:775–790
52. Pathak MAFitzpatrick TB (1992) The evolution of photochemotherapy with psoralens and UVA (PUVA): 2000 BC to 1992 AD. J Photochem Photobiol B Biol 14:3–22
53. Hönigsmann H, Jaschke E, Nitsche V, Brenner W, Rauschmeier W, Wolff K (1982) Serum levels of 8-methoxypsoralen in two different drug preparations. Correlation with photosensitivity and UVA dose requirements for photochemotherapy. J Invest Dermatol 79:233–236
54. Herfst MJ, De Wolff FA (1983) Intraindividual and interindividual variability in 8-methoxypsoralen kinetics and effect in psoriatic patients. Clin Pharmacol Ther 34:117–125
55. Brickl R, Schmid J, Koss FW (1984) Pharmacokinetics and pharmacodynamics of psoralens after oral administration: considerations and conclusions. Natl Cancer Inst Monogr 66:63–67
56. Dall'Acqua F (1986) Furocoumarin photochemistry and its main biological implications. In: Hönigsmann H, Stingl G (eds) Therapeutic photomedicine. Karger, Basel, pp 137–163 (Current problems in dermatology, vol 15)
57. Tessman JW, Isaacs ST, Hearst JE (1985) Photochemistry of the furan-side 8-methoxypsoralen-thymidine monoadduct inside the DNA helix. Conversion to diadduct and to pyrone-side monoadduct. Biochemistry 24:1669–1676
58. Schmitt I, Chimenti S; Gasparro F (1995) Psoralen-protein photochemistry – the forgotten field. J Photochem Photobiol B Biol 27:101–105
59. Averbeck D (1989) Recent advances in psoralen phototoxicity mechanism. Photochem Photobiol 50:859–882
60. Neuner P Neuner P; Charvat-B, Knobler R, Kirnbauer R, Schwarz A, Luger TA, Schwarz T (1994) Cytokine release by peripheral blood mononuclear cells is affected by 8-methoxypsoralen plus UV-A. Photochem Photobiol 59:182–188
61. Vallat V, Gilleaudeau P, Battat, L, Wolfe J, Nabeya R, Heftler N, Hodak E, Gottlieb AB, Krueger JG (1994) PUVA bath therapy strongly suppresses immunological and epidermal activation in psoriasis: a possible cellular basis for remittive therapy. J Exp Med 180:283–296
62. Johnson R, Staiano-Coico, L, Austin L, Cardinale I, Nabeya-Tsukifuji, R,Krueger JG (1996) PUVA treatment selectively induces a cell cycle block and subsequent apoptosis in human T-lymphocytes. Photochem Photobiol 63:566–571
63. Cripps DJ, Lowe NJ, Lerner AB (1982) Action spectra of topical psoralens: a re-evaluation. Br J Dermatol 107:77–82
64. Kaidbey KH (1985) An action spectrum for 8-methoxypsoralen-sensitized inhibition of DNA synthesis in vivo. J Invest Dermatol 85:98–101
65. Brücke J, Tanew A, Ortel B, Hönigsmann H (1991) Relative efficacy of 335 and 365 nm radiation in photochemotherapy of psoriasis. Br J Dermatol 124:372–374
66. Farr PM, Diffey BL, Higgins EM, Matthews JSN (1991) The action spectrum between 320 and 400 nm for clearance of psoriasis by psoralen photochemotherapy. Br J Dermatol 124:443–448
67. Ortel B, Gange RW (1990) An action spectrum for the elicitation of erythema in skin persistently sensitized by photobound 8-methoxypsoralen. J Invest Dermatol 94:781–785
68. Calzavara-Pinton PG (1997) Efficacy and safety of stand-up irradiation cubicles with UVA metal-halide lamps (and a new filter) or UVA fluorescent lamps for photochemotherapy of psoriasis. Dermatology 195:243–247

69. Hönigsmann H, Szeimies RF, Knobler R, Fitzpatrick TB, Pathak MA, Wolff K (1999) Photochemotherapy and photodynamic therapy. In: Freedberg IM, Eisen AZ, Wolff K, Austen KF, Goldsmith LA, Katz SI (eds) Fitzpatrick's dermatology in general medicine, 5th edn. McGrawHill, New York, pp 2880 – 2900
70. Henseler T, Wolff K, Hönigsmann H, Christopers E (1981) The European PUVA study (EPS) oral 8-methoxypsoralen photochemotherapy of psoriasis. A cooperative study among 18 European centres. Lancet 1:853 – 857
71. Melski JW, Tanenbaum L, Fitzpatrick TB, Bleich HL, Parrish JA (1977) Oral methoxsalen photochemotherapy for the treatment of psoriasis: a cooperative clinical trial. J Invest Dermatol 68:328 – 335
72. British Photodermatology Group (1994) British Photodermatology Group guidelines for PUVA. Br J Dermatol 130:246 – 255
73. Tanew A, Ortel B, Rappersberger K, Hönigsmann H (1988) 5-methoxypsoralen (Bergapten) for photochemotherapy. J Am Acad Dermatol 18:333 – 338
74. Carabott FM, Hawk JL (1989) A modified dosage schedule for increased efficiency in PUVA treatment of psoriasis. Clin Exp Dermatol 14:337 – 340
75. Green C George S, Lakshmipathi T, Ferguson J (1993) A trial of accelerated PUVA in psoriasis. Clin Exp Dermatol 18:297 – 299
76. Tanew A, Ortel B, Hönigsmann H (1999) Halfside comparison of erythemogenic versus suberythemogenic UVA doses in oral photochemotherapy of psoriasis. J Am Acad Dermatol 41: 408 – 413
77. Taylor CR, Kwangsukstith C, Wimberly J, Kollias N, Anderson RR (1999) Turbo-PUVA: dihydroxyacetone-enhanced photochemotherapy for psoriasis: a pilot study. Arch Dermatol 135:540 – 544
78. Fischer T, Alsins J (1976) Treatment of psoriasis with trioxsalen baths and dysprosium lamps. Acta Derm Venereol 56:383 – 390
79. Calzavara-Pinton PG, Ortel B, Carlino AM, Hönigsmann H, De Panfilis G (1993) Phototesting and phototoxic side effects in bath-PUVA. J Am Acad Dermatol 28:657 – 659
80. Cristofolini M, Recchia G, Boi S, Piscioli F, Bordin F, Baccichetti F, Carlassare F, Tamaro M, Pani B, Babudri N, Guiotto A, Rodighiero P, Vedaldi D, Dall'Acqua F (1990) 6-Methylangelicins: new monofunctional photochemotherapeutic agents for psoriasis. Br J Dermatol 122:513 – 524
81. Dubertret L, Averbeck D, Bisagni E, Moron J, Moustacchi E, Billardon C, Papadopoulo D, Nocentini S, Vigny P, Blais J, Bensasson RV, Ronfard-Haret JC, Land EJ, Zajdela F, Latarjet R (1985) Photochemotherapy using pyridopsoralens. Biochemie 67:417 – 422
82. Morison WL (1985) PUVA combination therapy. Photodermatol 2:229 – 236
83. Morison WL (1992) Phototherapy and photochemotherapy. Adv Dermatol 7:255 – 270
84. Petzelbauer P, Hönigsmann H, Langer K, Anegg B, Stroha, R, Tanew A, Wolff K (1990) Cyclosporin A in combination with photochemotherapy (PUVA) in the treatment of psoriasis. Br J Dermatol 123:641 – 647
85. Molin L, Larkö O (1997) Cancer induction by immunosuppression in psoriasis after heavy PUVA treatment (letter). Acta Derm Venereol 77(5):402
86. Van-de-Kerkhof PC, De-Rooij MJ (1997) Multiple squamous cell carcinomas in a psoriatic patient following high-dose photochemotherapy and cyclosporin treatment: response to long-term acitretin maintenance. Br J Dermatol 136(2):275 – 278
87. Fritsch PO, Hönigsmann H, Jaschke E, Wolff K (1978) Augmentation of oral methoxsalen-photochemotherapy with an oral retinoic acid derivative. J Invest Dermatol 70:178 – 182
88. Lauharanta J, Juvakoski T, Lassus A (1981) A clinical evaluation of the effects of an aromatic retinoid (Tigason), combination of retinoid and PUVA, and PUVA alone in severe psoriasis. Br J Dermatol 104:325 – 332

89. Hönigsmann H, Wolff K (1989) Results of therapy for psoriasis using retinoid and photochemotherapy (RePUVA). Pharmacol Ther 40:67–73
90. Hönigsmann H, Wolff K (1983) Isotretinoin-PUVA for psoriasis. Lancet 1:236
91. Saurat JH, Geiger JM, Amblard P, Beani JC, Boulanger A, Claudy A, Frenk E, Guilhou JJ, Grosshans E, Merot Y, Meynadier J, Tapernoux B (1988) Randomized double-blind multicenter study comparing acitretin-PUVA, etretinate-PUVA and placebo-PUVA in the treatment of severe psoriasis. Dermatologica 177:218–224
92. Tanew A, Guggenbichler A, Hönigsmann H, Geiger JM, Fritsch P (1991) Photochemotherapy for severe psoriasis without or in combination with acitretin: a randomized double-blind comparison study. J Am Acad Dermatol 25:682–684
93. Chou RC, Wyss R, Huselton CA, Wiegand UW (1992) A potentially new metabolic pathway: ethyl esterification of acitretin. Xenobiotica 22:993–1002
94. Maier H, Hönigsmann H (1996) Concentration of etretinate in plasma and subcutaneous fat after long-term acitretin. Lancet 348:1107
95. Stern RS (1994) Epidemiology of skin disease in HIV infection: a cohort study of health maintenance organization members. J Invest Dermatol 102:34S–37S
96. Duvic M, Rapini R, Hoots WK, Mansell PW (1987) Human immunodeficiency virus-associated vitiligo: expression of autoimmunity with immunodeficiency? J Am Acad Dermatol 17:656–662
97. Crane GA, Variakojis D, Rosen ST, Sands AM, Roenigk HH Jr (1991) Cutaneous T-cell lymphoma in patients with human immune deficiency virus infection. Arch Dermatol 127:989–994
98. Johnson TM, Duvic M, Rapini RP, Rios A (1985) Acquired immunodeficiency syndrome exacerbates psoriasis (letter). N Engl J Med 313:1415
99. Duvic M, Crane MM, Conant M, Mahoney SE, Reveille JD, Lehrman SN (1994) Zidovudine improves psoriasis in human immunodeficiency virus positive males. Arch Dermatol 130:447–451
100. Stingl G, Rappersberger K, Tschachler E, Garner S, Groh V, Mann DL, Wolff K, Popovic M (1990) Langerhans' cells in HIV-1 infections. J Am Acad Dermatol 22:1210–1217
101. Mahoney SE, Duvic M, Nickoloff BJ, Minshall M, Smith LC, Griffiths CE, Paddock SW, Lewis DE (1991) Human immunodeficiency virus transcripts identified in human immunodeficiency virus related psoriasis and Kaposi's sarcoma lesions. J Clin Invest 88:174–185
102. Kadunce DP, Krueger GG (1995) Pathogenesis of psoriasis, current concepts. Dermatol Clin 13:723–737
103. Ullrich SE (1996) Does exposure to UV radiation induce a shift to a Th-2-like immune reaction? Photochem Photobiol 64:254–258
104. Morrey JD, Bourn SM, Bunch TD, Jackson MK, Sidwell RW, Barrows LR, Daynes RA, Rosen CA (1991) In vivo activation of human immunodeficiency virus type I long terminal repeat by UV type A (UV-A) light plus psoralen and UV-B light in the skin of transgenic mice. J Virol 65:5045–5051
105. Wang CY, Brodland DG, Su WP (1995) Skin cancers associated with acquired immunodeficiency syndrome. Mayo Clin Proc 70:766–772
106. Meola T, Soter NA, Ostreicher R, Sanchez M, Moy JA (1993) The safety of UVB phototherapy in patients with HIV infection. J Am Acad Dermatol 29:216–220
107. Ranki A, Puska P, Mattinen S, Lagerstedt A, Krohn K (1991) Effect of PUVA on immunologic and virologic findings in HIV-infected patients. J Am Acad Dermatol 24:404–410
108. Horn TD, Morison WL, Farzadegan H, Zmudzka BZ, Beer JZ (1994) Effects of psoralen plus UVA radiation (PUVA) on HIV-1 in human beings: a pilot study. J Am Acad Dermatol 31:735–740
109. Zmudzka BZ, Miller SA, Jacobs ME, Beer JZ (1996) Medical UV exposures and HIV activation. Photochem Photobiol 64:246–253

110. Morison WL (1996) PUVA therapy is preferable to UVB phototherapy in the management of HIV-associated dermatoses. Photochem Photobiol 64:267–268
111. Cox NH., Jones SK, Downey DJ, Tuyp EJ, Jay JL, Moseley H, MacKie RM (1987) Cutaneous and ocular side-effects of oral photochemotherapy: results of an 8-year follow-up study. Br J Dermatol 116:145–152
112. Calzavara-Pinton PG, Carlino A, Manfredi E, Semerano F, Zane C, De Panfilis G (1994) Ocular side effects of PUVA-treated patients refusing eye sun protection. Acta Derm Venereol [Suppl] 186:164–165
113. Young AR (1996) Photochemotherapy and skin carcinogenesis: a critical review. In: Hönigsmann H, Jori G, Young AR (eds) The fundamental bases of phototherapy. OEMF, Milano, pp 77–87
114. Stern RS, Laird N for the Photochemotherapy Follow-up Study (1994) The carcinogenic risks of treatments for severe psoriasis. Cancer 73:2759–2764
115. Maier H, Schemper M, Ortel B, Binder M, Tanew A, Hönigsmann H (1996) Skin tumours in photochemotherapy for psoriasis. A single centre follow-up of 496 patients. Dermatology 193:185–191
116. Stern RS, Lunder EJ (1998) Risk of squamous cell carcinoma and methoxsalen (psoralen) and UV-A radiation (PUVA). A meta-analysis. Arch Dermatol 134(12):1582–1585
117. Stern RS, Liebman EJ, Vakeva L (1998) Oral psoralen and ultraviolet-A light (PUVA) treatment of psoriasis and persistent risk of nonmelanoma skin cancer. PUVA follow-up study. J Natl Cancer Inst 90:1278–1284
118. Henseler T, Christophers E, Hönigsmann H, Wolff K (1987) Skin tumors in the European PUVA study: eight year follow-up of 1643 patients treated with PUVA for psoriasis. J Am Acad Dermatol 16:108–116
119. Stern RS, Members of the photochemotherapy follow-up study (1990) Genital tumors among men with psoriasis exposed to psoralens and ultraviolet A (PUVA) radiation and ultraviolet B radiation. N Engl Med J 322:1093–1097
120. Wolff K, Hönigsmann H, (1991) Genital carcinomas in psoriasis patients treated with photochemotherapy. Lancet 1:439
121. Young AR, Magnus IA, Davies AC, Smith NP (1983) A comparison of the phototumorigenic potential of 8-MOP and 5-MOP in hearless albino mice exposed to solar simulated irradiation. Br J Dermatol 108:507–518
122. Gupta AK, Stern RS, Swanson NA, Anderson TF, the PUVA follow-up study (1988) Cutaneous melanomas in patients treated with psoralen plus ultraviolet A. J Am Acad Dermatol 19:67–76
123. Stern RS, Nichols KT, Vakeva LH (1997) Malignant melanoma in patients treated for psoriasis with methoxsalen (psoralen) and ultraviolet A radiation (PUVA). N Engl J Med 336:1041–1045
124. Wolff K(1997) Should PUVA be abandoned? Editorial. N Engl J Med 336:1090–1091
125. Gibbs NK, Hönigsmann H, Young AR (1986) PUVA treatment strategies and cancer risk. Lancet 1:150–151
126. Hannuksela-Svahn A, Sigurgeirsson B, Pukkala E, Lindelöf B, Berne B, Hannuksela M, Poikolainen K, Karvonen J (1999) Trioxsalen bath PUVA did not increase the risk of squamous cell skin carcinoma and cutaneous malignant melanoma in a joint analysis of 944 Swedish and Finnish patients with psoriasis. Br J Dermatol 141:497–501
127. Hannuksela M, Stenbäck F, Lahti A (1986) The carcinogenic properties of topical PUVA. A lifelong study in mice. Arch Dermatol Res 278:347–351
128. Hannuksela-Svahn A, Pukkala E, Koulu L, Jansén CT, Karvonen J (1999) Cancer incidence among Finnish psoriasis patients treated with 8-methoxypsoralen bath PUVA. J Am Acad Dermatol 40:694–696
129. Slaper H, Schothorst AA, Van der Leun JC (1986) Risk evaluation of UVB therapy for psoriasis: comparison of calculated risk for UVB therapy and observed risk in PUVA-treated patients. Photodermatol 3:271–283

130. Young AR (1995) Carcinogenicity of UVB phototherapy assessed. Lancet
     345:1431–1432
131. Morison WL, Baughman RD, Day RM, Forbes PD, Hönigsmann H, Krueger GG,
     Lebwohl M, Lew R, Naldi L, Parrish JA, Piepkorn M, Stern RS, Weinstein GD, Whit-
     more SE (1998) Consensus workshop on the toxic effects of long-term PUVA ther-
     apy. Arch Dermatol 134:595–598

4 Photo(chemo)therapy for Atopic Dermatitis

Jean Krutmann, Akimichi Morita

Contents

From Heliotherapy to Modern Phototherapy of Atopic Dermatitis

It has been appreciated for decades that ultraviolet (UV) radiation may be beneficial for patients with atopic dermatitis (reviewed in [28]). In 1929, the German dermatologist Buschke stated that the effect of sea climate on atopic dermatitis was "simply surprising," and in the 1940s Lomhold and Norrlind concluded that most patients with atopic dermatitis improved during the summer season [39]. In 1948 Nexman was the first to systematically assess the beneficial effects of phototherapy in atopic dermatitis patients, which in his study were exposed to radiation from a carbon arc lamp [46]. Modern fluorescent lamps with defined emission spectra for phototherapy of atopic dermatitis have been continually used from the end of the 1970s until today. During the last 5 years, several new phototherapeutic modalities including UVA-1 therapy [33, 34] as well as 311-nm UVB therapy [14] have been introduced. As a consequence, dermatologists may now select from a diversified spectrum of distinct phototherapeutic modalities the phototherapy of choice for their particular patient.

During the same period, substantial progress has been made in advancing our knowledge about the pathogenesis of atopic dermatitis. A modern approach to phototherapy of atopic dermatitis has to reflect treatment decisions on the background of recent pathogenetic concepts [36]. The following chapter will therefore briefly summarize current knowledge about the pathogenesis of atopic dermatitis.

Pathogenesis of Atopic Dermatitis

It is now generally believed that atopic dermatitis represents a T-cell-mediated immune response directed against inhalant allergens [25]. This concept is supported by the fact that the major clinical, histological, and immunohistochemical features of atopic dermatitis strongly resemble those observed in allergic contact dermatitis. Lesional skin of patients with atopic dermatitis contains an inflammatory infiltrate, which predominately consists of T-helper lymphocytes. Cytokines, which are produced in situ by these helper T-cells, considerably contribute to the generation and maintenance of skin lesions in atopic dermatitis patients. It has been learned that the quality of the cytokine profile expressed in lesional skin of patients with atopic dermatitis critically depends on the stage of this disease [21]. Biopsies that were taken either from acute atopic dermatitis or from eczematous skin lesions, which had been initiated under standardized conditions in atopic dermatitis patients by epicutaneous application of inhalant allergens and were analyzed at an early stage during their development (24 h after allergen application), revealed a preponderance of the Th2-like cytokine interleukin (IL)-4. At the same time, expression of the Th1-like cytokine interferon-γ decreased below background levels. At later points in time, that is, either in chronic, lichenified lesions of spontaneously evolving atopic eczema or in 48-h inhalant allergen patch-test-induced skin lesions, this cytokine pattern was reversed. At these later points, expression of the Th1-like cytokine interferon-γ predominated, whereas IL-4 expression was decreased [18, 19, 22]. Increased expression of interferon-γ appears to be responsible for the generation and maintenance of clinically apparent skin lesions in atopic dermatitis, since a close correlation between the clinical course of atopic dermatitis and in situ expression of interferon-γ in lesional atopic skin was observed. These findings may best be described by a two-phase model of the pathogenesis of atopic dermatitis, in which an initiation phase, which represents a Th2-like inflammatory response and develops without clinically apparent skin lesions, is switched into a second, eczematous phase, which is dominated by the Th1-like cytokine interferon-γ and clinically presents as eczema [24]. Recent studies indicate that the observed switch from a Th2- into a Th1-like cytokine pattern may be caused by an increased expression of the cytokine IL-12 (Fig. 1).

Concept-Linked Phototherapy for Atopic Dermatitis

Based on this two-phase model it is now possible to discriminate phototherapeutic strategies that are directed at the initiation phase of atopic dermatitis, and thus, in a more general sense, may be regarded as prophylactic, from phototherapies that are directed at the eczematous phase of this disease, and which provide symptomatic relief by downregulating interferon-γ expression in lesional atopic skin [36]. Symptomatic phototherapy of atopic dermatitis needs to be differentiated further into very potent phototherapeutic modalities, which may be used as a monotherapy for short periods of time to effectively treat patients

Fig. 1. Pathogenesis of atopic eczema

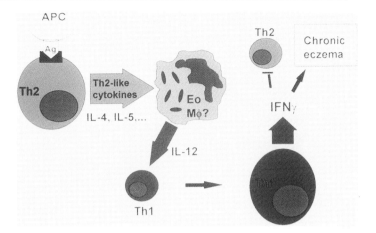

with acute, severe exacerbation of atopic dermatitis, and less-effective forms of phototherapy, which may be successfully employed as combination regimens over longer periods of time to treat patients with chronic forms of atopic dermatitis (Table 1). Current phototherapy of atopic dermatitis as conducted in daily practice is identical to symptomatic phototherapy.

Photo(chemo)therapy for Acute, Severe Atopic Dermatitis

In general, symptomatic phototherapy of acute, severe exacerbation of atopic dermatitis may be achieved with UVA-1, systemic psoralen plus UVA (PUVA), and extracorporeal photochemotherapy, whereas conventional UVA/UVB and narrowband UVB therapy represent phototherapeutic modalities that are primarily indicated for treatment of chronic stages of this disease (Table 1).

Table 1. Phototherapy for atopic dermatitis

Indication	Modality	Comment	Mode of action
Acute, severe	High-dose UVA-1, PUVA extracorporeal photopheresis	Monotherapy, alternative to glucocorticosteroids	Symptomatic, anti-eczematous
Chronic, moderate	311-nm, UVB, UVA/UVB, low-dose UVA-1, broadband UVB, broadband UVA	Combination therapy, to save glucocorticosteroids	Symptomatic, anti-eczematous, maintenance therapy

UVA-1 Phototherapy

The rationale for employing UVA-1 radiation, that is, long-wavelength UVA radiation (340–400 nm), in the treatment of patients with atopic dermatitis was based on immunological studies in which it was demonstrated that exposure of human skin to a single dose of 130 J/cm^2 UVA-1 radiation was associated with abrogation of epidermal Langerhans'-cell function to activate alloreactive T cells [3]. At the same time, evidence was accumulating that epidermal Langerhans' cells, by virtue of their capacity to bind IgE molecules, may play an important role in inhalant-allergen-mediated T-cell activation and thus be of critical importance for the pathogenesis of atopic dermatitis [6]. In addition, clinical studies comparing the efficacy of broadband UVB therapy versus UVA/UVB therapy in the management of patients with atopic dermatitis indicated that the therapeutic effectiveness of conventional UVB therapy may be significantly improved by increasing the UVA portion of the action spectrum (UVA/UVB therapy) [26].

The therapeutic effectiveness of UVA-1 irradiation in the management of patients with atopic dermatitis was first assessed in a pilot study in which patients with acute, severe exacerbation of atopic dermatitis were exposed once per day to a single dose of 130 J/cm^2 UVA-1 (high-dose UVA-1 therapy) for 15 consecutive days [34]. The therapeutic effectiveness of UVA-1 therapy was compared to that of a conventional UVA/UVB therapy by employing both modalities as a monotherapy, that is, additional treatment was restricted in both groups to the use of emollients. Therapeutic effectiveness was assessed by two means: an established clinical scoring system that had been originally developed by Costa et al. [10] consisting of a severity and a topographical score, and monitoring serum levels of eosinophil cationic protein. Serum levels of eosinophil cationic protein previously had been identified as sensitive parameters, which reflect disease activity in atopic dermatitis, and therefore were used as objective parameters to evaluate the therapeutic effectiveness of UVA-1 irradiation [11]. Assessment of clinical scores demonstrated that UVA-1 therapy was efficient in promptly inducing an improvement in clinical symptoms of patients with atopic dermatitis, and that in comparison to conventional UVA/UVB therapy significant differences in favor of UVA-1 therapy were observed after 6 and 15 exposures (Fig. 2). Similarly, elevated serum levels of eosinophil cationic protein in patients with atopic dermatitis were significantly decreased by UVA-1 therapy, but remained essentially unaltered in patients undergoing UVA/UVB therapy.

These preliminary but promising results indicated that UVA-1 therapy may represent a novel phototherapeutic modality that could be employed as a monotherapeutic approach to treat patients with acute, severe exacerbation of atopic dermatitis. Within the following years, these original observations have been confirmed by numerous reports, which mainly represent uncontrolled, open, and sometimes even non-comparative studies [1, 31, 32, 40, 66]. The pilot study by Krutmann et al. failed to provide a direct comparison of UVA-1 therapy with the topical use of glucocorticosteroids, which is the gold standard in the management of patients with acute, severe exacerbation of atopic dermatitis. In a subsequent multicenter trial, 53 patients were therefore randomly assigned to

Fig. 2. A patient with severe, acute exacerbation of atopic dermatitis before (a) and after (b) UVA1 phototherapy (10×130 J/cm^2)

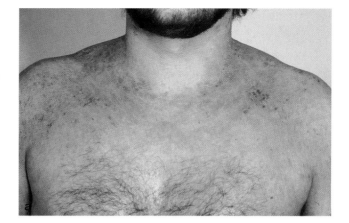

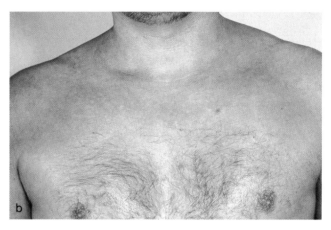

UVA-1 therapy (once daily, 130 J/cm^2, total of 10 days), conventional UVA/UVB therapy (once daily, minimal erythema dose (MED)-dependent, total of 10 days), or topical treatment with fluocortolone (once daily for 10 days) [37]. To date, this study is the only one to provide a multicentric evaluation of the efficacy of UVA-1 therapy in a controlled randomized fashion. It was observed that after ten treatments, patients in all three groups had improved, but the decrease in total clinical scores, and thus clinical improvement, was significantly greater in patients receiving either glucocorticosteroid or UVA-1 therapy, as compared to UVA/UVB therapy. Under these conditions, UVA-1 therapy, as compared to glucocorticosteroid treatment, was significantly better at day ten of therapy in reducing the total clinical score. These clinical observations were corroborated by laboratory assessments in which serum levels of eosinophil cationic protein as well as peripheral blood eosinophilia were compared before and after therapy between the three treatment groups. In aggregate, the multicenter-trial results indicate that UVA-1 therapy and glucocorticosteroid treatment are superior to conventional UVA/UVB therapy in the management of patients with acute, severe exacerbation of atopic dermatitis. UVA-1 therapy may thus be used as an alternative to glucocorticosteroids to treat severe atopic dermatitis.

UVA-1 therapy may not be performed in atopic dermatitis patients with UVA-1-sensitive atopic dermatitis or photodermatoses such as polymorphic light eruption [38]. It is necessary to exclude these diseases before the initiation of UVA-1 therapy. This can easily be accomplished by photoprovocation testing. Except for eczema herpeticum, no acute side effects have been observed in any of the atopic dermatitis patients treated with UVA-1. No other side effects have been observed, although its potential carcinogenic risk is a theoretical concern [38]. Exposure of hairless, albino Skh-hr1 mice to UVA-1 radiation has been shown to induce squamous cell carcinoma. The actual contribution of UVA-1 radiation to the development of malignant melanoma in humans is currently under debate and at this point cannot be excluded. Until more is known about UVA-1 therapy, its use should be limited to periods of severe, acute exacerbation and in general, one treatment cycle should not exceed 10–15 continuously applied exposures and should not be repeated more than once a year. Under no circumstances, UVA-1 phototherapy should be used for children (less than 18 years old) with atopic dermatitis [38]. In order to assess potential long-term side effects of UVA-1 phototherapy in a systematic manner, in Europe a prospective longitudinal study has been started to monitor patients treated with UVA-1 phototherapy for the development of skin cancer and photoaging (for details see chapter by H. Stege and R. Mang).

There is an ongoing debate whether therapeutic effectiveness of UVA-1 therapy is dose-dependent. Similar to a high-dose regimen with 130 J/cm^2, a medium UVA-1 dosage seems to be superior to UVA/UVB [31]. A direct comparison between a low-dose versus a high-dose UVA-1 regimen has recently been performed by J.C. Simon et al. (manuscript submitted for publication). In this open study, a high-dose protocol (130 J/cm^2) was superior to a medium-dose regimen (50 J/cm^2), which was more efficient than a low-dose schedule (20 J/cm^2). The latter observation is consistent with previous reports suggesting that a medium-dose regimen (50 J/cm^2) is superior to a low-dose regimen (20 J/cm^2) [27]. Also, UVA/UVB therapy was reported to be superior to a low-dose regimen (20 J/cm^2). It thus appears that a low-dose regimen does not offer any advantage over conventional phototherapeutic modalities. This is in contrast to medium- and high-dose UVA-1 phototherapy. In order to achieve an optimal and long-lasting therapeutic response, however, a high-dose regimen might be necessary [1].

Substantial progress has been made in understanding the photoimmunological mechanisms responsible for the therapeutic effectiveness of UVA-1 therapy in atopic dermatitis [35]. From these studies, it appears that UVA-1 therapy is capable of downregulating in situ expression of interferon-γ in lesional skin of patients with atopic dermatitis. This inhibitory effect was relatively specific since in the same biopsies, neither expression of the house-keeping gene β-actin nor of the cytokine IL-4 was reduced. Inhibition of interferon-γ expression in atopic eczema may not only be achieved by UVA-1 therapy, but could also be seen after topical application of glucocorticosteroids and most likely represents

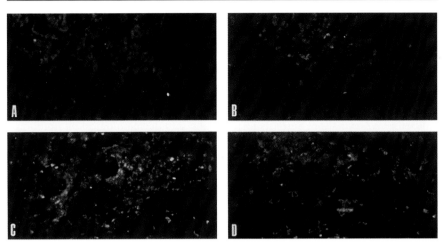

Fig. 3a–d. Apoptotic T cells in lesional skin of a patient with atopic eczema before (**A**) and after one (**B**), two (**C**), three (**D**) UVA-1 irradiations (single dose 130 J/cm²). Red, CD4$^+$ T cells (helper T cells); green, apoptotic TUNEL assay cells; orange, T cells

a general mechanism by which various treatment forms induce symptomatic relief in atopic dermatitis [18].

Downregulation of interferon-γ expression in atopic eczema is the consequence of direct effects of UVA-1 radiation on Th1-cells present within the dermal infiltrate [15, 16].

In vitro UVA-1 irradiation was found to be highly efficient in inducing apoptosis (programmed cell death) in human T cells. In vivo studies have revealed that UVA-1 phototherapy induced apoptosis in skin-infiltrating T cells (Fig. 3) and thereby caused a gradual reduction of the inflammatory infiltrate and a concomitant improvement of patients' skin disease [44]. These observations have stimulated interest in the use of UVA-1 phototherapy for other T-cell-mediated skin diseases as well [47].

In addition to directly affecting epidermal and dermal T cells, UVA-1 radiation may alter Th1-cell interferon-γ expression via indirect mechanisms, e.g., by inducing the production of anti-inflammatory cytokines such as IL-10 by epidermal keratinocytes, which in turn may act on T cells in a paracrine manner. In keeping with this concept are in vitro studies that demonstrate increased expression of IL-10 mRNA and secretion of IL-10 protein by cultured human keratinocytes following UVA-1 radiation exposure [20].

Immunohistochemical studies employing biopsies obtained from patients with atopic dermatitis undergoing UVA-1 therapy indicate that in addition to T cells and keratinocytes, epidermal Langerhans' cells and dermal mast cells represent target cells for UVA-1 radiation [18]. UVA-1 therapy, in contrast to UVA/UVB therapy, has reduced not only the relative number of IgE-bearing Langerhans' cells in the epidermis, but also the number of dermal CD1a$^+$ Langerhans' cells and mast cells. The latter observation prompted the use of UVA-1 therapy in the treatment of patients with urticaria pigmentosa, in which immediate and long-lasting remissions from cutaneous and systemic symptoms could be achieved [60].

PUVA Therapy

Systemic photochemotherapy (PUVA) combines the oral administration of psoralens with UVA radiation. Since its introduction into dermatological phototherapy some 30 years ago, PUVA has been found to be highly effective for the treatment of a variety of skin diseases (reviewed in [42]) including atopic dermatitis. Although there is no doubt that PUVA therapy may be successfully used not only for moderate, but also severe and even erythrodermic forms of atopic dermatitis, it has to be realized that PUVA therapy of this disease is associated with significant disadvantages [2, 4, 39, 42, 56, 57, 59, 64]. As compared to PUVA therapy of psoriasis, the actual number of treatments to clear atopic dermatitis was found to be relatively high. Even more important, cessation of PUVA therapy was associated with the occurrence of rebound phenomena in a high percentage of patients if photochemotherapy was not combined with systemic glucocorticosteroids, or if maintenance therapy was not continued for longer time intervals extending over several years [51]. Long-term use of PUVA is of particular concern in view of the relatively low age of patients with atopic dermatitis and recent reports indicate that long-term PUVA may be associated with an increased risk of developing skin cancer including malignant melanoma [62, 63]. Further disadvantages result from prolonged photosensitivity requiring protection by sunglasses to prevent cataract formation, and the occurrence of systemic side effects such as nausea in a relatively high percentage of patients (up to 20 %). PUVA therapy is thus of limited use for the treatment of patients with atopic dermatitis and does not represent an equivalent alternative to glucocorticosteroids or UVA-1 therapy in the management of severe exacerbation of atopic dermatitis.

Extracorporeal Photochemotherapy

Evidence exists that extracorporeal photopheresis may be of benefit for the management of patients with severe atopic dermatitis. Extracorporeal photopheresis consists of the passage of freshly drawn blood that contains photoactivatable psoralen (8-methoxypsoralen) through an extracorporeal UVA exposure system [13]. It is generally assumed that UVA radiation activates the pharmacologically inactive 8-methoxypsoralen, which then is thought to affect the lymphocytes within the blood preparation, and subsequently these "modulated" lymphocytes are re-infused into the patient.

Extracorporeal photopheresis has been used with some success in the treatment of patients with Sézary syndrome. There are also some indications that it might be used with benefit for the treatment of several immunologically based skin diseases such as graft-versus-host disease [65]. Prinz et al. were first to successfully use extracorporeal photochemotherapy for patients with atopic dermatitis [49]. They reported on three patients with severe atopic dermatitis with a life-long history of atopic dermatitis. Because their disease had finally become resistant to conventional therapies, extracorporeal photopheresis was started in these patients at 4-week intervals and found to induce clinical improvement of skin lesions associated with a reduction in serum levels of total IgE. Extracorporeal photopheresis was not used as a monotherapeutic approach but was combined with external use of topical prednicarbate, which, however, by itself was insufficient to control disease activity in these patients. These studies have been confirmed in an independent study in which three patients with previously intractable atopic dermatitis were subjected to extracorporeal photochemotherapy in a monotherapeutic design [54]. All patients showed prompt improvement, which was dependent on the frequency of treatment cycles (Fig. 4). When extracorporeal photochemotherapy was given at 2-week intervals, a rapid decrease in the overall skin score and in serum levels of eosinophil cationic protein and total IgE was observed. During free intervals from 2 to 4 weeks, however, these beneficial effects were rapidly lost, but they could be re-achieved after a renewed 2-week treatment schedule. In aggregate, these studies suggest that extracorporeal photopheresis is effective for the treatment of patients with atopic dermatitis, but controlled randomized studies, with a larger patients' collective, are required to confirm these preliminary observations. Also, this modality is expensive and time-consuming and therefore its use should be limited to atopic dermatitis patients in which other modalities have proven to be ineffective.

Photo(chemo)therapy for Chronic, Moderate Atopic Dermatitis

Broadband UVB therapy combined UVA/UVB therapy, 311-nm UVB therapy, broadband UVA therapy, or low dose UVA-1 therapy are effective treatments in mild and moderate atopic eczema but are not effective in patients with acute severe exacerbation of their disease [1, 9, 12, 14, 23–28, 32, 33, 41, 48, 50, 56]. These forms of UV phototherapy are not usually employed as monotherapeutic approaches but rather are used in combination with topical glucocorticosteroids in order to reduce need for corticosteroid application.

UVA/UVB Phototherapy

Recent studies indicate that combinations of UVB irradiation with UVA irradiation (UVA/UVB therapy) are superior to conventional broadband UVB, conventional UVA, and low-dose UVA-1 therapy in the management of chronic, moderate atopic dermatitis. In two paired comparison studies, Jekler and Larkö have shown UVB therapy to be superior to placebo. Intererstingly, UVB in high doses (0.8 MED) was equipotent to UVB in moderate doses (0.4 MED) [27]. The same authors, by employing a clinical scoring system, demonstrated in a paired comparison study statistically significant differences in favor of UVA/UVB therapy compared to broadband UVB therapy [26]. In this trial, patients were allowed to continue use of topical glucocorticosteroids, and, in addition, were irradiated 3 times per week for a maximum of 8 weeks in a UVB MED-dependent manner. These careful observations further prove the concept that UVA/UVB therapy is superior over UVB therapy in the management of patients with atopic dermatitis [36].

Narrowband UVB Phototherapy

Patients' most-frequent complaint in phototherapy for atopic dermatitis relates to worsening of itch and induction of sweating by heat, which may be associated with UV, in particular UVA therapy. In a recent study, George et al. have therefore incorporated air-conditioning into a 311-nm UVB irradiation unit [14]. By employing fifty TL-01 (100-W) lamps equipped with reflectors, a UVB output of 5 mW/cm^2 was achieved, which resulted in maximum treatment times of less than 10 min. In this well-designed study, steroid use by patients with moderate, chronic atopic dermatitis was monitored 12 weeks prior to phototherapy, during 12 weeks of phototherapy, and followed up for 24 weeks after cessation of phototherapy. The start of 311-nm UVB therapy not only decreased the total clinical score, but also substantially reduced the use of potent steroids. These beneficial effects were still present in the majority of patients 6 months after cessation of phototherapy.

These studies indicate that 311-nm UVB therapy may represent the phototherapeutic modality of choice to induce long-term improvement in patients with atopic dermatitis. They have recently been confirmed by an independent report, which suggested that no special cooling system is required in order to achieve the excellent therapeutic effects reported by George et al. [24].

In our hands, 311-nm UVB therapy has been found to be ideal in following UVA-1 therapy, which is used in the initial phase of treatment in order to manage acute, severe exacerbation of atopic dermatitis. UVA-1 therapy is then replaced by 311-nm UVB therapy, which is employed as an effective and presumably safe modality for maintenance therapy [68]. Because of the latter argument, it has also been advocated for children [9].

Photo(chemo)therapy for Chronic Vesicular Hand and Feet Eczema

Vesicular eczema of palms and soles is a common manifestation of atopic dermatitis that often runs a chronic course. Since clinical symptoms are limited to defined areas of the skin, whole-body UV irradiation would seem inappropriate. The recent development of cream-PUVA therapy offers the possibility to treat single, defined skin areas such as palms and soles without exposing nonlesional skin to UV radiation [61]. In addition, partial body UVA-1 irradiation has been proposed for this indication [58].

Cream-PUVA Photochemotherapy

For cream-PUVA a water-in-oil ointment containing 0.0006% 8-methoxypsoralen is applied to the area to be treated 1 h before UVA irradiation. Optimal phototoxicity is given 1–3 h after cream application and then rapidly falls of. In a first report, cream-PUVA therapy was found to be extremely beneficial

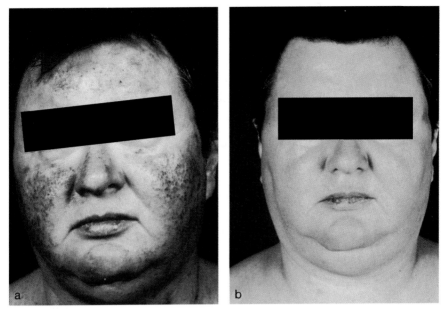

Fig. 4a, b. A patient with previously intractable atopic dermatitis before (**a**) and after (**b**) extracorporeal photochemotherapy (4 treatment cycles)

for patients with chronic hand and feet eczema [61]. After an average of 40 treatments, complete remission was observed in seven out of ten patients (Fig. 5). These observations have recently been confirmed in an independent study in

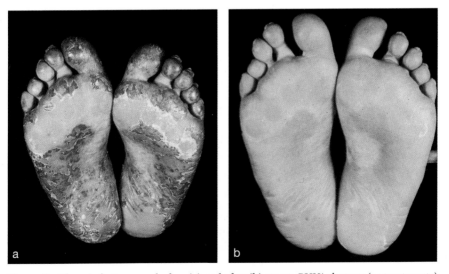

Fig. 5a, b. Chronic feet eczema before (**a**) and after (**b**) cream-PUVA therapy (34 treatments)

which cream-PUVA was reported to be superior to bath-PUVA for this indication [30]. This might be because the repetitive use of cream-PUVA, in contrast to bath-PUVA, does not cause exsiccation of eczematous skin. In addition, cream-PUVA, as compared with bath-PUVA, is easier, cheaper, and safer to perform.

Partial Body UVA-1 Phototherapy

In a recent study, the palms and backs of 12 patients with chronic dyshidrotic eczema were exposed to local UVA-1 phototherapy at a single dose of 40 J/cm^2 [58]. Local UVA-1 phototherapy was given as a monotherapy. After 15 treatments, there was a gradual improvement in 10 out of 12 patients. There was no relapse over a 3-month follow-up period. It has been suggested that the latter might be an advantage that local UVA-1 phototherapy might offer in comparison with local PUVA therapy. Controlled, comparative studies to prove this point, however, are currently unavailable.

Perspectives

In most instances photo(chemo)therapy for atopic dermatitis, in contrast to psoriasis, has been assessed in a monotherapeutic setting. Since atopic dermatitis, similar to psoriasis, is a chronic disease for which no curative treatment is available, therapeutic safety has to be a major concern. In this regard, combination regimens are of great interest because theoretically they allow combined modalities with different modes of action in order to enhance efficacy and safety at the same time. Controlled, randomized, comparative studies to assess the value of combining topical steroid treatment with new phototherapeutic modalities such as 311-nm UVB or UVA-1 phototherapy are therefore of significant practical relevance. The recent introduction of topical immunosuppressants for the management of patients with atopic dermatitis provides a completely new perspective for the symptomatic therapy of this disease. In this regard, combination regimens pose a major safety concern because immunosuppressive substances such as tacrolimus might increase the risk of developing skin cancer, in particular when used in combination with UV radiation. For a fair judgment of this problem, safety studies are an indispensable prerequisite.

Little is currently known about the possibility of using phototherapy in the prophylaxis of atopic eczema. A prophylactic phototherapeutic approach would be based on the capacity of ultraviolet radiation to specifically interfere with the initiation phase of this disease. In this regard it is of particular interest that repeated exposures of human skin to high doses of UVA-1 radiation is capable of suppressing the development of positive skin reactions in inhalant allergen patch tests of patients with atopic dermatitis [67]. Epicutaneous application of inhalant allergens, such as house dust-mite allergen, on the non-lesional skin of patients with atopic dermatitis, and proven sensitization against the allergen tested, has been found to induce eczematous skin lesions within 48 h after allergen application in about 45–50 % of patients tested [52, 53, 55]. Numerous immunohistochemical and, in particular, immunological studies have clearly established that the skin lesions induced are specifically caused by the inhalant allergen applied to the skin, and they do not merely represent an unspecific irritant reaction. As a consequence, the inhalant allergen patch test may therefore be regarded as a model for the initiation phase of atopic dermatitis, which, by definition, comprises the time in which the skin is hit by the aeroallergen to the time in which eczematous skin lesions start to develop. Within the same patient, that is, intraindividually, the induction of positive inhalant allergen patch test reactions has been a highly reproducible event, and this observation enabled us to ask whether UV radiation may have any effects on this system [67]. We have found that exposure of human skin to UVA-1 radiation is highly effective in completely suppressing the development of positive inhalant allergen patch tests. This inhibitory effect was relatively specific, since in the same patients, pre-irradiation of human skin with an equivalent dose of UVA-1 radiation failed to suppress the development of positive patch test reactions that were provoked by epicutaneous application of the irritant sodium lauryl sulfate. These preliminary observations indicate that repeated exposure of human skin to UVA-1 radiation may provide protection against initiation of atopic dermatitis lesions by inhalant allergens. This view is consistent with the clinical observation that cessation of high-dose UVA-1 therapy is not associated with rebound or immediate relapse of eczema in atopic dermatitis patients. Further studies are required to assess the underlying mechanisms responsible for the UVA-1 radiation-induced suppression of inhalant allergen patch test reactions. It will also be of interest to determine whether similar effects may be achieved by other wavelengths such as 311-nm UVB therapy. These studies may ultimately allow the development of phototherapeutic regimens in which patients with atopic dermatitis are irradiated at given intervals in order to provide maximal protection against re-exacerbation of their disease.

References

1. Abeck D, Schmidt T, Fesq H (2000) Long-term efficacy of medium dose UVA-1 phototherapy in atopic dermatitis. J Am Acad Dermatol 42:254–257
2. Atherton DJ, Carabott F, Glover MT, Hawk JM (1988) The role of psoralen photochemotherapy (PUVA) in the treatment of severe atopic eczema in adolescents. Br J Dermatol 118:791–795
3. Baadsgard O, Lisby S, Lange-Wantzin G, Wulf HC, Cooper KD (1989) Rapid recovery of Langerhans cell alloreactivity, without induction of autoreactivity, after in vivo ultraviolet A, but not ultraviolet B exposure of human skin. J Immunol 142:4213–4217
4. Binet O, Aron-Brunetiere C, Cuneo M, Cesaro M-J (1982) Photochimiotherapie par voie orale et dermatite atopique. Ann Dermatol Venereol 109:589–590
5. Bos JD, Wierenga EA, Smitt JHS, van der Heijden FL, Kapsenberg ML (1992) Immune dysregulation in atopic eczema. Arch Dermatol Res 128:1509–1514
6. Bruijnzeel-Koomen C (1986) IgE on Langerhans cells: new insights into the pathogenesis of atopic dermatitis. Dermatologica 172:181–184
7. Bruijnzeel-Koomen CAFM, van Wichen DF, Spry CJF, Venge P, Bruynzeel PLB (1988) Active participation of eosinophils in patch test reactions to inhalant allergens in patients with atopic dermatitis. Br J Dermatol 118:222–233

8. Buckely CC, Ivison C, Poulter LW, Rustin MHA (1992) FceR11/CD23 receptor distribution in patch test reactions to aeroallergens in atopic dermatitis. J Invest Dermatol 99:184–188
9. Collins P, Ferguson J (1995) Narrowband (TLO1) UVB airconditioned phototherapy for atopic eczema in children. Br J Dermatol 133:653–654
10. Costa C, Rillet A, Nicolet M, Saurat JH (1989) Scoring atopic dermatitis: the simpler the better. Acta Derm Venereol (Stockh) 69:41–47
11. Czech W, Krutmann J, Schöpf E, Kapp A (1992) Serum eosinophil cationic protein is a sensitive measure for disease activity in atopic dermatitis. Br J Dermatol 126:351–355
12. Falk ES (1985) UV-light therapies in atopic dermatitis. Photodermatol Photoimmunol Photomed 2:241–246
13. Gasparro F, Edelson RL (1995) Extracorporeal photochemotherapy. In: Krutmann J, Elmets CA (eds) Photoimmunology. Blackwell Scientific, Oxford, pp 231–245
14. George SA, Bilsland DJ, Johnson BE, Fergusson J (1993) Narrow-band (TL01) UVB air-conditioned phototherapy for chronic severe adult atopic dermatitis. Br J Dermatol 128:49–56
15. Godar DE (1996) Preprogrammed and programmed cell death mechanisms of apoptosis: UV-induced immediate and delayed apoptosis. Photochem Photobiol 63:825–830
16. Godar DE (1999) UVA 1 radiation mediates singlet-oxygen and superoxide-anion production which trigger two different final apoptotic pathways: the S and P site of mitochondria. J Invest Dermatol 112:3–12
17. Grabbe J, Welker P, Humke S, Grewe M, Schöpf E, Henz BM, Krutmann J (1996) High-dose UVA-1 therapy, but not UVA/UVB therapy, decreases IgE binding cells in lesional skin of patients with atopic eczema. J Invest Dermatol 107:419–423
18. Grewe M, Gyufko K, Schöpf E, Krutmann J (1994) Lesional expression of interferon-γ in atopic eczema. Lancet 343:25–26
19. Grewe M, Walther S, Gyufko K, Czech W, Schöpf E, Krutmann J (1995) Analysis of the cytokine pattern expressed in situ in inhalant allergen patch test reactions of atopic dermatitis patients. J Invest Dermatol 105:407–410
20. Grewe M, Gyufko K, Krutmann J (1995) Interleukin-10 production by cultured human keratinocytes: regulation by ultraviolet B and A1 radiation. J Invest Dermatol 104:3–6
21. Grewe M, Bruijnzeel-Koomen CAFM, Schöpf E, Thepen T, Langeveld-Wildschuh AG, Ruzicka T, Krutmann J (1998) A role for Th1 and Th2 cells in the immunopathogenesis of atopic dermatitis. Immunol Today 19:359–361
22. Hamid Q, Boguniewicz M, Leung DYM (1994) Differential in situ cytokine gene expression in acute versus chronic atopic dermatitis. J Clin Invest 94:870–876
23. Hannuksela M, Karvonen J, Husa M, Jokela R, Katajamäki L, Leppisaari M (1985) Ultraviolet light therapy in atopic dermatitis. Acta Derm Venereol (Stockh) 114:137–139
24. Hudson-Peacock MJ, Diffey BL, Farr PM (1996) Narrow-band UVB phototherapy for severe atopic dermatitis. Br J Dermatol 135:332
25. Jekler J, Larkö O (1988) UVB phototherapy of atopic eczema. Br J Dermatol 119:697–705
26. Jekler J, Larkö O (1990) Combined UV-A-UV-B versus UVB phototherapy for atopic dermatitis. J Am Acad Dermatol 22:49–53
27. Jekler J, Larkö O (1991) Phototherapy for atopic dermatitis with ultraviolet A (UVA), low-dose UVB and combined UVA and UVB: two paired comparison studies. Photodermatol Photoimmunol Photomed 8:151–156
28. Jekler J (1992) Phototherapy of atopic dermatitis with ultraviolet radiation (dissertation). Graphics Systems AB, University of Göteborg, Göteborg, 1992, 10
29. Kavli G (1978) Fotokjemoterapi med psoralen og langbolget ultrafiolett lys. 1 1/2 ars erfaring fra hudavdelingen in Tromso. Tidsskr Nor Lageforen 98:269–271

30. Kerscher M (1998) Creme-PUVA und Bade-PUVA. In: Plewig G, Wolff H (eds) Fortschritte der Dermatologie und Venerologie. Springer, Heidelberg, pp 135–139
31. Kobyletzki G, Pieck C, Hoffmann K, Freitag M, Altmeyer P (1999) Medium-dose UVA-1 cold-light phototherapy in the treatment of severe atopic dermatitis. J Am Acad Dermatol 41:931–937
32. Kowalzick L, Kleinhenz A, Weichenthal M, Ring J (1995) Low dose versus medium dose UVA-1 treatment in severe atopic dermatitis. Acta Derm Venereol (Stockh) 75:43–45
33. Krutmann J, Schöpf E (1992) High-dose UVA1 therapy: a novel and highly effective approach for the treatment of patients with acute exacerbation of atopic dermatitis. Acta Derm Venereol (Stockh) 176:120–122
34. Krutmann J, Czech W, Diepgen T, Niedner R, Kapp A, Schöpf E (1992) High-dose UVA1 therapy in the treatment of patients with atopic dermatitis. J Am Acad Dermatol 26:225–230
35. Krutmann J (1995) UVA1-induced immunomodulation. In: Krutmann J, Elmets CA (eds) Photoimmunology. Blackwell Scientific, Oxford, pp 246–256
36. Krutmann J (1996) Phototherapy for atopic dermatitis. Dermatol Ther 1:24–31
37. Krutmann J, Diepgen TL, Luger TA, Grabbe S, Meffert H, Sönnichsne N, Czech W, Kapp A, Stege H, Grewe M, Schöpf E (1998) High-dose UVA1 therapy for atopic dermatitis: Results of a multicenter trial. J Am Acad Dermatol 38:589–593
38. Krutmann J (1999): Therapeutic photomedicine: Phototherapy. In: Freedberg IM, Eisen AZ, Wolff K, Austen KF, Goldsmith LA, Katz SI, Fitzpatrick TB (eds) Fitzpatrick's dermatology in general medicine, 5th edn. McGraw-Hill, New York, pp 2870–2879
39. Lomhold S (1974) Hudsygdommene og deres behandling, 2nd edn. Copenhagen 97:425
40. Meffert H, Sönnichsen N, Herzog M, Hutschenreuther A (1992) UVA-1 cold light therapy of severe atopic dermatitis. Dermatol Monatsschr 78:291–296
41. Midelfart K, Stenvold S-E, Volden G (1985) Combined UVB and UVA phototherapy of atopic eczema. Dermatologica 171:95–98
42. Morison WL, Parrish JA, Fitzpatrick TB (1978). Oral psoralen photochemotherapy of atopic eczema. Br J Dermatol 98:25–30
43. Morison WL (1985) Phototherapy and photochemotherapy of skin disease, 2nd edn. Raven, New York, pp 148–152
44. Morita A, Werfel T, Stege H, Ahrens C, Karmann K, Grewe M, Grether-Beck S, Ruzicka T, Kapp A, Klotz O, Sies H, Krutmann J (1997) Evidence that singlet oxygen-induced human T-helper cell apoptosis is the basic mechanism of ultraviolet-A radiation phototherapy. J Exp Med 186:1763–1768
45. Norrling R. Prurigo Besnier (1946) A clinical-experimental study of its pathogenesis with special reference to acute infections of the respiratory tract (dissertation). Acta Derm Venereol (Stockh) [Suppl] 13:86–91
46. Nexman P-H (1948) Clinical studies of Besnier's prurigo (dissertation). Rosenkilde and Bagger, Copenhagen
47. Plettenberg H, Stege H, Megahed M, Ruzicka T, Hosokawa Y, Tsuji T, Morita A, Krutmann J (1999) Ultraviolet A1 (340–400 nm) phototherapy for cutaneous T-cell lymphoma. J Am Acad Dermatol 41:47–50
48. Potekaev NS, Sevidova LY, Vladimirov VV, Kochergin NG, Shinaev NN (1987) Selective phototherapy and dimociphon immunocorrective therapy in atopic dermatitis. Vestn Dermatol Venereol 9:39–42
49. Prinz B, Nachbar F, Plewig G (1994) Treatment of severe atopic dermatitis with extracorporeal photopheresis. Arch Dermatol Res 287:48–52
50. Pullmann H, Möres E, Reinbach S (1985) Wirkungen von Infrarot- und UVA-Strahlen auf die menschliche Haut und ihre Wirksamkeit bei der Behandlung des endogenen Ekzems. Z Hautkr 60:171–177

51. Rajka G (1980) Recent therapeutic events: cimetidine and PUVA. Acta Derm Venereol (Stockh) [Suppl] 92:117–118
52. Ramb-Lindhauer CH, Feldmann A, Rotte M, Neumann CH (1991) Characterization of grass pollen reactive T-cell lines derived from lesional atopic skin. Arch Dermatol Res 283:71–76
53. Reitamo S, Visa K, Kähönen K, Stubb S, Salo OP (1986) Eczematous reactions in atopic patients caused by epicutaneous testing with inhalant allergens. Br J Dermatol 114:303–308
54. Richter H, Billmann-Eberwein C, Grewe M, Stege H, Berneburg M, Ruzicka T, Krutmann J (1998) Successful monotherapy of severe and intractable atopic dermatitis by photopheresis. J Am Aacad Dermatol 38:585–588
55. Sager N, Feldmann A, Schilling G, Kreitsch P, Neumann C (1992) House dust-mite specific T cells in the skin of subjects with atopic dermatitis: frequency and lymphokine profile in the allergen patch test. J Allergy Clin Immunol 89:801–807
56. Salo O, Lassus A, Juvaksoski T, Kanerva L, Lauharanta J (1983) Behandlung der Dermatitis atopica und der Dermatitis seborrhoica mit selektiver UV-Phototherapie und PUVA. Dermatol Monatsschr 169:371–375
57. Sannwald C, Ortonne JP, Thivolet J (1979) La photochimiotherapie orale de l'eczema atopique. Dermatologica 159:71–77
58. Schmidt T, Abeck D, Boeck K, Mempel M, Ring J (1998) UVA1 irradiation is effective in treatment of chronic vesicular dyshidrotic hand eczema. Acta Derm Venereol (Stockh) 78:318–319
59. Soppi E, Viander M, Soppi A-M, Jansen CT (1982) Cell-mediated immunity in untreated and PUVA-treated atopic dermatitis. J Invest Dermatol 79:213–217
60. Stege H, Schöpf E, Krutmann J (1995) High-dose UVA1 therapy in the treatment of patients with urticaria pigmentosa. J Invest Dermatol 105:499A
61. Stege H, Berneburg M, Ruzicka T, Krutmann J (1997) Cream-PUVA-Photochemotherapy. Hautarzt 48:89–93
62. Stern RS and members of the Photochemotherapy Follow-Up Study (1990) Genital tumors among men with psoriasis exposed to psoralen and ultraviolet A radiation (PUVA) and ultraviolet B radiation. N Engl J Med 322:1093–1096
63. Stern RS, Nichols KT, Vakeva LH (1997) Malignant melanoma in patients treated for psoriasis with methoxsalen (psoralen) and ultraviolet A radiation (PUVA). N Engl J Med 336:1041–1045
64. Vaatainen N, Hannuksela M, Karvonen J (1979) Local photochemotherapy in nodular prurigo. Acta Dermatol 59:544–547
65. Volcz-Platzer B, Hönigsmann H (1995) Photoimmunology of PUVA and UVB therapy. In: Krutmann J, Elmets CA (eds) Photoimmunology. Blackwell Scientific, Oxford, pp 265–273
66. von Bohlen F, Kallusky J, Woll R (1994) The UVA1 cold light treatment of atopic dermatitis. Allergologie 17:382–384
67. Walter S, Grewe M, Gyufko K, Czech W, Kapp A, Stege H, Schöpf E, Krutmann J (1994) Inhalant allergen patch tests as a model for the induction of atopic dermatitis: analysis of the in situ cytokine pattern and modulation by UVA1. Abstract. Arch Dermatol Res 286:220
68. Young AR (1995) Carcinogenicity of UVB phototherapy assessed. Lancet 345:1431–1432

5 Phototherapy and Photochemotherapy of the Idiopathic Photodermatoses

Adrian Tanew, James Ferguson

Contents

Introduction

The term idiopathic photodermatoses denotes dermatological diseases that occur in otherwise healthy individuals as a result of exposure to natural or artificial light without the intervention of an external photosensitizer. This group of diseases includes polymorphic light eruption, hydroa vacciniforme, actinic prurigo, solar urticaria, and chronic actinic dermatitis. All these diseases have two factors in common: first, they are precipitated by electromagnetic radiation in the ultraviolet or visible range; second, the exact pathomechanism leading to the clinical manifestation of these diseases remains to be elucidated, but presumably it is immunologic in nature. In particular, it is still entirely unknown which chromophore(s) are responsible for the initiation of the photochemical reactions that ultimately lead to the inflammatory reaction in the skin. Diagnosis of the photodermatoses is mainly based on clinical features and phototesting, whereas histopathological or laboratory investigations play a subordinate role.

Essentially all photodermatoses represent well-established indications for phototherapy and photochemotherapy [psoralen plus UVA (PUVA)]. The aim of treatment is to prevent the outbreak of disease by increasing the patients' tolerance to sunlight. In the following, the use of phototherapy and photochemotherapy in each of the photodermatoses will be discussed. After a short description of the disease, the protocols and specific phototherapeutic considerations will be outlined along with an overview on achievable results.

Polymorphic Light Eruption

Contrary to all other photodermatoses, polymorphic light eruption (PLE) is extremely common. The prevalence of PLE is reported to range between 3 % and 21 % with a strong female preponderance and a marked latitude gradient. Patients with PLE may have a positive family history. An autosomal dominant inheritance with incomplete penetration is assumed, however, a higher prevalence of specific HLA types in PLE patients has not been demonstrated.

PLE is characterized by seasonal occurrence and usually starts to appear in late spring or during holidays in sunny regions. The time interval between the beginning of sun exposure and the outbreak of the skin eruption may range from less than an hour to a few days. The main symptom is intense itching, which usually precedes the appearance of a papular, vesicular, or plaque-like rash in sun-exposed skin areas [22]. Other less common morphologic variants of PLE are erythema multiforme-like or hemorrhagic lesions. Pruritus without clinical signs has also been described.

The most important diagnostic tool is phototesting. Once the minimal erythema dose (MED) of UVA and UVB has been determined, previously affected regions of the skin are repeatedly exposed to erythemogenic doses of both spectra with the aim of inducing specific lesions. This photoprovocation test is performed to confirm the diagnosis of PLE, which otherwise is often only based on the patient's history. Photoprovocation also provides information on the individual action spectrum for PLE induction, which is relevant for preventive measures. Phototesting of large groups of patients have shown that PLE is caused by UVA in about 50 % – 75 %, by UVB in 10 % – 15 % and by UVA and UVB in 15 % – 35 % of patients, respectively [21, 37]. The disease, which may spontaneously resolve [18], shows a wide range of clinical severity, with the majority managed simply with careful light avoidance and broad-spectrum sunscreen use. For a minority, such measures are inadequate; in this group desensitization with either UVB or PUVA can be considered.

Phototherapy of Polymorphic Light Eruption

At first glance it seems a paradox to use phototherapy to prevent a condition that is caused by light. However, many patients report that the rash occurs less frequently or entirely disappears during the course of the summer months. This gradually increasing tolerance towards sunlight is termed "hardening effect."

The presumed mechanisms of action underlying this effect are an enhanced filtering effect of the skin as a result of increased melanin formation and thickening of the stratum corneum and an altered immunological reactivity of the skin.

Photoprevention or photochemoprevention of PLE is likely to be based on the same mechanisms. A short course of radiation is usually sufficient to achieve a hardening effect. To avoid PLE provocation by this procedure, two strategies can be considered. One is to use the UV spectrum for prophylaxis that failed to induce PLE during phototesting, and the other is to administer therapeutic doses of responsible wavelengths that are below the threshold of induction.

Based on these considerations, desensitization with broadband UVB is especially suitable for patients whose PLE is precipitated by UVA. Several studies have shown that 12–15 treatments at a frequency of 3–5 exposures per week increase the patients' tolerance to sunlight and is effective in preventing or attenuating the occurrence of PLE [35, 36]. It is believed unnecessary to administer erythemogenic UVB doses although evidence is lacking. Treatment-induced pigmentation is not a reliable indication of therapeutic effect since patients with skin types I and II who only tan poorly may experience good PLE prevention.

Table 1. Examples of UVB and PUVA treatment protocols for PLE desensitization

	Treatment Protocol
UVB desensitization (broad- or narrowband)	Determination of minimal erythema dose (MED) with readings at 24 h Initial irradiation dose – 70 % of MED 20 % increments at each visit if no erythema[a] and no provoked PLE[b] Outpatients – 3 times weekly for 5 weeks (total 15 treatments) Inpatients – daily for 2 weeks (total 10 treatments)
PUVA desensitization	8-MOP or 5-MOP Determination of minimal phototoxic dose (MPD) with readings at 72 h Initial dose – 70 % of MPD 20 % increments at each visit if no erythema[a] and no provoked PLE[b] 3 times weekly for 4 weeks (total 12 treatments)
If erythema	Grade 1 – previous dose repeated Grade 2 – postpone one treatment and same dose repeated, followed by 20 % increments Grade 3/4 – no treatment until recovery, then dose reduced by half followed by 10 % increments
If provoked PLE	Itch or mild PLE – topical steroid if required Moderate – same dose and moderate/potent topical steroid, followed by 10 % increments Severe – postpone 1 or 2 treatments, potent topical steroid and restart with penultimate dose followed by 10 % increments

[a] As the alternative, refer to "If erythema" section.
[b] As the alternative, refer to "If provoked PLE" section.

Despite widespread use, treatment regimens vary greatly between centers [7] (Table 1). In some units, narrowband (TL-01) UVB has gradually replaced broadband UVB and PUVA and is considered the treatment of first choice for PLE desensitization. In those centers, PUVA is reserved for those who fail to gain satisfactory protection. In a recent controlled, observer-blind randomized study comparing narrowband UVB with PUVA in 25 patients both treatments were found to be not only equally effective in preventing PLE but also were equally capable of provoking PLE during the treatment course [4]. In this solitary work the management of PLE by narrowband UVB appeared to be superior to broadband UVB which is known to be less effective than PUVA.

The advantages of broad- and narrowband UVB over PUVA include
1. absent psoralen sensitization and associated gastrointestinal upset,
2. avoidance of the need for eye photoprotection during the post-treatment period,
3. the ability to use in children and during pregnancy,
4. easier and cheaper administration, and perhaps most importantly for those requiring yearly desensitization courses,
5. it is believed that both broadband and TL-01 UVB are safer than PUVA in terms of the risk of non-melanoma cutaneous malignancy [8, 49].

Photochemotherapy of Polymorphic Light Eruption

Since photochemotherapy of PLE involves the administration of a photosensitizers only small doses of UVA are required. Such doses are in general much lower than those required to cause PLE but still have the potential to induce pigmentation and to modulate immune responses in the skin. The first reports on the successful use of PUVA in the prevention of PLE appeared in the late 1970s. In one study PUVA hardening resulted in complete protection of 5/5 patients [16], whereas in another trial the occurrence of PLE was markedly attenuated in 9/10 patients [38]. All study patients had a long history of severe PLE and had used sunscreens without success. The efficacy of photochemotherapy in the prevention of PLE was confirmed in four other clinical studies with comparably good therapeutic results [2, 32, 36, 37]. Moreover, photochemotherapy proved to be substantially more effective than broadband UVB. While PUVA provides for almost complete or complete prevention of symptoms in 90 %–100 % of patients, the therapeutic response rate to broadband UVB is between 60 % and 80 %.

PUVA hardening is indicated in selected patients with severe PLE that cannot be prevented by the use of sunscreens or UVB phototherapy. Treatment is given 3 times weekly over a period of 4 weeks. Both 8-methoxypsoralen (8-MOP) and 5-methoxypsoralen (5-MOP) can be used as photosensitizer, however, 5-MOP is preferable for two reasons. First, gastrointestinal and central nervous side effects that are common with 8-MOP almost never occur with 5-MOP. Second, 5-MOP is more pigmentogenic than 8-MOP.

For the therapeutic effect suberythemogenic UVA doses are generally sufficient. Photoprotection can thus be achieved by low cumulative UVA doses and treatment beyond these protective threshold doses appears to offer no further benefit [32].

Despite the low UVA doses used for irradiation, some patients do develop abortive eruptions of PLE during the initial phase of PUVA hardening. This indicates that PUVA-specific mechanisms of PLE induction exist. Interruption of the treatment or reduction of the UVA dose is rarely required in such cases. Usually, brief symptomatic treatment with topical corticosteroids is sufficient.

The therapeutic value of preventive photochemotherapy for PLE has to be balanced against the potential long-term side effects of this treatment modality. A host of follow-up data on psoriatic patients treated with PUVA has shown that a cumulative exposure of more than 200 treatments can significantly increase the risk of squamous cell carcinoma [46, 47]. Given the fact that very few treatments and low cumulative UVA doses (ranging from 15 to 40 J/cm^2 per treatment course, depending on skin type and photosensitizer) are required for photoprotection and that PLE can severely impair patients in their outdoor activities, PUVA treatment of PLE is justified when other preventive measures have failed.

Practical Aspects of Desensitization

When discussing a desensitization course with a patient (Table 2), it is important to highlight that a history of natural "hardening" is not required to produce a therapeutic effect and that each patient can expect to respond differently and as such treatment will be individualized. In the case of PLE management, study work suggests that at least one episode of mild PLE can be expected in half of those patients desensitized. The first course is exploratory and patients should be forewarned that although their eruption may be provoked, it should not prevent continuing treatment. In those cases where PLE episodes are more troublesome, greater caution with incremental dose steps, along with the use of post-photo(chemo)therapy potent topical steroid, usually allows treatment to continue to completion. For those patients who only desire to expose their arms, legs and face during the summer months, treatment can be localized by advising

Table 2. Desensitization: practical points worth consideration

---

A history of natural hardening is not a prerequisite
Each patient will respond differently
The first course is exploratory
Consider treatment of sunlight exposed sites only, i.e., arms, legs, face
In severe cases, topical steroid use post-phototherapy may help
In those patients wearing clothing in the cubicle, remember to wear the same thick cotton/UV opaque clothing at the same position at each treatment
Post-desensitization, encourage patients to cautiously seek sunlight exposure to maintain hardening effect during summer months. Provide a post-desensitization information sheet
Patients who have had three successful courses with good results should be encouraged to miss a year. Spontaneous resolution does occur

---

the patient to wear the same thick cotton short-sleeved shirt and shorts at each treatment. The clothing must be worn in exactly the same position on each occasion to prevent sunburn reactions in those areas not previously treated. After completion of the desensitization course, patients should be encouraged to cautiously seek sunlight exposure to keep their artificially induced photoprotection topped up. The risk of not doing so is that the beneficial effects may be lost within 4–6 weeks [37]. One possible explanation for poor responders is that the treatment course may have been given too early in spring which, when combined with a poor early summer sunshine, may result in a loss of photoprotection. The effects of desensitization, whether PUVA or UVB, are temporary, and treatment needs to be repeated on a yearly basis. There appears to be no loss of benefit with subsequent treatment courses, and it is a useful practice for those patients who have had 3–4 years of successful desensitization to be encouraged to try a year without treatment.

Long-term risk, e.g., photodamage and nonmelanoma skin cancer, of repeated yearly phototherapy courses in children or adults who suffer from abnormal photosensitivity, is a potential problem. If necessary, does the clinician advise repeating the treatment for 20 or 30 years? Probably yes, for in PLE the cumulative lifetime solar exposure is likely to be no greater, and probably less, than in normal subjects, suggesting that where there is a significant benefit this will outweigh a slightly increased risk [29].

Hydroa Vacciniforme

Hydroa vacciniforme is a very rare photodermatosis characterized by light-induced papulovesicular eruptions affecting mainly the face, chest, forearms, and hands. The lesions progress into serous-hemorrhagic blisters with a necrotic epidermis that heal with crusting and lead to varioliform scars. The eyes may also be involved in the form of conjunctivitis with concomitant photophobia or corneal ulceration. The disease usually starts in childhood and takes a chronic recurrent course. Spontaneous remission often occurs in early adulthood. Men are more frequently affected than women.

In several studies the action spectrum of hydroa vacciniforme was found to lie within the UVA range [10, 14, 17, 27, 30]. Reproduction of lesions can be achieved by repeated irradiation with UVA doses between 30 and 60 J/cm^2.

Management of hydroa vacciniforme is generally much more difficult than that of PLE. Conventional sunscreens have a limited filtering effect against UVA radiation and in most cases do not provide adequate protection. The same is true for beta-carotene and antimalarial agents. This emphasizes the value of phototherapy and photochemotherapy in the treatment of hydroa vacciniforme.

Phototherapy of Hydroa Vacciniforme

Owing to the low prevalence of hydroa vacciniforme, only anecdotal reports exist on the use of photoprevention therapy [17]. In a summary of ten patients who had received different treatments, Sonnex and Hawk [45] state that two patients had remained free of symptoms in the summer months following UVB phototherapy.

Data concerning treatment with narrowband UVB are equally scarce. In an investigation on the efficacy of narrowband UVB in the prevention of photodermatoses, Collins and Ferguson [5] treated four patients with hydroa vacciniforme. Of these, two responded well to treatment with good photoprotection during the summer months.

Photochemotherapy of Hydroa Vacciniforme

The first report of a patient with hydroa vacciniforme successfully treated with PUVA was published in 1981 by Jaschke and Hönigsmann [27]. After twelve exposures the patient had remained free of symptoms throughout the whole summer period. In another patient who received 12 and 8 PUVA exposures in two consecutive years, respectively, treatment did not entirely prevent the outbreak of disease but reduced the symptoms [14].

In Vienna we have performed photochemotherapy for several years in four patients with considerable success. While the healthy skin of the patients remained entirely free of symptoms after photochemotherapy, discrete lesions developed in the scarred areas of the skin. The therapy regimen is similar to that used in PLE, consisting of three PUVA exposures per week for a total of 4–6 weeks.

Actinic Prurigo

Actinic prurigo is another rare and probably underdiagnosed photodermatosis [1, 12, 23]. It is a chronic disease that starts in childhood and mainly affects women. Often patients have a positive family history of atopy or photosensitivity. A strong HLA association with the DR4 allele, in particular the rare subtype DRB1*0407, has been reported recently [15]. The clinical manifestation is distinct, consisting of pruriginous skin lesions located mainly, but not exclusively, in sun-exposed areas of the skin. Usually the face is also affected with characteristic involvement of the distal part of the nose. Another common feature is exfoliative cheilitis of the lower lip. The acute reaction to sunlight appears as edematous erythema that subsequently develops into pruriginous lesions. The disease is initially seasonal but eventually becomes perennial with marked aggravation in the summer months. In adulthood the patients may experience attenuation of the symptoms or even spontaneous remission.

Phototesting reveals normal or reduced erythema thresholds in the UVB and UVA range. Specific skin lesions can be induced by photoprovocation. The action spectrum comprises the entire ultraviolet range but mostly lies within the UVA region [23].

Phototherapy for Actinic Prurigo

In an open study, phototherapy with narrowband UVB was assessed and found to be highly effective in six patients with actinic prurigo, increasing their daily tolerance of sunlight to 6 h or more over the following summer season [5]. In two of these six patients also, previous treatment with broadband UVB had been successful, while four patients who had received PUVA treatment achieved a similar degree of success. Narrowband UVB therapy was used either 3 times per week for 5 weeks or, if hospitalized, 5 times per week for 2 weeks. Pruritus was recorded in five patients and provocation of lesions in four. If severe, potent topical steroids can be applied with further phototherapy increments restricted to 10 %.

Photochemotherapy for Actinic Prurigo

Farr and Diffey [11] treated five patients with PUVA twice weekly for a total of 15 weeks. A decrease in photosensitivity was observed at 4 weeks of treatment. After the end of treatment and a mean cumulative UVA dose of 58 J/cm^2 all patients were free of symptoms throughout the summer although spending up to several hours in the sun. Photochemotherapy was well tolerated except for sporadic erythema reactions.

Solar Urticaria

Solar urticaria is a rare disease characterized by a whealing reaction in response to exposure to sunlight or artificial radiation, e.g., solaria. The urticarial lesions usually develop within a few minutes, are confined to the light-exposed areas of the skin, and are accompanied by strong itching. In cases of pronounced photosensitivity and extensive light exposure, patients might develop generalized urticaria and signs of anaphylactic shock. A less severe form of this photodermatosis is fixed solar urticaria in which the urticarial reaction is confined to circumscribed areas of the skin [42]. As with other members of the idiopathic photodermatoses, spontaneous resolution may occur but is not the rule.

The action spectrum differs from person to person, extending from short-wave ultraviolet light to the visible range. Since nearly all patients react to UVA or visible light, sunscreens are, as a rule, ineffective. The phenomenon of photo-inhibition, which denotes the suppression of light-induced urticaria by subsequent exposure to radiation of longer (in rare cases shorter) wavelengths has been documented in a few patients [26].

Phototesting in solar urticaria is of major diagnostic and therapeutic relevance [44]. Irradiation with gradually increasing doses of UVB, UVA, and visible light is performed to determine the minimal urticarial dose (MUD). This serves as a guideline for the therapeutic dose that can be tolerated by the patients at the beginning of phototherapy or photochemotherapy. Patients with solar urticaria should also be examined for the presence of a photoreactive factor in the plasma [24]. To this purpose, plasma is obtained from the patient and irradiated ex vivo with the activating light spectrum. The irradiated plasma is then injected into the dermis of the patient's skin together with unirradiated plasma as a control. In case of a whealing reaction to the light-activated plasma, the elimination of the circulating photoreactive factor by plasmapheresis can be considered [9].

Phototherapy for Solar Urticaria

Following an urticarial eruption the skin remains refractory to subsequent light exposure for several hours, which provides the basis for the concept of desensitization. The aim of desensitization is to keep the patients in a chronic refractory state by means of repeated exposure to the wavelengths that precipitate solar urticaria [41]. This form of therapy usually employs UVA, which is part of the action spectrum in most patients. However, the induction of tolerance with UVB has also been reported [28]. In the initial phase of desensitization, one or more irradiations are given daily using doses that are below the MUD. Thereafter, the interval between the treatments as well as the irradiation dose are increased until the individual's maximum tolerance is achieved. It is hypothesized that the irradiation causes the photoallergen to block the binding sites of mast cell-bound IgE antibodies, thereby preventing further mast cell degranulation [31].

Bernhard et al. [3] reported the use of UVA alone using the dose below the MUD being given 3–5 times weekly for up to 6 weeks. Three of the five patients reported benefit lasting for most of the subsequent summer months. A similar experience of prolonged benefit following UVA phototherapy has been reported in two patients suffering from severe solar urticaria. Treatment in these cases was twice daily for 2–3 weeks. Monochromator phototesting demonstrated persistent benefit 3 months after phototherapy [6].

A different concept of phototherapy for solar urticaria is UVB irradiation of patients whose disease is precipitated by the UVA or visible range [33]. Here the strategy is to avoid the activating spectrum rather than using it to induce refractoriness. The therapeutic intention aims at increasing the light filtering properties of the patients' skin by means of pigmentation and epidermal hyperplasia.

Data concerning the use of narrowband UVB phototherapy in solar urticaria are scarce. In one study, a small number of highly UVA/visible light sensitive patients was treated, but the therapeutic effect persisted only for 3–4 weeks [5].

Photochemotherapy for Solar Urticaria

The efficacy of photochemotherapy in solar urticaria was documented in several studies in the 1980s [1, 39, 40]. PUVA has the advantage over phototherapy that the treatment-induced protection is in general of much longer persistence.

PUVA is administered 3 times weekly using 8-MOP at a dose of 0.6 mg/kg. Treatment with 5-MOP requires higher irradiation doses and is not indicated in patients with pronounced photosensitivity in the UVA range. The initial UVA dose should be just below the threshold dose for erythema and urticaria induction. In highly UVA-sensitive patients a short pretreatment with UVA phototherapy has been used to facilitate subsequent irradiation with PUVA [43]. Hudson-Peacock et al. [25] reported one patient with a detectable photoallergen in the plasma in whom PUVA treatment could not be performed because the MUD_{UVA} was as low as 0.05 J/cm^2. After five courses of plasmapheresis, the MUD_{UVA} had increased to 1.3 J/cm^2 and PUVA therapy could be initiated.

In the first phase of treatment, the patients' tolerance to sunlight is gradually increased until they are able to resume outdoor activities without experiencing eruptions of solar urticaria. In this phase of treatment, the frequency of irradiation is kept constant at 3 times per week while the UVA dose is continuously increased. As soon as adequate desensitization is achieved, patients are placed on a maintenance schedule. In that phase of treatment 1–2 weekly exposures are usually sufficient.

The mechanisms of action of PUVA in solar urticaria are not fully understood. In addition to PUVA-induced pigmentation, effects on mast-cell degranulation, antigen-IgE interaction and downregulation of IgE production have been implicated in the therapeutic effect.

Practical Aspects of Desensitization

During photo(chemo)therapy there is a risk of inducing urticaria which, if extensive, may result in anaphylaxis. It is therefore mandatory to determine the MUD prior to any desensitization treatment and to use antihistamine cover even if the patient's solar urticaria is only partially responsive. Limited sites such as arms and face might be treated initially to minimize the risk of shock, which may occur with generalized solar urticaria induction.

Chronic Actinic Dermatitis

This condition, which is not as rare as once thought, predominantly affects males who represented 90% of a case study group of 370 [13]. Although the under 50-year-old age group is occasionally affected, 90% of cases are between the ages 50 and 70 years. The majority suffer from a non-specific dermatitis that predominantly involves sunlight-exposed skin but may spread to covered areas. A severe pseudolymphomatous variant of chronic actinic dermatitis is termed actinic reticuloid and is characterized by nodules that may coalesce into plaques. Classical investigative findings include marked UVB and UVA sensitivity with extension of half of the cases into the visible region. In addition, many patients have associated contact or photocontact allergy. Management involves behavioral sunlight avoidance combined with the use of thick woven cotton clothing and sun protective agents in combination with freedom from known contact allergens.

Photo(chemo)therapy for Chronic Actinic Dermatitis

In 1979, Morison et al. [34] reported successful management with 8-MOP PUVA initially administered under systemic prednisolone and later as a maintenance monotherapy. Hölzle et al. [20] induced long-term remission in two patients with severe UV sensitivity. At the beginning of treatment, very low UVA doses were employed and only parts of the patients' body were irradiated. In a further study, four patients using PUVA with potent topical steroid applied immediately post-irradiation, produced a good result in all studied [19]. Although there is a lack of further data, there is a feeling that mild and moderate subjects do well, while those severely affected fail to tolerate even the lowest increments of PUVA. More recently, Toonstra et al. [48] reported a good response in 13 patients with actinic reticuloid using small increments of UVB irradiation from a high-pressure mercury arc lamp. Further work to assess this approach is required, particularly when one considers the severe degree of UVB sensitivity that many of these patients demonstrate.

Conclusion

Although the mechanisms of artificial hardening in the idiopathic photodermatoses are not clearly understood, work is underway to help probe these which, when more clearly defined, should help design future therapy. There is no doubt that these forms of treatment currently do present a satisfactory if, for some patients, a time-consuming management approach.

References

1. Addo HA, Frain-Bell W (1984) Actinic prurigo – a specific photodermatosis? Photodermatology 1:119–s128
2. Addo HA, Sharma SC (1987) UVB phototherapy and photochemotherapy (PUVA) in the treatment of polymorphic light eruption and solar urticaria. Br J Dermatol 116:539–547
3. Bernhard JD, Jaenicke K, Momtaz-T K, Parrish JA (1984) Ultraviolet A phototherapy in the prophylaxis of solar urticaria. J Am Acad Dermatol 10:29–33
4. Bilsland D, George SA, Gibbs NK, Aitchison T, Johnson BE, Ferguson J (1993) A comparison of narrow band phototherapy (TL-01) and photochemotherapy (PUVA) in the management of polymorphic light eruption. Br J Dermatol 129:708–712
5. Collins P, Ferguson J (1995) Narrow-band UVB (TL-01) phototherapy: an effective preventive treatment for the photodermatoses. Br J Dermatol 132:956–963
6. Dawe RS, Ferguson J (1997) Prolonged benefit following ultraviolet A phototherapy for solar urticaria. Br J Dermatol 137:144–148
7. Dawe RS, MacKie RM, Ferguson J (1998) The Scottish phototherapy audit: the need for evidence based guidelines? Br J Dermatol 139 [Suppl 51]:17
8. de Gruijl FR (1998) What do we know about skin cancer risk? PUVA vs UVB vs TL01. In: Hönigsmann H, Knobler RM, Trautinger F, Jori G, (eds) Landmarks in photobiology. OEMF spa, Milano, pp 448–450
9. Duschet P, Leyen P, Schwarz T, Höcker P, Greiter J, Gschnait F (1987) Solar urticaria – effective treatment by plasmapheresis. Clin Exp Dermatol 12:185–188

10. Eramo LR, Garden JM, Esterly NB (1986) Hydroa vacciniforme. Diagnosis by repetitive ultraviolet-A phototesting. Arch Dermatol 122:1310–1313
11. Farr PM, Diffey BL (1989) Treatment of actinic prurigo with PUVA: mechanism of action. Br J Dermatol 120:411–418
12. Ferguson J (1990a) Polymorphic light eruption and actinic prurigo. Curr Probl Dermatol 19:130–147
13. Ferguson J (1990b) Photosensitivity dermatitis and actinic reticuloid syndrome (chronic actinic dermatitis). Semin Dermatol 9:47–54
14. Galosi A, Plewig G, Ring J, Meurer M, Schmoeckel C, Schurig V, Dorn M (1985) Experimentelle Auslösung von Hauterscheinungen bei Hydroa vacciniformia. Hautarzt 36:566–572
15. Grabczynska SA, McGregor JM, Kondeatis E, Vaughan RW, Hawk JLM (1999) Actinic prurigo and polymorphic light eruption: common pathogenesis and the importance of HLA-DR4/DRB1×0407. Br J Dermatol 140:232–236
16. Gschnait F, Hönigsmann H, Brenner W, Fritsch P, Wolff K (1978) Induction of UV light tolerance by PUVA in patients with polymorphous light eruption. Br J Dermatol 99:293–295
17. Halasz CLG, Leach EE, Walther RR, Poh-Fitzpatrick MB (1983) Hydroa vacciniforme: induction of lesions with ultraviolet A. J Am Acad Dermatol 8:171–176
18. Hasan T, Ranki A, Jansen CT, Karvonen J (1998) Disease associations in polymorphous light eruption: a long-term follow up study of 94 patients. Arch Dermatol 134:1081–1085
19. Hindson C, Spiro J, Downey A (1985) PUVA therapy of chronic actinic dermatitis. Br J Dermatol 113:157–160
20. Hölzle E, Hofmann C, Plewig G (1980) PUVA-treatment for solar urticaria and persistent light reaction. Arch Dermatol Res 269:87–91
21. Hölzle E, Plewig G, Hofmann C, Roser-Maass E (1982) Polymorphous light eruption. Experimental reproduction of skin lesions. J Am Acad Dermatol 7:111–125
22. Hölzle E, Plewig G, von Kries R, Lehmann P (1987) Polymorphous light eruption. J Invest Dermatol 88:32s–38s
23. Hölzle E, Rowold J, Plewig G (1992) Aktinische Prurigo. Hautarzt 43:278–282
24. Horio T, Minami K (1977) Solar urticaria: photoallergen in a patient's serum. Arch Dermatol 113:157–160
25. Hudson-Peacock MJ, Farr PM, Diffey BL, Goodship THJ (1993) Combined treatment of solar urticaria with plasmapheresis and PUVA. Br J Dermatol 128:440–442
26. Ichihashi M, Hasei K, Hayashibe K (1985) Solar Urticaria. Further studies on the role of inhibition spectra. Arch Dermatol 121:503–507
27. Jaschke E, Hönigsmann H (1981) Hydroa vacciniforme – Aktionsspektrum. UV-Toleranz nach Photochemotherapie. Hautarzt 32:350–353
28. Kalimo K, Jansen C (1986) Severe solar urticaria: active and passive action spectra and hyposensitizing effect of different UV modalities. Photodermatology 3:194–195
29. Larkö O, Diffey BL (1983) Natural UV-B radiation received by people with outdoor, indoor, and mixed occupations and UV-B treatment of psoriasis. Clin Exp Dermatol 8:279–285
30. Leenutaphong V (1991) Hydroa vacciniforme: an unusual clinical manifestation. J Am Acad Dermatol 25:892–895
31. Leenutaphong V, Hölzle E, Plewig G (1990) Solar urticaria: studies on mechanisms of tolerance. Br J Dermatol 122:601–606
32. Leonard F, Morel M, Kalis B, Amblard P, Avenel-Audran M, Beani JC, Bonnetblanc JM, Leroy D, Marguery MC, Peyron JL, Rouchouze B, Thomas P (1991) Psoralen plus ultraviolet A in the prophylactic treatment of benign summer light eruption. Photodermatol Photoimmunol Photomed 8:95–98
33. Machet L, Vaillant L, Muller C, Henin P, Brive D, Lorette G (1991) Traitement par UVB thérapie d'une urticaire solaire induite par les UVA. Ann Dermatol Venereol 118:535–537

34. Morison WL, White HAD, Gonzalez E, Parrish JA, Fitzpatrick TB (1979) Oral methoxsalen photochemotherapy of uncommon photodermatoses. Acta Derm Venereol (Stockh) 59:366–368
35. Morison WL, Momtaz K, Mosher DB, Parrish JA (1982) UV-B phototherapy in the prophylaxis of polymorphous light eruption. Br J Dermatol 106:231–233
36. Murphy GM, Logan RA, Lovell CR, Morris RW, Hawk JLM, Magnus IA (1987) Prophylactic PUVA and UVB therapy in polymorphic light eruption – a controlled trial. Br J Dermatol 116:531–538
37. Ortel B, Tanew A, Wolff K, Hönigsmann H (1986) Polymorphous light eruption: action spectrum and photoprotection. J Am Acad Dermatol 14:748–753
38. Parrish JA, Le Vine MJ, Morison WL, Gonzalez E, Fitzpatrick TB (1979) Comparison of PUVA and beta-carotene in the treatment of polymorphous light eruption. Br J Dermatol 100:187–191
39. Parrish JA, Jaenicke KF, Morison WL, Momtaz K, Shea C (1982) Solar urticaria: treatment with PUVA and mediator inhibitors. Br J Dermatol 106:575–580
40. Plewig G, Hölzle E, Lehmann P (1986) Phototherapy for photodermatoses. Curr Probl Dermatol 15:254–264
41. Ramsay CA (1977) Solar urticaria treatment by inducing tolerance to artificial radiation and natural light. Arch Dermatol 113:1222–1225
42. Reinauer S, Leenutaphong V, Hölzle E (1993) Fixed solar urticaria. J Am Acad Dermatol 29:161–165
43. Roelandts R (1985) Pre-PUVA UVA desensitization for solar urticaria. Photodermatology 2:174–176
44. Ryckaert S, Roelandts R (1998) Solar urticaria. A report of 25 cases and difficulties in phototesting. Arch Dermatol 134:71–74
45. Sonnex TS, Hawk JLM (1988) Hydroa vacciniforme: a review of ten cases. Br J Dermatol 118:101–108
46. Stern RS, Laird N (1994) The carcinogenic risk of treatments for severe psoriasis. Cancer 73:2759–2764
47. Studniberg HM, Weller P (1993) PUVA, UVB, psoriasis, and nonmelanoma skin cancer. J Am Acad Dermatol 29:1013–1022
48. Toonstra J, Henquet CJM, van Weelden H, van der Putten SCJ, van Vloten WA (1989) Actinic reticuloid: a clinical, photobiologic, histopathologic, and follow-up study of 16 patients. J Am Acad Dermatol 21:205–214
49. Young AR (1995) Carcinogenicity of UVB assessed. Lancet 345:1431–1432

6 Photo(chemo)therapy for Cutaneous T-Cell Lymphoma

Herbert Hönigsmann, Adrian Tanew, Paul R. Bergstresser

Contents

Cutaneous T-cell lymphoma (CTCL) encompasses a heterogeneous group of non-Hodgkin lymphomas that present primarily with cutaneous involvement [1, 2]. Quite commonly, the term CTCL is used to refer only to mycosis fungoides (MF), which is the most common form within this group, and to its rare leukemic variant, the Sézary syndrome (SS). Both are low-grade malignant T-helper cell lymphomas. So far phototherapy and photochemotherapy are the established treatment options for only the MF and SS type of CTCL. Therefore this chapter will focus on the treatment of these two disorders.

Mycosis fungoides usually runs a protracted course after presenting initially as erythematous or eczematous patches and plaques of the skin. Eventually these lesions may progress to become tumors and then ulcers, and the disease may disseminate to lymph nodes and internal organs, accompanied by a poor prognosis. The Sézary syndrome is the leukemic variant of MF, and it presents as erythroderma with generalized lymphadenopathy and circulating atypical T lymphocytes having large hyperconvoluted nuclei (Sézary cells). In its most severe form, Sézary syndrome manifests with leonine facies, hyperkeratosis and fissuring of the palms and soles, and severe pruritus. Histopathologically, mycosis fungoides and Sézary syndrome are characterized by infiltration of the skin with small T lymphocytes with cerebriform nuclei displaying the T-helper phenotype (CD4$^+$). Once the diagnosis is made, patients are staged according to the TNM system, which is based on the type and extent of skin lesions and on the presence or absence of involvement of lymph nodes, blood, and internal organs

[3, 4]. The natural course of MF usually is divided according to the National Institute of Health (NIH) classification into an early disease stage (stage IA, IB, IIA) and an advanced disease stage (stage IIB, III, IV) [3, 4]. This distinction widely correlates with the response to phototherapy and photochemotherapy. Whereas early stages respond well and show long periods of remission, common experience indicates that the presence of tumors worsens the prognosis and that complete remission is exceptional and of short duration. Thus, besides its prognostic implications, staging of CTCL is essential to the development of therapeutic strategies for the individual patient.

Since in most patients with early stage MF the disease is confined to the skin, topical therapy including ultraviolet light (UVB and psoralen plus UVA), topical chemotherapy (mechlorethamine and carmustine), and electron beam alone may be sufficient.

There has been an ongoing debate for many years about whether aggressive treatment should be instituted as early as possible in the course of the disease to induce a permanent cure, or whether one should keep this option for advanced stages of CTCL. Ultimately, Kaye et al. [5], in a randomized trial, compared electron-beam therapy and chemotherapy with conservative topical therapy. Whereas complete response rates were significantly higher with early aggressive treatment, disease-free intervals and overall survival did not differ significantly between the two groups. Consequently, a conservative and stage-adjusted treatment approach, with increasing aggressiveness, is now widely accepted [6]. In addition to topical chemotherapy and the use of total-skin electron-beam therapy, in the last 25 years photochemotherapy and UVB phototherapy have become established as efficient and well-tolerated treatment modalities for patients with early stage CTCL.

UVB Phototherapy

It was common knowledge that MF lesions often occur in non-sun-exposed areas of the body, and that patients with early stage MF benefit from exposure to natural sunlight. For this reason, conventional UV lamps were long used for MF treatment before modern high-intensity lamps became available.

The introduction of oral photochemotherapy in 1974 [7] not only started a new era in dermatological therapy but also sparked interest in photobiological research in general. This, in turn, led to the development of high-intensity ultraviolet lamps, which greatly improved UVB phototherapy, making whole body treatment within reasonably short exposure times feasible. A first report on home ultraviolet phototherapy of early MF appeared in 1982 [8]; 31 patients with stage I MF were treated with fluorescent lamps (Westinghouse FS 40) emitting broadband ultraviolet radiation between 280 and 350 nm. Threshold erythemogenic doses were applied to patients every other day until clearing occurred, and thereafter alternate-day maintenance therapy was continued for several months. Of the patients, 61 % cleared completely after a median treatment period of 4 months, and another 23 % had responses of more than 50 %. In contrast to the apparent complete clinical responses, control skin biopsies from

18 patients revealed in all instances a mild residual lymphocytic infiltrate in the papillary dermis. Four patients with relatively short maintenance therapy (3–7 months) relapsed within a few months after discontinuation, whereas maintenance treatment over 1 year or longer provided prolonged remissions.

In a long-term follow-up, 74 % of the same patient cohort remained in complete remission after a median treatment period of 5 months [9]. Responses to phototherapy were better in patients with eczematous (patch) stage MF than in patients with the plaque stage, whereas the extent of skin involvement did not influence the outcome. After discontinuing maintenance treatment, 23 % of the patients stayed free of lesions for a median of more than 90 months.

With a similar treatment protocol, Ramsay et al. found complete clearing in 83 % of patients with early stage CTCL, after a median period of 5 months [10]. With prolonged maintenance therapy, the median duration of remission within the observation period was 22 months. Twenty percent of patients with complete responses had recurrences of their disease. The four patients with plaque disease did not respond to UVB treatment.

The proposed mechanisms of UVB phototherapy for CTCL include impairment of epidermal Langerhans' cell function and alterations in cytokine production and adhesion molecule expression by keratinocytes [11].

In conclusion, UVB phototherapy seems to be efficient in early eczematous (patch)-stage CTCL and may be performed as home treatment under physician's guidance. Prolonged maintenance exposure is necessary to prevent early relapses. In general, it can be stated that UVB phototherapy is a safe therapeutic option for stage I MF. The outcome appears to be determined rather by the depth of the malignant infiltrate than by the extent of body surface involvement. UVB treatment is not indicated in patients with plaque stage or more advanced stages of CTCL.

Practical Aspects of UVB Phototherapy

UVB phototherapy is easy to perform and does not require special precautions other than eye protection with UV-absorbing goggles. Treatment should be given in threshold erythemogenic doses at least thrice weekly. As starting dose 50 % of the minimal erythema dose is recommended; thereafter, gradual dose increments should be performed to induce and maintain faint erythema reactions. Once clearing is achieved, alternate-day treatments should be continued for several months.

Acute side effects of UVB treatment are few, and they occur primarily as mild overdose reactions or dryness of the skin. The risk of long-term side effects, such as skin cancer development, is presumably much lower than that which occurs with photochemotherapy (PUVA) (see below). On the other hand, UVB phototherapy is clearly less efficient than PUVA, and the duration of treatment in the clearing and maintenance phases is longer, and thus it requires higher patient compliance.

Whether patients would benefit from adding UVA, as is sometimes recommended, remains questionable, and narrowband UVB (311–313 nm radiation,

Philips TL-01 lamp) and broadband UVB therapy have not been compared in MF. Recently, a pilot study documented the efficacy of medium- to high-dose UVA-1 therapy in patients with stage IA and IB (Plettenberg et al. (1999) J Am Acad Dermatol 41:47–50)

Photochemotherapy (PUVA)

Gilchrest et al. in 1976 were the first to report the successful use of psoralen plus UVA (PUVA) photochemotherapy in treating CTCL [12]. Based on the known beneficial effects of sunlight on MF, these investigators hypothesized that PUVA treatment would be therapeutically effective. Nine patients with unsatisfactory responses to other treatments and histologically confirmed plaque-, tumor-stage, or the erythrodermic form of CTCL were subjected to photochemotherapy. Of these nine patients, four achieved complete remissions, and five experienced significant improvement. The effect of treatment was clearly shown by shielding one forearm from UVA exposure throughout the initial phase of treatment. Whereas complete clearing occurred in all other areas, the disease even worsened in the control arm, thus ruling out the possibility that spontaneous remission had occurred. The absence of a treatment response in the control arm also clearly indicated that the therapeutic effect of PUVA in CTCL was local rather than systemic.

This first trial was followed by numerous clinical, histopathological, and experimental studies (for references see [13, 14]) addressing the rates of initial response and average duration of remission in relation to the stage of CTCL, the efficacy of PUVA compared with other established treatment options, the efficacy of combination treatments, the mechanisms responsible for the therapeutic effects, and the risk of short- and long-term hazards.

Response Rates and Duration of Remission in Relation to CTCL Stage

Several studies on large patient cohorts have provided information on the response rates of initial PUVA treatment in relation to the disease stage [15–20]. Different treatment protocols, psoralen preparations, and light sources used in these studies may have contributed to some heterogeneity in the results. The percentage of patients who achieved complete remission during the first course of PUVA treatment was reported to be 75 % – 100 % for stage IA, 47 % – 100 % for stage IB, 67 % – 83 % for stage IIA, 40 % – 100 % for stage IIB, and 33 % – 100 % for stage III. Very few patients in stage IV have been treated with PUVA monotherapy because in this stage it is generally considered to be of palliative or adjunctive therapeutic value alone. Herrmann et al. [14] have summarized the outcome of five of these studies, comprising 244 patients. They have calculated the following average complete initial response rates: stage IA (90 %), stage IB (76 %), stage IIA (78 %), stage IIB (59 %), and stage III (61 %).

Of major relevance to predicting long-term outcome are data on relapse rates and mean disease-free intervals. In the first follow-up study of 44 PUVA-treated patients, 56 % (5/9) with stage IA disease and 39 % (10/26) with stage IB disease remained in remission during a mean follow-up period of 44 months [17]. Patients who experienced relapses had mean disease-free intervals of 20 months for stage IA and 17 months for stage IB. All patients (7/7) with stage IIB disease had multiple recurrences, and of the 2 patients with stage III disease, both of whom were initially brought into remission, one relapsed during maintenance therapy and one was lost from follow-up.

In a recent study of 82 patients who were followed over a median period of 43 months, 53 % (10/19) were in stage IA, 37 % (13/49) in stage IB, 50 % (3/6) in stage IIA, and the only one in stage IVA remained without recurrences after complete clearing. One stage IIB patient and two of six stage III patients were initially cleared; however, they all eventually relapsed [16].

In summary, published data thus far indicate that PUVA is an excellent treatment option for early stage (IA–IIA) CTCL because high rates of complete clearing can be achieved, and a substantial percentage of patients remains free of disease for many years. In advanced stages (IIB–IVB), PUVA is not sufficient as monotherapy, but as adjunctive treatment it can reduce the tumor burden in the skin and can increase the quality of life for patients.

Comparison with Other Established Treatment Methods

Other widely used treatments for CTCL include topical mechlorethamine (HN2), topical carmustine (BCNU), and total skin electron-beam radiation therapy (EBRT) [21–24]. Unfortunately, randomized trials that compare short-term efficacy, freedom-from-relapse periods, and survival rates of these modalities have not been performed. In an early non-randomized study on 42 patients, EBRT was found to be slightly more effective than HN2, but with considerably higher relapse rates [25]. Recently, retrospective analysis of a large patient cohort with stage IA disease showed EBRT to be superior to HN2 in rates of both complete clearing and freedom from relapse. However, no significant difference was observed in the 10-year survival rates [26]. When the results of PUVA therapy were compared with those of previous studies using HN2 and BCNU, no statistically significant differences in complete response rates or long-term survival were found for patients in stages IA and IB [16]. Due to the lack of comparable data, duration of remission could not be compared with HN2, but it was clearly better for PUVA than for BCNU in patients with stage IA and IB disease at 2 and 5 years.

Combination Treatments

Combination with Retinoids (RePUVA)

The effectiveness of retinoids in CTCL may be related to its immunomodulatory, antineoplastic, antiproliferative, and anti-inflammatory properties. In addition, reduced epidermal thickness of retinoid-treated skin may enhance UVA skin penetration.

A number of clinical studies have demonstrated benefit from the retinoid drugs in the treatment of MF and the Sézary syndrome [27–31]. When given as monotherapy, both isotretinoin and etretinate rarely cause durable remissions, and thus far their main use in CTCL is as an adjunctive agent to the more established treatments, such as systemic chemotherapy, interferons or photochemotherapy. The essential question, whether retinoids plus PUVA leads to better results than PUVA therapy alone, was addressed in an open study by the Scandinavian MF group in 69 patients with plaque stage mycosis fungoides. The combined administration of retinoids and PUVA did not yield higher response rates than PUVA alone, although the cumulative PUVA dose at the time of remission was significantly lower in patients receiving retinoids. However, maintenance treatment with retinoids seemed to prolong the duration of remission [32]. The combination of etretinate in a dose of 1.0–1.5 mg/kg with PUVA produced complete clearing in 80 % (32/40) of patients with MF (stages IB to IVA) and in 75 % (6/8) of patients with the Sézary syndrome [33]. Histopathological examination of biopsies from patients who had cleared clinically did, however, reveal the persistence of atypical lymphocytes in deeper layers of the dermis.

Combination with Interferon-α

The first report on the successful use of high-dose interferon (IFN)-α in patients with advanced refractory cutaneous T-cell lymphoma appeared in 1984 [34]. Since then, several clinical trials, mostly using IFN-α-2a, confirmed the validity of this therapeutic approach for all stages of CTCL. They provided data on efficacy, dose regimens, predictors of response, and side effects [35, 36]. Based on the promising results obtained with interferon monotherapy, it seemed logical to combine PUVA and interferon, with the aim of enhancing the efficacy of both regimens. In a phase I trial on 15 patients with CTCL (stages IB to IVB), Kuzel et al., using a thrice weekly combination of PUVA and IFN-α-2a ($6 - 30 \times 10^6$ IU), achieved complete remission in 80 % (12/15) and an overall (complete or partial) response rate of 93 % (14/15). In addition, the combined treatment provided for faster and more durable responses than were seen with either modality alone [37]. Upon recent reevaluation of their original patient cohort and 24 patients enrolled subsequently who had received IFN-α-2a up to a maximum dose of 12×10^6 IU/m^2 [38], the complete response rate was 62 % (24/39) and the overall response rate 90 % (35/39). The lower percentage of patients with complete responses in comparison to the initial trial was attributed to the enrollment of new patients who were, in part, at higher stages. The median duration of remission for complete responders was 60 months and that of partial responders, 13 months.

Less-favorable treatment results were found in 11 patients (1 stage IB, 2 stage IIA, 5 stage IIB, 2 stage III, 1 stage IVA) with PUVA 4 times weekly and IFN-α-2a in an initial dosage of 9×10^6 IU 3 times weekly [39]. Complete clearing was achieved in 45 % (5/11) and partial clearing (improvement of 50 %) in 55 % (6/11) of the patients, respectively. Three patients relapsed within a mean follow-up period of 7.5 months. In another study, PUVA plus low-dose IFN-α ($3–6 \times 10^6$ IU/ day) resulted in complete remissions for 5 patients who were previously refractory to PUVA monotherapy and it also reduced the cumulative UVA dose required for clearing [40].

The efficacy of IFN-α (9×10^6 IU thrice weekly) plus PUVA (2–5 times weekly) compared with IFN-α (9×10^6 IU thrice weekly) plus acitretin (0.5 mg/ kg body weight/day) was investigated in a recent randomized multicenter trial [41]. Forty patients (30 stage I, 10 stage II) receiving IFN-α and PUVA and 38 patients (30 stage I, 8 stage II) receiving IFN-α and acitretin were evaluated. Complete response was found in 83 % (25/30) of stage I patients and 20 % (2/10) of stage II patients with IFN-α plus PUVA versus 53 % (16/30) of stage I patients and 0 % (0/8) of stage II patients with IFN-α plus acitretin. The median duration until complete response was 21 weeks in patients receiving IFN-α plus PUVA and 62 weeks in patients receiving IFN-α plus acitretin. Treatment had to be discontinued because of severe side effects in 8 patients receiving IFN-α plus acitretin but in only 2 patients on IFN-α plus PUVA [41].

An important aspect is the fact that patients can develop anti-interferon antibodies during IFN-α treatment, which can impair the treatment response. Suppression of anti-IFN-α antibody formation by PUVA treatment in patients with MF has been reported [42]. In a recent study, the occurrence of neutralizing IFN-α antibodies was again found to be significantly lower in patients receiving PUVA; however, an even higher than expected incidence of clinically relevant binding IFN-α antibodies was detected [43]. Consequently, patients treated with a combination of IFN-α and PUVA should be monitored regularly for IFN-α antibodies.

Practical Aspects of Photochemotherapy

Before initiating therapy, a thorough clinical and histopathological examination, including immunophenotyping and application of molecular biological techniques, is required, and the patient must be staged according to the TNM classification. In patients with stage IA–IIA disease, we usually start with PUVA monotherapy, which most often induces complete and durable remissions within an acceptable time. PUVA alone has the advantage of a lower toxicity profile compared with combination regimens. With the treatment protocol detailed below, an average of 20–30 exposures and a cumulative UVA dose of 50–150 J/cm^2 are required for clearing. Combination treatment is used in patients who are slow or incomplete responders to PUVA monotherapy or who relapse during or soon after discontinuation of maintenance therapy. In patients with advanced stages (IIB–IV), we recommend PUVA as an adjunctive treatment in combination with ionizing radiation, systemic chemotherapy, or for patients with Sézary syndrome, extracorporeal photopheresis.

Photochemotherapy of CTCL generally is performed according to the same guidelines as in psoriasis (see Chap. 3, this volume). Most investigations have used 8-methoxypsoralen because 5-methoxypsoralen is not widely available, in particular, not in the United States. Trioxsalen and 8-methoxypsoralen bath-PUVA treatment for CTCL is performed in Scandinavia. Bath PUVA may not be ideal because the face and the scalp can hardly be treated adequately, and new lesions can occur in these areas during treatment. Both 8- and 5-methoxypsoralen are suitable photosensitizers, and they appear to give comparable results, provided that adequate doses of UVA radiation are employed. 5-Methoxypsoralen causes fewer adverse reactions and is less phototoxic than 8-methoxypsoralen, but considerably higher UVA doses are required [44]. It appears advisable to use 5-methoxypsoralen primarily in patients who have 8-methoxypsoralen intolerance or to facilitate dosimetry in patients with pronounced photosensitivity.

There are no comparative data to provide meaningful conclusions about whether the United States or European PUVA protocol is superior for patients with CTCL. In psoriasis the more aggressive European approach has been shown to result in faster clearing of the disease, with lower a cumulative UVA dose [45]. The major differences between the two treatment protocols concern the determination of a patient's sensitivity to PUVA and the choice of an initial UVA irradiation dose, subsequent dose increments, treatment frequency in the clearing and maintenance phases of treatment, and the duration of maintenance treatment (for details see Chap. 3, this volume).

The United States treatment protocol employs a starting dose that is based on the patient's skin type and the degree of pigmentation before therapy, and it usually ranges between 1.5 and 3 J/cm^2 [46]. Treatment is given 2–3 times weekly with UVA dose increments of 0.5 J/cm^2 or more, depending on the presence of erythema. When complete remission is achieved clinically and confirmed histologically, maintenance treatment is initiated, with decreasing frequency down to one monthly exposure over several months or indefinitely.

In the European protocol, before treatment, each patient's sensitivity to PUVA is determined by MPD (minimal phototoxicity dose) testing after administering the photosensitizer [47]. The MPD, or a dose just below the MPD, is then taken as the starting dose. Exposure is 4 times weekly, and the dose is adjusted regularly to maintain a faint erythema reaction in each patient's skin. As with the United States protocol, biopsies from previously involved skin sites are taken after complete clearing to exclude a persisting malignant infiltrate in the deeper dermis [48]. There is no clear answer to the question of how to proceed if there is no remaining clinical evidence of disease, but histologically some dermal infiltrates are present. We recommend in such cases to start with maintenance treatment. This is given twice weekly for 1 month and once weekly for another month. In this phase of treatment the UVA dose is usually kept constant. If a patient remains free from disease after 2 months of maintenance, treatment is discontinued. If relapse occurs, the initial treatment frequency of four exposures per week is resumed and the UVA dose is increased if erythema is no longer apparent. So far, no information is available on the optimal length of maintenance therapy or if maintenance therapy does indeed prolong survival.

Cautious dosimetry is warranted in patients with CTCL because quite often their thresholds for erythema is unusually low [48, 49]. When pronounced photosensitivity is evident by MPD testing, a short concomitant course of systemic corticosteroids (prednisolone) may enable patients to tolerate PUVA treatment, without developing severe phototoxic reactions [50]. Increased photosensitivity is also a commonly recognized side effect of IFN-α administration [37, 39].

Another specific finding in the initial phase of PUVA treatment is the appearance of previously invisible subclinical lesions in some patients. It is for this reason that patients with only a few lesions should also receive whole body exposure and that bath-PUVA may not be sufficient. Special attention and care is required to expose evenly all body sites to the UVA radiation including the intertriginous areas. Otherwise, clearing in light-shielded regions, such as the groin and axillae, will be retarded or incomplete [51]. Regions not accessible to UVA radiation, such as the hairy scalp or the interdigital areas, require additional treatment, such as topical mechlorethamine or ionizing radiation. It is reasonable to keep a record of patients' cumulative irradiation doses and to consider combination or rotational therapies when the total UVA dose exceeds 1,000 J/cm^2. However, long-term side effects related to the cumulative UVA dose may be regarded less important in the treatment of a malignant disease, in particular, as other treatment options such as mechlorethamine or ionizing radiation are also known carcinogens.

Regular follow-up examinations are mandatory for all patients, and they should include a careful clinical evaluation for the development of cutaneous malignancies. Suspicious lesions must be removed without delay and examined histologically.

The Action Mechanisms of PUVA in Mycosis Fungoides

The mechanisms by which PUVA induces clearing of the malignant T-cell infiltrate from skin are still under investigation. PUVA affects a variety of different targets in skin, and it is likely that the concerted interaction of several PUVA-induced cellular alterations is responsible for this therapeutic effect. The cytotoxic effect that PUVA exerts on infiltrating T cells in the epidermis and superficial dermis is within this context. The recent observation that PUVA selectively eliminates T-lymphocyte populations by induction of apoptosis indicates that this effect may play a major role [52]. PUVA may also act by interfering with epidermal cytokine production and by directly downregulating homing receptors on epidermotropic malignant T cells. Finally, PUVA treatment causes a functional impairment of CDla$^+$ Langerhans' cells, which are thought to be involved in the pathogenesis of CTCL by perpetuating the epidermal affinity of infiltrating T cells [11].

Short-Term and Long-Term Hazards Associated with Photochemotherapy

The range of acute side effects of PUVA in patients with CTCL is, in principle, the same as in patients with other PUVA-responsive diseases (such as psoriasis). The most frequent acute adverse reaction is phototoxicity that presents as painful erythema, edema, and occasional blister formation. In contrast to lesional skin in psoriasis, in which hyperkeratosis and epidermal thickening may decrease the penetration of UVA radiation, increased phototoxicity can be occasionally observed in plaques and tumors of MF, sometimes leading to erosions and superficial ulcerations. The emergence of previously invisible erythematous and eczematoid lesions of MF is not uncommon during the first treatments and must not be attributed to UVA overdose [53]. Other side effects include pruritus, intolerance reactions to 8-methoxypsoralen such as nausea or dizziness and, rarely, disseminated eruptions of herpes simplex.

The most serious concern with respect to long-term hazards of PUVA treatment relates to the development of cutaneous malignancies. It is now widely accepted from numerous follow-up studies of patients with psoriasis that PUVA may act as complete carcinogen and that it is associated with a dose-dependent increased risk for squamous cell carcinomas and keratoacanthomas [54–56]. Higher than expected rates of non-melanoma skin cancer and anecdotal cases of metastatic squamous cell carcinomas have also been reported in PUVA-treated CTCL patients; however, all of these patients had also received other carcinogenic treatments, including ionizing radiation, topical nitrogen mustard, or systemic chemotherapy [57, 58]. In the long-term follow-up study by Herrmann et al. [16]), 10 % of patients showed chronic actinic damage, with PUVA-induced lentigines and actinic keratoses, and 3 of 82 patients (3.7 %) had developed squamous cell carcinomas. Most of these chronic changes occurred in patients who had been receiving PUVA for more than 10 years with cumulative UVA doses of more than 2,000 J/cm^2 [16].

Taken together, there is clear evidence that the combined or sequential use of different therapies for CTCL may increase synergistically the risk of squamous cell carcinomas, whereas it is currently impossible to accurately estimate the risk for CTCL patients having been treated with PUVA monotherapy. More information on long-term risks of PUVA is provided in Chap. 3 (this volume). Certainly, the impact of this risk has to be balanced against the therapeutic benefit, but as stated above, this may be meaningless in a potentially life-threatening disease such as CTCL as opposed to psoriasis.

Perspectives

Several issues remain to be answered by future controlled studies. The most important question is whether photochemotherapy, given either alone or in combination with other treatments, has the capacity to induce a permanent remission or even cure in patients with early stage disease. In Sweden, the death rate in MF has dropped significantly since the introduction of PUVA treatment, towards the end of the 1970s. According to the death statistics of dermatological diseases of the Swedish National Central Bureau of Statistics in Stockholm, it seems probable that PUVA is the reason for this decrease of the death rate [59]. More data are also needed to delineate the optimal PUVA treatment protocol for CTCL, which should provide for maximum efficacy with lowest UVA dose requirements. In this regard, the refinement of combination therapies will certainly result in major improvements. Finally, with increasing understanding of the immunopathogenetic events leading to CTCL, markers for therapeutic responses will eventually be identified and help to individualize therapeutic strategies.

References

1. Koh HK, Charif M, Weinstock MA (1995) Epidemiology and clinical manifestations of cutaneous T-cell lymphoma. Hematol Oncol Clin North Am 9:943–960
2. Willemze R, Beijaards RC, Meijer CJLM (1994) Classification of primary cutaneous T-cell lymphomas. Histopathology 24:405–415
3. Bunn PA Jr, Lamberg SI (1979) Report of the committee on staging and classification of cutaneous T-cell lymphomas. Cancer Treat Rep 63:725–728
4. Lamberg SI, Green SB, Byar DP et al (1984) Clinical staging for cutaneous T-cell lymphoma. Ann Intern Med 100:187–192
5. Kaye FJ, Bunn PA Jr, Steinberg S et al (1989) A randomized trial comparing combination electron-beam radiation and chemotherapy with topical therapy in the initial treatment of mycosis fungoides. N Engl J Med 321:1784–1790
6. Jörg B, Kerl H, Thiers BH, Bröcker EB, Burg G (1994) Therapeutic approaches in cutaneous lymphoma. Dermatol Clin 12:433–441
7. Parrish JA, Fitzpatrick TB, Tanenbaum L, Pathak MA (1974) Photochemotherapy of psoriasis with oral methoxsalen and longwave ultraviolet light. N Engl J Med 291:1207–1211
8. Milstein HI, Vonderheid EC, Van Scott EJ, Johnson WC (1982) Home ultraviolet phototherapy of early mycosis fungoides: Preliminary observations. J Am Acad Dermatol 6:355–362
9. Resnik KS, Vonderheid EC (1993) Home UV phototherapy of early mycosis fungoides: long-term follow-up observations in thirty-one patients. J Am Acad Dermatol 29:73–77
10. Ramsay DL, Lish KM, Yalowitz CB, Soter NA (1992) Ultraviolet-B phototherapy for early-stage cutaneous T-cell lymphoma. Arch Dermatol 128:931–933
11. Volc-Platzer B, Hönigsmann H (1995) Photoimmunology of PUVA and UVB therapy. In: Krutmann J, Elmets CA (ed) Photoimmunology. Blackwell Science, Oxford, pp 265–273
12. Gilchrest BA, Parrish JA, Tanenbaum L, Haynes HA, Fitzpatrick TB (1976) Oral methoxsalen photochemotherapy of mycosis fungoides. Cancer 38:683–689
13. Hönigsmann H, Szeimies RF, Knobler R, Fitzpatrick TB, Pathak MA, Wolff K (l999) Photochemotherapy and photodynamic therapy. In: Freedberg IM, Eisen AZ, Wolff K, Austen KF, Goldsmith LA, Katz SI, Fitzpatrick TB (eds) Fitzpatrick's dermatology in general medicine, 5th edn. McGraw-Hill, New York, pp 2880–2900
14. Herrmann Jr, Roenigk HH Jr, Hönigsmann H (1995) Ultraviolet radiation for treatment of cutaneous T-cell lymphoma. Hematol Oncol Clin North Am 9:1077–1088
15. Abel EA, Sendagorta E, Hoppe RT, Hu CH (1987) PUVA treatment of erythrodermic and plaque-type mycosis fungoides. Arch Dermatol 123:897–901
16. Herrmann Jr, Roenigk HH Jr, Hurria A et al (1995) Treatment of mycosis fungoides with photochemotherapy (PUVA): long-term follow-up. J Am Acad Dermatol 33:234–242
17. Hönigsmann H, Brenner W, Rauschmeier W, Konrad K, Wolff K (1984) Photochemotherapy for cutaneous T cell lymphoma. J Am Acad Dermatol 10:238–245
18. Powell FC, Spiegel GT, Muller SA (1984) Treatment of parapsoriasis and mycosis fungoides: the role of psoralen and long-wave ultraviolet light A (PUVA). Mayo Clin Proc 59:538–546
19. Rosenbaum MM, Roenigk HH Jr, Caro WA, Esker A (1985) Photochemotherapy in cutaneous T cell lymphoma and parapsoriasis en plaque. J Am Acad Dermatol 13:613–622
20. Vella Briffa D, Warin AP, Harrington CI, Bleehen SS (1980) Photochemotherapy in mycosis fungoides. Lancet 2:49–53
21. Holloway KB, Flowers FP, Ramos-Caro FA (1992) Therapeutic alternatives in cutaneous T-cell lymphoma. J Am Acad Dermatol 27:367–378

22. Hoppe R (1991) The management of mycosis fungoides at Stanford – standard and innovative treatment programs. Leukemia 5 [Suppl 1]:46–48

23. Vonderheid EC, Tan ET, Kantor AF, Shrager L, Micaily B, van Scott EJ (1989) Long-term efficacy, curative potential, and carcinogenicity of topical mechlorethamine chemotherapy in cutaneous T cell lymphoma. J Am Acad Dermatol 20:416–428

24. Zackheim HS, Epstein EH Jr, Crain WR (1990) Topical carmustine (BCNU) for cutaneous T cell lymphoma: a 15-year experience in 143 patients. J Am Acad Dermatol 22:802–810

25. Hamminga B, Noordijk EM, van Vloten WA (1982) Treatment of mycosis fungoides. Total-skin electron-beam irradiation vs topical mechlorethamine therapy. Arch Dermatol 118:150–153

26. Kim YH, Jensen RA, Watanabe GL, Varghese A, Hoppe RT (1996) Clinical stage la (limited patch and plaque) mycosis fungoides. A long-term outcome analysis. Arch Dermatol 132:1309–1313

27. Claudy AL, Rouchouse B (1985) Treatment of cutaneous T cell lymphoma with retinoids. In: Saurat JH (ed) Retinoids: new trends in research and therapy. Retinoid symposium, Geneva 1984. Karger, Basel, pp 335–340

28. Kessler JF, Jones SE, Levine N, Lynch PJ, Rohman Both A, Meyskens L Jr (1987) Isotretinoin and cutaneous helper T cell lymphoma (mycosis fungoides). Arch Dermatol 123:201–204

29. Mahrle G, Thiele B (1987) Retinoids in cutaneous T cell lymphomas. Dermatologica 175 [Suppl 1]:145–150

30. Molin L, Thomsen K, Volden G et al (1987) Oral retinoids in mycosis fungoides and Sézary syndrome: a comparison of isotretinoin and etretinate. Acta Derm Venereol (Stockh) 67:232–236

31. Thomsen K, Molin L, Volden G, Lange Wantzin G, Hellbe L (1984) 13-cis-retinoic acid effective in mycosis fungoides. Acta Derm Venereol (Stockh) 64:563–566

32. Thomsen K, Hammar H, Molin L, Volden G (1989) Retinoids plus PUVA (RePUVA) and PUVA in mycosis fungoides, plaque stage. Acta Derm Venereol (Stockh) 69:536–538

33. Serri F, De Simone C, Venier A, Rusciani L, Marchetti E (1990) Combination of retinoids and PUVA (Re-PUVA) in the treatment of cutaneous T-cell lymphomas. Curr Probl Dermatol 19:252–257

34. Bunn PA Jr, Foon KA, Ihde DC et al (1984) Recombinant leukocyte A interferon: An active agent in advanced cutaneous T-cell lymphomas. Ann Intern Med 101:484–487

35. Olsen EA, Bunn PA (1995) Interferon in the treatment of cutaneous T-cell lymphoma. Hematol Oncol Clin North Am 9:1089–1107

36. Thestrup-Pedersen K (1990) Interferon therapy in cutaneous T-cell lymphoma. Curr Probl Dermatol 19:258–263

37. Kuzel TM, Gilyon K, Springer E et al (1990) Interferon alfa-2a combined with phototherapy in the treatment of cutaneous T-cell lymphoma. J Natl Cancer Inst 82:203–207

38. Kuzel TM, Roenigk HH Jr, Samuelson E et al (1995) Effectiveness of interferon alfa-2a combined with phototherapy for mycosis fungoides and the Seizure syndrome. J Clin Oncol 13:257–263

39. Otte HG, Herges A, Stadler R (1992) Kombinationstherapie mit Interferon α2a und PUVA bei kutanen T-Zell-Lymphomen. Hautarzt 43:695–699

40. Mostow EN, Neckel SL, Oberhelman L, Anderson TF, Cooper KD (1993) Complete remissions in psoralen and UVA (PUVA)-refractory mycosis fungoides-type cutaneous T-cell lymphoma with combined interferon alfa and PUVA. Arch Dermatol 129:747–752

41. Stadler R, Otte HG, Luger T, Henz BM, Kuhl P, Zwingers T, Sterry W (1998) Prospective randomized multicenter clinical trial on the use of interferon – 2α plus acitretin versus interferon – 2α plus PUVA in patients with cutaneous T-cell lymphoma stages I and II. Blood 92:3578–3581

42. Kuzel TM, Roenigk HH Jr, Samuelson E, Rosen ST (1992) Suppression of anti-interferon α-2a antibody formation in patients with mycosis fungoides by exposure to longwave UV radiation in the A range and methoxsalen ingestion. J Natl Cancer Inst 84:119–121
43. Rajan GP, Seifert B, Prümmer O, Joller-Jemelka HI, Burg G, Dummer R (1996) Incidence and *in-vivo* relevance of antiinterferon antibodies during treatment of low-grade cutaneous T-cell lymphomas with interferon alpha-2a combined with acitretin or PUVA. Arch Dermatol Res 288:543–548
44. Tanew A, Ortel B, Rappersberger K, Hönigsmann H (1988) 5-Methoxypsoralen (Bergapten) for photochemotherapy. J Am Acad Dermatol 18:333–339
45. Henseler T, Wolff K, Hönigsmann H, Christophers E (1981) Oral 8-methoxypsoralen photochemotherapy of psoriasis. Lancet i:853–857
46. Roenigk HH Jr (1977) Photochemotherapy for mycosis fungoides. Arch Dermatol 113:1047–1051
47. Wolff K, Gschnait F, Hönigsmann H, Konrad K, Parrish JA, Fitzpatrick TB (1977) Phototesting and dosimetry for photochemotherapy. Br J Dermatol 96:1–10
48. Lowe NJ, Cripps DJ, Dufton PA, Vickers CFH (1979) Photochemotherapy for mycosis fungoides. A clinical and histological study. Arch Dermatol 115:50–53
49. Volden G, Thune PO (1977) Light sensitivity in mycosis fungoides. Br J Dermatol 97:279–284
50. Molin L, Volden G (1987) Treatment of light-sensitive mycosis fungoides with PUVA and prednisolone. Photodermatol Photoimmunol Photomed 4:106–107
51. Du Vivier A, Vollum DI (1980) Photochemotherapy and topical nitrogen mustard in the treatment of mycosis fungoides. Br J Dermatol 102:319–322
52. Johnson R, Staiano-Coico L, Austin L, Cardinale I, Nabeya-Tsukifuji, Krueger JG (1996) PUVA treatment selectively induces a cell cycle block and subsequent apoptosis in human T-lymphocytes. Photochem Photobiol 63:566–571
53. Hönigsmann H, Tanew A, Wolff K (1987) Treatment of mycosis fungoides with PUVA. Photodermatol Photoimmunol Photomed 4:55–58
54. Maier H, Schemper M, Ortel B, Binder M, Tanew A, Hönigsmann H (1996) Skin tumors in photochemotherapy for psoriasis. A single center follow-up of 496 patients. Dermatology 193:185–191
55. Stern RS, Laird N (1994) The carcinogenic risk of treatments for severe psoriasis. Cancer 73: 2759–2764
56. Studniberg HM, Weller P (1993) PUVA, UVB, psoriasis, and nonmelanoma skin cancer. J Am Acad Dermatol 29:1013–102
57. Abel EA, Sendagorta E, Hoppe RT (1986) Cutaneous malignancies and metastatic squamous cell carcinoma following topical therapies for mycosis fungoides. J Am Acad Dermatol 14:1029–1038
58. Smoller BR, Marcus R (1994) Risk of secondary cutaneous malignancies in patients with long-standing mycosis fungoides. J Am Acad Dermatol 30:201–204
59. Swanbeck G, Roupe G, Sandström MH (1994) Indications of a considerable decrease in the death rate in mycosis fungoides by PUVA treatment. Acta Derm Venereol (Stockh)74:465–466

7 Phototherapeutic Options for Vitiligo

Bernhard Ortel, Claudia Alge, Amit Pandy

Contents

Introduction

Ultraviolet radiation-based therapies of vitiligo are the most potent options for its treatment. This chapter shall provide detailed information about the role and application of phototherapeutic regimens. Initially, the disease will be defined and compared to other conditions in the differential diagnosis. The main portion of this chapter will concentrate on ultraviolet phototherapy and photochemotherapy. Adjunctive and combined therapeutic modalities are discussed, as well as alternative treatment options.

Diagnosis

Vitiligo is an acquired pigmentary disorder, clinically characterized by the development of white macules, which are caused by the destruction of melanocytes in the affected skin [44, 48]. The prevalence of the disease in the United States and in Europe has been estimated at around 1%. A predominance of women has been suggested, but this observation may well reflect a greater willingness of women in many cultures to express concern about cosmetic problems. Half of all patients develop the disease before the age of 20. Onset at an old age occurs but is unusual, and should raise concern about underlying disorders or associated diseases. Generalized vitiligo is the most common clinical presentation and commonly involves the face and acral areas. Depigmentation in these very visible areas leads to cosmetic disfigurement and may be a source of severe psychological distress for the patient.

Clinical Features

The primary lesion is a white, sharply defined macule with convex margins. In individuals with fair skin, it may be difficult to distinguish between hypopigmentation and the complete absence of melanin (leukoderma) as seen in vitiligo. The use of a Wood's lamp (see "Differential Diagnosis") helps to distinguish hypopigmented from depigmented macules. Wood's light examination is also useful in viewing sun-protected areas of individuals with darker complexion where the skin is less tanned. Occasionally, vitiligo lesions display an elevated, erythematous margin, which may be pruritic. These changes are features of inflammatory infiltration [8]. Another rare presentation of the disease is trichrome vitiligo, named after three shades of pigmentation, representing normal skin, partial depigmentation, and complete pigment loss [37]. The hair within vitiligo patches may remain normally pigmented, but in older lesions the hair is often amelanotic (leukotrichia) [36].

Distribution

Depigmentation occurs in three different patterns. (1) Generalized vitiligo is the most common type, showing widespread depigmentation in a remarkably symmetrical distribution. The macules develop over the extensor surfaces of joints and bony prominences, on the face (especially in periorificial areas such as around the mouth and eyes), neck, anogenital region, and the acral areas of the extremities. (2) Segmental vitiligo is characterized by distribution in an asymmetric, dermatomal distribution. (3) Focal vitiligo represents localized lesions in a non-dermatomal arrangement.

Course and Prognosis

Vitiligo is a chronic disorder and its course is unpredictable. Most often, depigmentation is a gradually progressive process, but in generalized vitiligo, patients may report a sudden onset with rapid spread of vitiligo over a period of a few months [59]. Subsequently, the disease may remain quiescent for many years. Up to 30 % of the patients report "spontaneous" repigmentation, which appears in perifollicular and marginal areas of sun-exposed lesions during the summer months. Complete sunlight-induced repigmentation is extremely rare. Independently of the initial course of the disease, vitiligo may come to a halt and remain stable for decades. Focal and segmental vitiligo usually do not extend beyond their initial regional distribution, and once the expansion stops, they tend to be quite stable. Segmental vitiligo can also occur as a distinctive part of generalized disease and may precede its onset.

Differential Diagnosis

Several dermatoses result in a decrease or loss of melanin pigmentation of the epidermis [61, 97]. Therefore, the first and most important step toward treatment of vitiligo is to confirm the diagnosis. Some dermatoses that resemble vitiligo are easy to treat (e.g., tinea versicolor), while some require definite treatment (e.g., leprosy), and others do not respond to standard treatment of vitiligo (e.g., piebaldism). Examination with ultraviolet A (UVA) radiation (320 – 400 nm, e.g., a Wood's light or black light) facilitates distinction between hypopigmentation and depigmentation. It has been claimed that the fluorescence of pathologically increased biopterin metabolites accentuates the difference between normal and vitiliginous skin under UVA illumination [80]. Careful inspection of the anogenital region is helpful for confirming the diagnosis of generalized vitiligo. This area shows constitutive hyperpigmentation and is usually involved in generalized vitiligo. Dopa staining of a biopsy from the border of a lesion can demonstrate the absence of tyrosinase-positive melanocytes in the affected skin.

Table 1 provides a list of differential diagnoses. The most important clinical criteria for a diagnosis of generalized vitiligo are symmetrical, acral, and periorificial distribution of progressive lesions. Congenital forms of leukoderma and hypomelanoses often display a typical distribution pattern (e.g., piebaldism) and their lesions are stable. However, they need not be apparent at birth. Postinflammatory hypopigmentation is frequently seen in patients with dark complexion following flares of atopic eczema, lupus erythematosus, or psoriasis, with lesions showing irregular mottling of hyperpigmented and hypopig-

Table 1. Differential diagnosis of vitiligo

Chemically induced leukoderma
Tinea versicolor
Piebaldism
Waardenburg syndrome
Vogt-Koyanagi-Harada syndrome
Tuberous sclerosis
Postinflammatory hypopigmentation
(e.g., psoriasis, lupus erythematosus, atopic dermatitis)
Incontinentia pigmenti achromians
Postinfectous hypopigmentation
(e.g. leprosy, syphilis, leishmaniasis)
Idiopathic guttate hypomelanosis
Nevus depigmentosus
Nevus anemicus

mented areas. It is important to rule out hypopigmentation that is caused by
leprosy, as the anesthetic macules of leprosy can mimic vitiligo. Leprosy is
mostly prevalent in hot and humid climates. Within the U.S. it is endemic in
Texas, southern Louisiana, Hawaii, and California. Patients with leprosy may be
encountered in areas with large numbers of immigrants from endemic areas of
the world. Post-syphilitic leukoderma has become rare but must be included in
the diagnostic considerations. Probably the most common infectious cause of
hypopigmentation is Malassezia furfur, the organism that causes tinea versicolor. It is important to rule out chemically induced leukoderma to help avoid further exposure to the causative agent (such as phenol and its derivatives). Due to
the great similarities between vitiligo and chemical leukoderma, it may be very
difficult or impossible to distinguish between these two.

Associated Findings

Vitiligo can be associated with a number of phenomena. Some are diagnosti-
cally important while others give important clues regarding pathogenesis. There
are reports of familial aggregation and approximately 20 % of people with vitiligo have at least one first-degree relative also afflicted with vitiligo [54]. Vitiliginous lesions can develop at sites subjected to trauma, an effect known as
Koebner's phenomenon [56]. A typical feature is the onset or exacerbation of
vitiligo following the specific trauma of severe sunburn. Vitiligo may be associated with autoimmune diseases in the patients or their relatives, and it has been
suggested that this association is stronger for childhood onset [32]. However,
autoantibodies (e.g., directed against thyroid antigens, mitochondria, parietal
cells of the gastric mucous membranes, etc.) can also be present without clinical
relevance. Therefore, the diagnostic impact of autoantibodies alone in vitiligo is
very limited [79]. Table 2 shows disorders that have been frequently found in
association with vitiligo. Although the majority of patients will turn out to be

Table 2. Disorders associated with vitiligo

Thyroid disease[a]
Diabetes mellitus type I[a]
Pernicious anemia[a]
Myasthenia gravis[a]
Addison's disease[a]
Hypoparathyroidism[a]
Alopecia areata
Lichen simplex
Morphea
Melanoma[a]
Halo nevus[a]

[a] Specific autoantibodies may be detected.

otherwise healthy, initial examination should include careful evaluation of the patient's history and of clinical signs of potentially associated autoimmune diseases. In the absence of clinical findings, extensive serological screening is not necessary. New data even suggest that vitiligo is not truly associated with autoimmune endocrine disorders [60].

Depigmented areas in the pigment epithelium of the retina and the choroid occur in up to 40 % of patients [5]. Moreover, the incidence of uveitis in vitiligo patients is elevated; therefore, ophthalmologic evaluation is warranted [62]. Melanocytic nevi surrounded by a concentric ring of depigmentation, known as halo nevi, may herald the onset of vitiligo, but can be an isolated finding as well.

The simultaneous presentation of vitiligo and melanoma might be caused by an autoimmune mechanism and is seen as a favorable symptom in metastasizing melanoma [21]. At the same time, it is recommended that one carefully examines vitiligo patients for melanoma, especially those with onset at an older age.

Pathogenesis

Three mechanisms have been proposed to explain the destruction of melanocytes in vitiligo. The concept with the most support is the autoimmune hypothesis [21, 47, 55]. Serological and clinical associations with autoimmune phenomena as well as the efficiency of immunomodulating treatments lend support to this concept. Segmental vitiligo seems to be based on a primarily neuronal disorder [4, 42]. This hypothesis is supported by the fact that the clinical course of patients with segmental vitiligo is different from patients with generalized vitiligo [34]. The similarity in the clinical presentation of chemically induced leukoderma and generalized vitiligo renders support to the autocytotoxicity hypothesis, which proposes that melanocytes might be destroyed by toxic intermediates formed during normal melanin biosynthesis. Recently, it has been postulated that a specific metabolite of tetrahydrobiopterin inhibits the phenylalanine hydroxylase reaction and ultimately may initiate depigmentation in patients with vitiligo [80]. It is important to consider that multiple mechanisms could play a role in the pathogenesis of vitiligo [46, 60].

Psychosocial Impact of Vitiligo

Vitiligo is not merely a cosmetic problem. Although it is relatively harmless regarding mortality and physical morbidity, vitiligo can cause profound psychological and social disturbance [69, 76]. The majority of patients develop the disease during puberty, at an age in which cosmetic problems cause severe distress for the developing personality. Visibility of the lesions, which are frequently located in socially interactive sites such as the face and fingertips, makes patients feel that they are the object of frequent staring. The suffering of the patients may appear disproportionate to others, a fact that patients often view as a lack of understanding and compassion. Some patients report that serious psychological trauma, such as the loss of a family member, led to the onset or re-exacerbation of their disease.

It is extraordinarily important that the physician respect the feelings of vitiligo patients, otherwise the physician may contribute to the suffering. It is of equal importance to reassure the patient of the overall benign and non-life-threatening course of the disease, but the consultation should not end at this point. Patients may find it helpful to meet other people affected by vitiligo and to exchange their experiences. Patient forums that provide information and support exist in many countries, and the Internet has made them easily accessible.

Treatment of Vitiligo

Vitiligo poses no threat to the patient's life and treatment is not necessary to prevent physical harm, although the depigmented areas are susceptible to actinic damage. The overall aim of dealing with vitiligo is to improve the cosmetic appearance using three strategies including hiding the areas of vitiligo, repigmentation of the lesions, and irreversible depigmentation of the unaffected epidermis [44]. While phototherapeutic approaches are most effective, other modalities will first be reviewed, since treatment of vitiligo frequently combines or sequentially utilizes several approaches [7, 27].

Sun Protection

The avoidance of sun exposure and permanent use of sunscreen protection with a sun protection factor of more than 15 is of substantial importance for every vitiligo patient. Due to the lack of melanin pigmentation, the vitiliginous skin is much more susceptible to UV radiation and develops painful sunburns even after brief sun exposure. In patients who are prone to koebnerization, a sunburn may lead to exacerbation of the disease. Sunlight-induced tanning of normal skin also enhances the contrast to affected skin. Therefore, opaque sunscreens or those that contain UVA and UVB filters are recommended. These are more effective at reducing tanning induced by the UVA portion of the sunlight. Thorough information on sun protection includes advice on adequate clothing choices and strategies of sun avoidance. In fair skinned individuals, conscientious sun protection by itself may be perfectly adequate for disease management.

Camouflage

In patients with low constitutive melanin pigmentation, the use of regular makeup may be sufficient to conceal vitiligo. A more intense contrast between unaffected skin and vitiligo requires special preparations. Specialized makeup products for efficient camouflage can be individually matched to most skin hues, even with seasonal variations in color. Another property of these medical cosmetics is that they are waterproof. This reduces the frequency of time-consuming application procedures. Some patients prefer professional makeup of the type used in movies and on stage.

"Sunless" tanning agents that contain dihydroxyacetone (DHA) are available from many cosmetic companies. DHA induces a chemical reaction with proteins in the stratum corneum, which leads to a brown coloration that does not wash off. Due to the localization of the reaction products in the stratum corneum and its continuous loss during the epidermal renewal process, repeated applications are required. Chemical tanning alone does not provide sufficient sun protection and should therefore be combined with regular sun protection measures.

A certain orange or brownish skin coloration can also be achieved by ingestion of beta-carotene, canthaxanthin or both. Usually this specific hue is not considered optimal, but for individuals with skin types I and II, oral carotenes may be considered an alternative to repigmentation therapy if combined with sun protection.

Repigmentation Therapies

Table 3 shows an overview of therapeutic strategies to restore normal pigmentation in vitiligo.

Immunomodulation

The therapeutic use of immunosuppressive drugs is based on the hypothesis that vitiligo is an autoimmune disorder. The efficiency of these drugs supports this point of view. Corticosteroids can be applied topically and systemically [12, 40, 71]. All modalities of steroid use involve specific side effects. Topical class 3 or class 4 corticosteroids are often a first-line therapeutic choice in previously untreated patients. In order to reduce the side effects of prolonged corticosteroid treatment, systemic steroids are usually administered as pulse therapy in

Table 3. Therapies for the repigmentation of vitiligo

Application	Systemic	Topical
Phototherapy		+
Photochemotherapy		
Psoralens	+	+
Khellin	+	+
Phenylalanine	+	
Corticosteroids	+	+
Cyclophosphamide	+	
Isoprinosine	+	
Levamisole	+	
Cyclosporin A	+	
P. leukotomos extract	+	
5-Fluouracile		+
Melagenina		+
Pseudo-catalase		+
Melanocyte transfer		+

vitiligo, or in combination with cytotoxic drugs. Cyclosporin A [13], cyclophosphamide [28], 5-fluouracile [91, 96], Levamisole [72], and Isoprinosine have all been used to treat vitiligo by modifying the immune response. These therapeutic approaches showed greatly variable therapeutic efficacy. Severe side effects, which may occur with systemic immunosuppressive regimens, require careful analysis of the benefit-risk ratio. Because vitiligo is a pigmentary disorder, potential serious side effects caused by long-term systemic steroids and immunosuppressives may not justify their use in this condition.

Melanocyte Transfer

The principle of this therapy is to transfer autologous melanocytes from normal patient skin to vitiliginous areas [9]. This modality may be considered in inactive, non-progressive, segmental, or focal vitiligo. Acral or periorificial areas that remain unresponsive at the conclusion of otherwise successful non-surgical repigmentation therapy are good locations for melanocyte transfer. The therapeutic principle is the removal of lesional epidermis, which is replaced by normal autologous epidermis. A variety of techniques have been developed for both removal of the vitiliginous skin and the harvest and transfer of normal epidermis, or, alternatively, in vitro-cultured epidermal cells or melanocytes [25, 26, 49]. On the scalp, eyebrows, and eyelids, single hair grafting has been successfully used for repigmentation [53]. Conversely, leukotrichia has been reversed with autologous grafting [3].

Alternative Modalities of Treatment

Either primarily or after failures of well-established medical treatment, some patients seek cure from alternative methods. Although there are reports of excellent responses to some of these treatments, the unavailability of controlled studies makes a fair or quantitative evaluation of these methods difficult. In addition, side effects may not be well established. Although presented as alternative treatments, some herbal drugs may contain undeclared quantities of psoralens or corticosteroids. Among these alternative treatment modalities is a product known as melagenina. This therapy was developed in Cuba by physicians, but its chemical composition is only poorly defined. The purity of this human placenta-derived agent with respect to infectious (e.g., virus) particles is not guaranteed, and no large controlled studies have been conducted [58]. Therapeutic effects have been documented in a few independent reports but these effects did not fulfill the promises of the proponents of the therapy. It seems that the overall efficacy of melagenina has been shown to be much lower than that achieved with psoralen plus UVA [90]. In addition, the cost of melagenina treatment is high, and it is extremely time-consuming. Thus, melagenina is not recommended by most experts as a treatment option.

Depigmentation

The induction of a universal, chemically induced leukoderma is generally irreversible and therefore should be considered only in selected patients. This option is only applicable with very extensive vitiligo covering more than 50 % of the body surface in patients who have failed, reject, or cannot use repigmentation therapy. Besides the use of chemical depigmentation, the ruby laser has shown efficacy.

Phototherapeutic Options for the Repigmentation of Vitiligo

History

Phototherapy for vitiligo is based on the observation that in many patients sun-exposed lesions tend to show follicular repigmentation during the summer months. With the increased sensitivity of vitiligo to sunburn and the unpredictable dosimetry with natural sunlight, solar phototherapy has not evolved into a true therapeutic option. On the other hand, first descriptions of vitiligo treatment with what can be considered photochemotherapy date back about 4,000 years, which makes PUVA one of the oldest therapeutic principles that are still in use in the twenty-first century [73]. The beneficial effect of topical plant extract applications combined with subsequent sun exposures was observed in several parts of the world. Some of these phototherapeutic treatment regimens are still being practiced as popular/ethnic medicine on the Indian subcontinent and North Africa. It can be assumed that these preparations contain psoralens or related photosensitizers (Fig. 1e). Photochemotherapy of vitiligo was revived for modern medicine half a century ago when El Mofty published the success of his therapeutic trials and subsequently identified the psoralens as the active compounds [24]. Today, PUVA may still be the most effective monotherapy for vitiligo.

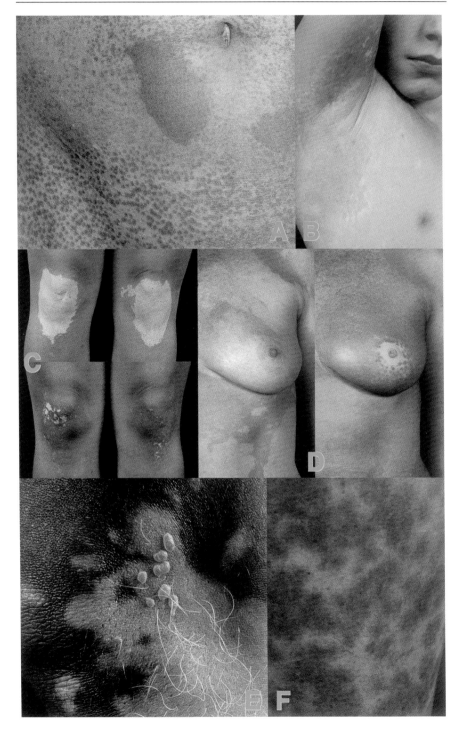

Before Getting Started

Once the diagnosis of vitiligo is established, and the patient decides to attempt repigmentation, phototherapy can be considered. Before phototherapy or photochemotherapy is initiated, the patient needs extensive counseling concerning the specifics of the treatments. One should provide the patient with written information about the disease, phototherapies, and treatment alternatives. The expectations from either side need to be carefully evaluated. Unless patients are strongly motivated, compliance will be poor and treatment should not be initiated. Patients need to be aware of therapy-associated inconveniences and should be ready to cope with these. Phototherapy and photochemotherapy of vitiligo require 100–300 irradiation treatments, and patients will face a major time commitment as well as considerable costs. Longer-lasting interruptions of therapy are disadvantageous because they may halt the progression of the repigmentation process. Another issue concerns individuals with darker skin complexion: the contrast between lesional and surrounding uninvolved skin becomes accentuated due to the phototherapy-induced tanning of normal epidermis. This makes lesions even more visible until they are repigmented. Additional measures, such as camouflage cosmetics (see the section on camouflage above) may be useful to cover exposed lesions during this period. However, any substance blocking or absorbing UVA needs to be removed before each treatment. After discussing phototherapy-related issues, patients are asked to sign a consent form that summarizes this information including the specific regimen and possible adverse effects.

UVB Phototherapy

Many patients experience follicular repigmentation in sun-exposed areas during the summer months. This effect of solar UV exposure is usually reversible, but also repeatable. Because of seasonal and weather-dependent variations of sunlight intensity in moderate climates, the sun as the only light source may not suffice to induce complete repigmentation. On the other hand, a study with topical khellin and sunlight showed that control areas, which got only sun exposure, achieved satisfactory therapeutic results [64]. Although PUVA may be the

Fig. 1a–f. Clinical effects of phototherapy and photochemotherapy. **a** Peri-follicular repigmentation during systemic PUVA using TMP. **b** Almost complete, inhomogenous repigmentation after 4 months of phototherapy using narrow-band (311 nm) UVB. **c** Repigmentation after 1 year of oral 5-MOP+UVA. Lack of repopulation of the scar area. **d** Repigmentation of large trunk areas, while the areolae remain unpigmented. **e** Phototoxic reaction with blister formation in vitiliginous skin. **f** Stationary state of pigmentation on the lower calf after long-term PUVA. (Courtesy of Prof. H. Höningsmann, University of Vienna) most commonly employed phototherapeutic modality in vitiligo therapy, consistent treatment with UVB irradiation delivered by artificial light sources for a sufficiently long period can also achieve a good therapeutic effect. There are only a few publications about UVB phototherapy for vitiligo. A study by Koster and Wiskemann [43] showed good results of whole-body broadband UVB phototherapy. More recently, localized UVB phototherapy of segmental vitiligo showed excellent results in a controlled study [50]. In a study comparing whole-body narrowband (311-nm) UVB irradiations with PUVA using topical unsubstituted psoralen, 311-nm UVB was as effective as PUVA but had fewer side effects [98]. UVB is also used for stimulating repigmentation as part of combination therapy, which is discussed at the end of this chapter. UVA alone is of limited benefit, and is mainly used with photosensitizers or in combination therapy.

Phototesting and Treatment Start

During phototherapy for vitiligo it is necessary to keep exposures within the narrow dose range that induces minimally perceptible erythema, which is assumed to indicate optimal dosimetry. More intense erythema causes discomfort or pain, and may potentially lead to worsening of the disease. In order to avoid unwanted UVB-induced phototoxicity in affected skin, phototherapy must be initiated with caution. The erythema threshold in unpigmented areas may be drastically reduced. Therefore, it is of great importance to initially assess individual UVB sensitivity by determining the minimal erythema dose (MED). A vitiliginous area, which is not sun exposed under normal circumstances (usually the buttocks, lower back or abdomen – as opposed to e.g., the dorsal forearm), should be chosen for MED determination. Repeated sun exposures lead to adaptive changes even in unpigmented skin, resulting in reduced UVB sensitivity (higher MED) [51, 93]. To avoid phototoxic reactions in the early treatment phase, the initial dose should not be measured in such adapted areas. Doses for the MED test are to be chosen in the lower range such as those usually employed for skin phototype I. If a vitiligo patient has a history of pronounced photosensitivity, even lower doses may be needed.

Treatment Schedules

The initial exposure is 70 % of the MED in lesional skin. The subsequent doses are chosen according to the clinical response in the vitiligo areas. The goal is to induce a just-perceivable erythema. This minimal erythema is practically the only parameter useful for individually determining increments. On the other hand, more prolonged or intense erythema should be avoided. An alternative option is to increase the dose once weekly by 10 % – 20 % of the preceding dose.

Most commonly, three treatments per week are given. Schedules with 2 irradiations per week may not be sufficient for optimal treatment success, but this has not been rigorously tested. Unfortunately, there are not enough controlled studies available to favor any one particular phototherapy regimen over another.

Light Sources and Dosimetry

Any light source that is suitable for phototherapy (e.g., for treatment of psoriasis) can be used for treatment of vitiligo. Fluorescent lamps are most frequently applied, but metal halide lamps and SUP (selective ultraviolet phototherapy) lamps may also be used. According to our own experience [66] (Fig. 1b), and as recently demonstrated in a controlled study, the 311-nm narrowband UVB fluorescence bulb (Philips TL-01) is very efficient in the phototherapy of vitiligo [98]. As for the phototherapy of psoriasis, the disparity of the ultraviolet action spectra for erythema and antipsoriatic activity has theoretically and practically justified the use of narrowband UVB. The action spectrum for the phototherapy of vitiligo is not known, but this controlled study would favor narrowband UVB among the UVB sources. Most recently, a study in childhood vitiligo demonstrated safety and quite impressive efficacy of narrowband UVB [57]. These two studies clearly encourage more extensive use of narrowband UVB in the treatment of vitiligo.

UVB dosimetry is more demanding with vitiligo than with other indications because of the increased photosensitivity of vitiliginous skin. The initial treatment phase is most critical because UVB-induced adaptation of the vitiligo areas subsequently reduces their sensitivity. It is important to control the output of the irradiation units on a regular basis and to keep careful records of the applied doses, not just the exposure times. Built-in dosimeters, which are available with many commercial irradiation units, are helpful but are no substitute for regular checks with a well-calibrated, hand-held dosimeter. Particular attention has to be paid to any changes in the treatment routine. Lamp replacement, a change to a different unit within the office, or a move to a different treatment center all imply the risk of delivering excessive irradiation and consequently causing phototoxic side effects.

Adverse Effects

The most frequent side effect is UVB-induced erythema. Environmental UVB exposure has to be considered, and sun protection is recommended on days of therapeutic exposures. One possible consequence of strong phototoxic reactions is a deterioration of the disease due to a Koebner reaction. Regular monitoring of the clinical response and the early symptoms of phototoxicity such as itch and burning sensations helps avoid severe acute side effects. Therapy of UVB-induced burns includes symptomatic measures and topical steroids. With severe phototoxicity that may occur with accidental overexposure, systemic non-steroidals and corticosteroids may be needed. Long-term treatment with UVB may produce accelerated photoaging [19], cutaneous and systemic immunosuppression [10], and an increased risk of skin cancer [22]. Detailed investigations regarding these effects on larger groups of vitiligo patients are not available and therefore we can only speculate about the magnitude of these risks. A few reports on patients receiving long-term UVB treatment suggest that these risks are not of great clinical significance [88, 89].

Table 4. Choice of photosensitizers

Photosensitizer	General		In children		With sunlight	
	Topical	Oral	Topical	Oral	Topical	Oral
8-MOP	+	+	+			
5-MOP	+	+				+
TMP	+	+		+		+
Khellin	+	+	+		+	+
Phenylalanine		+		+		+

Photochemotherapy

The combination of a photosensitizer and UVA radiation makes more variations in treatment regimens possible than phototherapy with UVB. These choices make photochemotherapy more versatile. Options with photochemotherapy comprise topical or systemic application of different photosensitizers and the choice of different light sources (Table 4). As mentioned above, it is extremely important that patient and physician develop a clear understanding of treatment goals and side effects and evaluate whether the expected therapeutic effect justifies time commitment and expense. Treatment should only be initiated if patients are strongly motivated and if the lesions are in locations that are known to respond to photochemotherapy. Acral vitiligo and the so-called lip-tip variant respond minimally to photochemotherapy.

Initiation of Therapy

A detailed explanation of the treatment plan should be given to the patient. Ideally, the patients should gain some understanding of the principles of photochemotherapy, which enables them to appreciate therapy-associated risks and avoid them. In addition to an explanation by the physician, the patient should obtain detailed written information about the treatment, the chances of repigmentation, and short- and long-term side effects. This material may be reviewed on an informed consent form. Patients should be instructed to wear UVA absorbing sunglasses and avoid direct and filtered sunlight for 24 h after treatment. The same precautions are to be taken in vitiligo as in photochemotherapy of other diseases. Contraindications are the same as in psoriasis and include age below 12 years, pregnancy, and nursing. Topical photochemotherapy may be used in children below age 12.

It is crucial that the patient understands that PUVA, like other vitiligo therapies, may require months or even years to achieve a satisfactory result. All-too-optimistic prognoses regarding therapeutic efficacy and time to produce adequate repigmentation should be avoided. The patients must be aware that the treatments stimulate the pigmentation of normal skin, which will heighten the contrast between normal and vitiliginous skin.

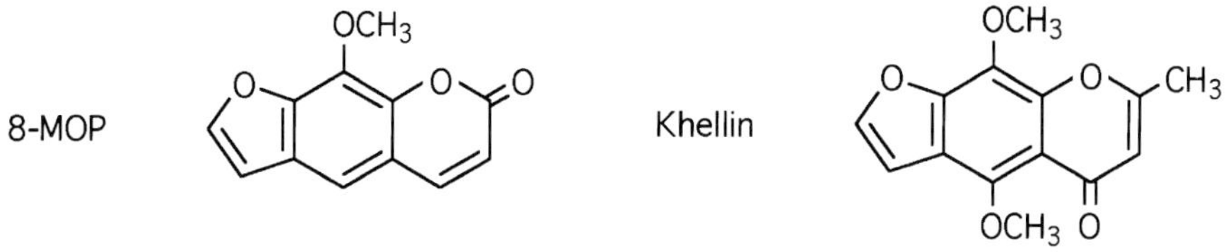

Fig. 2. Chemical structures of 8-MOP and khellin

Systemic Photochemotherapy

In systemic photochemotherapy the photosensitizer is generally ingested, although other routes of administration such as enemas have been explored [85]. The furocoumarins psoralen, 8-methoxypsoralen (8-MOP, Fig. 2), 5-methoxypsoralen (5-MOP), and trimethylpsoralen (TMP) have been successfully used in several studies [35, 73, 74]. Other photosensitizers are available for vitiligo treatment as well. Khellin is a furanochromone with structural similarity to psoralen and is activated by UVA [52]. The amino acid L-phenylalanin combined with UVA irradiation also shows some success in the treatment of vitiligo [19]. Analogous to 'PUVA' for psoralen plus UVA, the acronyms 'KUVA' and 'PAUVA' have been suggested for these alternative regimens.

PUVA

Oral doses of psoralens used for vitiligo treatment are usually smaller than those used for e.g., psoriasis (i.e., 0.3–0.6 mg/kg 8-MOP and 0.6–0.8 mg/kg of 5-MOP and TMP). The period of time between ingestion of the photosensitizer and irradiation depends on the drug used but also on the galenical preparation. For example, 8-MOP is available in a crystalline form, a micronized crystalline preparation, and as liquid capsules. All these preparations yield different plasma levels regarding absolute values, delay times, and reproducibility of maximal concentrations.

With the use of 8-MOP and 5-MOP determination of the minimal phototoxicity dose (MPD)is strongly recommended to avoid phototoxic side effects. As for determination of the UVB MED, the test should preferentially be carried out in the most sensitive lesions.

Treatment has to be started at low UVA doses, such as 50 % of the MPD. Increments must be made with great caution and not more frequently than once a week. Treatments are given 3 times a week, as less than two weekly exposures may not have a beneficial effect. With 5-MOP and 8-MOP, the UVA dose is increased until a light pink erythema is induced in the vitiliginous areas, and further increases are only made to maintain this degree of minimal erythema response. Although it is not clear whether this pink erythema really is a good indicator for optimal dosimetry, it seems to be the only clinical parameter suitable for individualized UVA dosimetry. Further increases have not been found to be useful. Some centers established maximal UVA doses, which are used as a maintenance dose even in the absence of pink erythema. This dose depends on the skin phototype and ranges between 5 and 15 J/cm^2.

Symptomatic erythema must be avoided because excess phototoxicity may produce a Koebner reaction. If PUVA induces an undesired erythematous reaction, treatment has to be interrupted until these signs of overdose have resolved. Treatment should be resumed with lower UVA doses. Repeated episodes of phototoxicity may be an indication that the psoralen dose needs to be reduced, although this is a much less common cause of phototoxicity.

TMP never induces a clinical phototoxic reaction because the blood levels are very low compared to other psoralens and acutely phototoxic levels are not reached. Therefore, MPD tests are not necessary with TMP, and dosimetry follows a fixed regimen. Irradiation starts at $1-2$ J/cm^2 with weekly increases of 1 J/cm^2 until a maintenance dose of $10-15$ J/cm^2 is attained.

KUVA

Khellin (Fig. 2) was discovered for photochemotherapy in Egypt and initially used with solar radiation for the therapy of vitiligo [1]. Treatment with artificial light sources at a frequency of 3 times a week confirmed the effectiveness of this modification of photochemotherapy. Khellin is administered orally at a standard dose of 100 mg per treatment and reaches reliable plasma levels after 2.5 h [68]. One of the greatest advantages is that oral khellin never induces clinical phototoxic reactions [67]. Therefore, irradiation can be started at higher UVA doses than in PUVA, and more rapid increments are possible. Another advantage is that the sun can be used as light source. During summer months treatments can be performed outdoors as long as sunlight is strong enough. With the sun as light source, UVB-induced erythema that is independent of khellin becomes a limiting factor for exposure times. Despite these advantages and good therapeutic results, khellin has not gained lasting acceptance. Khellin has been used at high doses in the treatment of angina pectoris for several years, but currently no pure pharmacological preparations are available, and it is not likely that khellin will be approved for the treatment of vitiligo. In addition, 30 % of vitiligo patients developed reversible increases in liver transaminases that remain to be explained [23, 68]. Under special circumstances, KUVA may be considered an alternative to conventional photochemotherapy.

PAUVA

PAUVA is the combination of the amino acid L-phenylalanine with UVA irradiation. The use of a physiological instead of a xenobiotic photosensitizer makes this form of photochemotherapy conceptually attractive [19]. L-phenylalanine is taken in fixed doses of $50-200$ mg/kg and ingested $0.5-1$ h before irradiation (3 times a week) [19, 84]. No serious adverse effects of L-phenylalanine loading have been reported, but a potential for side effects at such high doses has been discussed [15].

Similar to khellin, L-phenylalanine produces no clinical phototoxic side effects and UVA dosimetry is therefore unproblematic. The UVA doses are usually increased up to a maximal level of 12 J/cm^2. Early reports described good therapeutic results, but the overall efficacy remains controversial [78]. Most recently, an uncontrolled trial was reported that used a combination of topical and systemic phenylalanine [18].

Topical Photochemotherapy

Photochemotherapy with topical 8-MOP can be used in patients with small lesions (less than 5 % total body surface area) or in children younger than 12 years in whom systemic PUVA is contraindicated. The therapy must be done in an office setting, since home treatment involves a high risk of severe phototoxic side effects. Topical 8-MOP preparations have been used in concentrations of up to 1 %. Such high concentration resulted in a higher incidence of phototoxic side effects but did not give better therapeutic results than lower concentration such as 0.1 % [30]. We recommend a starting concentration of 0.05 % or 0.1 % 8-MOP in ethanolic solution. In order to avoid variations of the 8-MOP concentration in the skin it is crucial that the photosensitizer preparation is applied evenly on the treatment area. Fifteen to 30 min after application the skin is exposed to UVA radiation, with an initial dose of 0.25 J/cm^2. Exposure times are increased weekly in steps of 0.25 J/cm^2 unless erythema becomes excessive. Treatments are recommended twice per week, but should not be done on consecutive days. Once a dose of 5 J/cm^2 is reached, a slightly higher concentration of psoralen is prescribed and the same frequency of treatments is followed. This procedure is repeated until a dose and exposure time are attained that produce a just-perceptible erythema but do not result in burning. Patients need to wash off the remaining 8-MOP with water and soap immediately after the irradiation and apply UVA-protective sun block to avoid phototoxic side effects by environmental sun exposure. TMP and 5-MOP can also be used for topical PUVA but are more phototoxic than 8-MOP. For topical application, the vehicle plays a major role for delivery and resulting cutaneous psoralen levels. For example, unsubstituted psoralen is efficacious at 0.005 % in a gel preparation [98].

Photochemotherapy with topical khellin does not result in clinical phototoxicity. This makes topical KUVA a low-risk combination with solar radiation. As with oral khellin, the UVB portion of the sunlight has to be considered (see "Systemic Photochemotherapy"). Topical preparations of khellin in concentrations of 5 % proved to be effective. As there is no clinical phototoxicity, higher concentrations may be used [6, 65]. As with psoralens, there is evidence that drug availability and clinical response does not only depend on khellin concentration, but that the vehicle may be of critical importance [64]. Because topical KUVA involves no risk for the patient, it can be used with solar UVA-radiation. The efficacy of topical KUVA in comparison with oral PUVA or other therapeutic modalities has not been established.

Radiation Sources and Dosimetry

Regular broadband UVA lamps, which are manufactured for PUVA therapy, serve as light sources for the photochemotherapy of vitiligo. These are either fluorescent bulbs or metal halide lamps. If metal halide lamps are used, a UVB filter is required to eliminate the shorter wavelength portion of the emission spectrum. As already discussed for phototherapy, the dosimetry of photochemotherapy of vitiligo needs always to be done with special care because overexposure may result in serious adverse reactions.

Photochemotherapy with Solar Irradiations

PUVASol is the combination of psoralens with the sun as source of UVA radiation. For this treatment modality it is of great importance that the patient is thoroughly instructed. The therapy is usually carried out without constant supervision by the physician, which makes it crucial that the patient understands the principles of therapy and possible sources of unwanted psoralen phototoxicity. Before the initiation of treatment, the same work-up as for standard PUVA is recommended.

TMP and low-dose 5-MOP (0.6 mg/kg) are the oral drugs of choice. Systemic 8-MOP cannot be recommended without close supervision, since its phototoxicity after ingestion is too high. For the same reason, psoralens should not be used topically in combination with sunlight. Khellin plus sunlight, however, can be used with topical as well as with systemic application [1, 6]. Systemic L-phenylalanine and systemic plus topical L-phenylalanine have also been used with solar radiation [45].

The UVB portion of the solar spectrum can induce sunburn independently of the treatment-induced effect. This can be avoided by application of UVB-protective sunscreens, which still allow penetration of UVA radiation. Most patients are aware of how long they can stay in the sun without being burned. Especially in the first weeks, while treatment-induced sun tolerance builds up, exposure times should be increased slowly, beginning with 5-min exposures for either body side (between 11:00 A.M. and 2:00 P.M. in a moderate climate), followed by weekly increments of 2–5 min until a maximum of 45 min for either side is reached.

These exposure-time guidelines have to be reduced in regions with more intense solar radiation. Treatment 2 or 3 times a week should be used, but when using psoralens treatments should be avoided on consecutive days. Patients should be seen frequently and should keep exact records of their medication, exposure times, and side effects.

Home Treatment

Home treatment using artificial radiation sources is only an option for patients with appropriate motivation and a sufficient understanding of the therapy. Similar to PUVASol, TMP, 5-MOP, khellin, and L-Phenylalanin may be employed as photosensitizers. We strongly advise against any topical applications of psoralens. Home tanning equipment with UVA fluorescence bulbs can be used as source of UVA radiation. Dosimetry and dose increments have to be carefully discussed and carried out. One should never rely on energy output information provided with the radiation source. Low levels of energy or units which are too small require long sessions for therapeutically efficient exposures. UVA units with metal halide lamps usually yield higher output but they are also more expensive and require UVB filtering. In some of these lamps, the field of irradiation is small and inhomogeneous but may suffice for smaller areas, as in segmental vitiligo. In the initial treatment phase, regular follow-ups may help the patient avoid phototoxic side effects but still reach therapeutically relevant doses in reasonable time.

Adverse Reactions

The most important acute side effect of phototherapy or photochemotherapy is excessive phototoxicity. Symptoms are pruritus, redness, edema, blisters (Fig. 1e), and with massive PUVA overdose, skin necrosis. Treatment consists of topical steroids. In case of massive and extensive phototoxicity, non-steroidal anti-inflammatory drugs and systemic steroids should be used for symptomatic relief. Photochemotherapy has to be interrupted and is continued with lower doses after the signs of overdose have resolved.

Long-term side effects of PUVA, as with prolonged use of other phototherapeutic modalities, includes premature photoaging of the skin. This may be more of a concern with khellin, L-phenylalanine, and systemic TMP, because of the higher UVA doses used in these regimens. Long-term treatment of vitiligo with PUVA may induce xerosis and PUVA keratoses [38] and lentigines ("PUVA lentigines"). PUVA-induced hypertrichosis has been reported in few cases [20].

Studies in the USA and Europe documented an increased incidence of squamous cell carcinoma after long-term PUVA with 8-MOP in the treatment of psoriasis (see Chap. 14, this volume). The incidence of squamous cell carcinomas in psoriatics correlates with the cumulative total UVA dose, but during vitiligo treatment cumulative doses are usually much lower, therefore vitiligo patients undergoing photochemotherapy may have a lower risk of developing skin cancer [100].

Keratoses and skin carcinomas in PUVA-treated vitiligo patients have been reported [14, 92, 101] possibly indicating that a subset of vitiligo patients may be susceptible to PUVA-induced carcinogenesis.

It has been shown in psoriatics that with adequate precautions serious ocular side effects from PUVA can be prevented [17, 77]. Ocular hazards may become an issue if patients want to treat periocular vitiligo. In this case, eyes need to be completely shut during irradiation, and UVA protective glasses need to be worn after treatment. Because of the possible involvement of the eyes and standard photochemotherapy recommendations, eye exams should be performed initially, and repeated at least annually.

In addition to the side effects that are associated with photochemotherapy, individual therapeutic modalities may cause regimen-specific adverse reactions. Local PUVA can cause intense hyperpigmentation in marginal areas due to exposure of normal surrounding skin. Ingestion of photosensitizers may lead to gastrointestinal and central nervous symptoms, which are more frequently observed with 8-MOP and khellin than with 5-MOP or TMP. For L-phenylalanine, no specific side effects have been described so far. Oral khellin therapy induces reversible increase of liver function parameters in 30 % of patients (see section on systemic KUVA).

Therapeutic Effect of Photochemotherapy

There are no parameters that allow a reliable prognosis for an individual patient. The skin phototype correlates to some extent with response to treatment, with darker-skinned patients more likely to achieve an acceptable degree of repigmentation. Treatment is more efficient in generalized vitiligo than in the focal or segmental variant, which often do not respond satisfactorily. Lesions of the face, neck, and trunk respond more quickly than those in acral sites. Even if a good overall response is obtained, periungual areas, scars, genitalia, nipples, and palms and soles tend to remain unpigmented (Fig. 1c,d). Long-standing vitiligo responds less favorably than early disease. The initial rate of repigmentation may not correlate with the overall treatment success and therefore cannot be used as a prognostic factor.

The course of repigmentation in phototherapy and photochemotherapy is very similar. In the beginning only the unaffected skin shows a response to treatment, which will heighten the contrast with the vitiliginous skin and make the disease even more visible. This effect is most pronounced with psoralens, which enhance the UVA effect. With KUVA and PAUVA, which do not result in clinical phototoxicity, this effect is much weaker. Simultaneously, the vitiliginous skin develops some protection from further irradiation that is unrelated to pigmentation. This protective effect is common to phototherapy and photochemotherapy and is much appreciated by many patients, since it results in decreased sun sensitivity. Termed "Lichtschwiele" in German, this UV barrier is partly due to epidermal hyperplasia and hyperkeratosis.

Course of Repigmentation

The actual improvement of vitiligo can be first seen as early as after 15 – 20 irradiations, when perifollicular and marginal repigmentation appears (Fig. 1a). This newly formed pigmentation is darker than the tanned unaffected skin (Fig. 1a,b). Ideally, these first signs of therapeutic efficacy are followed by a relatively rapid spread of the repigmentation, which after several months to years can result in complete confluency of the follicular areas (Fig. 1b,c). More often, however, gradual retardation or a complete stagnation (Fig. 1d,f) follows the initial spread of pigment, before repigmentation is complete. If such a reduction of therapeutic response is encountered, it is usually futile to further increase the UVA doses because this will rather result in phototoxic reactions rather than an improved therapeutic result. It is more promising to change to a different photosensitizer (e.g., from khellin or 8-MOP to 5-MOP) or to use a drug combination (e.g., 8-MOP plus TMP) [74].

Not uncommonly, patients have a more optimistic view of the improvement of the treated area than the therapist. These patients may not want to terminate the treatment even though actual success may not justify continuation of the therapy.

Long-Term Results

Not many reports are available that have recorded the long-term efficacy of vitiligo therapies, including phototherapeutic modalities. It has been demonstrated that after PUVA treatment the majority of the patients retain PUVA-induced repigmentation for many years [39]. This seems especially true for patients who were treated until stagnation of repigmentation occurred. Another study, however, reports recurrence of vitiligo in 40 % of the patients after finishing PUVA treatment [100]. For UVB phototherapy and other photochemotherapy regimens, sufficient data are not available to allow evaluation of long-term efficacy.

Mechanisms

Neither the pathogenesis of vitiligo nor the mechanisms of repigmentation by phototherapies are completely understood. UVB as well as PUVA stimulate melanogenesis in melanocytes of normal skin, which results in tanning. This effect, however, seems to be independent of those mechanisms, which induce repigmentation of vitiligo skin. Controlled experiments with oral KUVA treatment demonstrated that, while both UVA alone and KUVA stimulated pigmentation of normal skin, only KUVA induced follicular repigmentation in affected skin. This suggests that local phototoxic mechanisms may be crucial for therapeutic efficacy or, that a putative systemic effect of photochemotherapy alone does not suffice to induce repigmentation [68].

The efficacy of immune-suppressive therapy in vitiligo supports the concept of autoimmune pathogenesis. Local and systemic immune suppression by UVB and PUVA are well established, and this book includes an extensive review of their effects on cutaneous immune mechanisms. Growth factor expression is also modulated by UVB and PUVA exposure, which may contribute to the therapeutic efficacy.

Photochemotherapy in Children

Children younger than 12 years old should not undergo PUVA treatment because the spectral properties of the anterior segment of the eye allow UVA penetration. Systemic treatments with a risk of adverse effects should generally be avoided in children. First-line treatment of vitiligo consists of topical steroids. Due to the high risk of phototoxic side effects using topical 8-MOP application, this form of PUVA is only indicated in localized forms of vitiligo and should be performed by an experienced phototherapist. Topical khellin treatment (5 % [65]) can be used without phototoxicity and can also be employed in larger areas without burn hazard. Because of its potential to cause hepatotoxicity, oral khellin should only be used with great caution and under regular measurement of liver function parameters. With systemic khellin, phototoxicity is not encountered. Combination of oral L-phenylalanine and UVA has been recommended for children without reports of serious side effects [82]. Systemic TMP has been successfully used in combination with both office treatment and sunlight [83].

Combination Therapies

Combined therapies aim at a higher efficacy, which may result in a quicker treatment response, a reduction of the unwanted treatment effects, or both. In combined regimens for vitiligo therapy, a phototherapeutic modality is usually included. Phototherapy and photochemotherapy are efficient by themselves, with relatively few side effects. PUVA has an exquisite stimulating effect on pigmentation of normal skin and repigmentation of vitiligo. In combination treatments, the phototherapeutic component contributes its stimulatory effects on melanocytes. At this time, there are no established combination therapies, but some experimental strategies may find their place in vitiligo treatment in the future.

A multicenter study was initiated which evaluates the combined use of UVB and a topical modifier of metabolism (so-called pseudocatalase). UVB has the function to induce repigmentation, whereas the topical treatment is meant to stop the activity of the disease. A first report of the results was very promising [81] and further studies are awaited. Anapsos (Difur) is a herbal-derived drug. For 200 years, South American popular medicine employed the fern Polypodium leucotomos and its extracts such as anapsos in a variety of diseases. Recently, the immunomodulating effects of aqueous P. leucotomos extracts have been described [11]. The P. leucotomos preparation anapsos (7–10 mg/kg) has been used for treatment of vitiligo for quite some time and first reports document good results [29], but larger controlled studies are needed for validation. It could also be demonstrated that combination with sunlight, and especially PUVA, enhances anapsos-induced immunomodulation and accelerates the therapeutic effect. The repigmentation of vitiligo with autologous split skin grafts may be accelerated if the centrifugal spread of the transplanted melanocytes is stimulated by PUVA [86]. When PUVA-treated patients had small remaining leukodermas resurfaced with a pulsed CO_2 laser, the laser-treated, but not the other vitiligo areas repigmented under continued photochemotherapy [41]. Studies in small groups of patients have also shown efficacy of combinations of PUVA with minoxidil or calcipotriol [70, 87]. The combination of UVA with topical corticosteroids was more effective than either component alone [99]. These reports indicate a potential for future validation in larger studies. They also demonstrate that there is always a way of improving established therapies by increasing efficacy and reducing side effects.

Conclusion

Phototherapy and photochemotherapy with psoralens are among the most effective treatment modalities for the repigmentation of vitiligo. The choice of the photosensitizer and the treatment regimen depends on clinical parameters, such as extent of the lesions, age of the patient, and radiation source. When used in combination with other therapeutic modalities, phototherapy or photochemotherapy contribute to the therapeutic effect, which leads to repigmentation of the affected skin.

References

1. Abdel-Fattah A, Aboul-Enein MN, Wassel GM, El-Menshawi BS (1982) An approach to the treatment of vitiligo by khellin. Dermatologica 165:136–140
2. Agarwal G (1998) Vitiligo: an under-estimated problem. Family Practice 15 [Suppl 1:]S19–23
3. Agrawal K, Agrawal A (1995) Vitiligo: surgical repigmentation of leukotrichia. Dermatol Surg 21:711–715
4. Al'Abadie MS, Senior HJ, Bleehen SS, Gawkrodger DJ (1994) Neuropeptide and neuronal marker studies in vitiligo. Br J Dermatol 131:160–165
5. Albert DM, Nordlund JJ, Lerner AB (1979) Ocular abnormalities occurring with vitiligo. Ophthalmology 86:1145–1160
6. Alomar A (1992) Some new treatment of vitiligo vulgaris: phototherapy with topical khellin. 18th world congress of dermatology. Dermatology: progress and perspectives, New York, pp 517–520
7. Antoniou C, Katsambas A (1992) Guidelines for the treatment of vitiligo. Drugs 43:490–498
8. Badri AM, Todd PM, Garioch JJ, Gudgeon JE, Stewart DG, Goudie RB (1993) An immunohistological study of cutaneous lymphocytes in vitiligo. J Pathol 170:149–155
9. Behl PN, Bhatia RK (1973) Treatment of vitiligo with autologous thin Thiersch's grafts. Int J Dermatol 12:329–331
10. Beissert S, Schwarz T (1999) Mechanisms involved in ultraviolet light-induced immunosuppression. J Invest Dermatol Symp Proc 4:61–64
11. Bernd A, Ramirez-Bosca A, Huber H, Diaz Alperi J, Thaci D, Sewell A, Quintanilla Almagro E, Holzmann H (1995) In vitro studies on the immunomodulating effects of polypodium leucotomos extract on human leukocyte fractions. Arzneimittelforschung 45:901–904
12. Bleehen SS (1976) The treatment of vitiligo with topical corticosteroids. Light and electronmicroscopic studies. Br J Dermatol 94 [Suppl 12]:43–50
13. Brown MD, Gupta AK, Ellis CN, Rocher LL, Voorhees JJ (1989) Therapy of dermatologic disease with cyclosporin A. Adv Dermatol 4:3–27; discussion 28
14. Buckley DA, Rogers S (1996) Multiple keratoses and squamous carcinoma after PUVA treatment of vitiligo. Clin Exp Dermatol 21:43–45
15. Burkhart CG, Burkhart CN (1999) Phenylalanine with UVA for the treatment of vitiligo needs more testing for possible side effects (letter; comment). J Am Acad Dermatol 40:1015
16. Calanchini-Postizzi E, Frenk E (1987) Long-term actinic damage in sun-exposed vitiligo and normally pigmented skin. Dermatologica 174:266–271
17. Calzavara-Pinton PG, Carlino A, Manfredi E, Semeraro F, Zane C, De Panfilis G (1994) Ocular side effects of PUVA-treated patients refusing eye sun protection. Acta Derm Venereol Suppl 186:164–165
18. Camacho F, Mazuecos J (1999) Treatment of vitiligo with oral and topical phenylalanine: 6 years of experience (letter). Arch Dermatol 135:216–217
19. Cormane RH, Siddiqui AH, Westerhof W, Schutgens RB (1985) Phenylalanine and UVA light for the treatment of vitiligo. Arch Dermatol Res 277:126–130
20. Cox NH, Jones SK, Downey DJ, Tuyp EJ, Jay JL, Moseley H, Mackie RM (1987) Cutaneous and ocular side-effects of oral photochemotherapy: Results of an 8-year follow-up study. Br J Dermatol 116:145–152
21. Cui J, Bystryn JC (1995) Melanoma and vitiligo are associated with antibody responses to similar antigens on pigment cells. Arch Dermatol 131:314–318
22. de Gruijl FR (1999) Skin cancer and solar UV radiation (review; 69 refs.) Eur J Cancer 35:2003–2009

23. Duschet P, Schwarz T, Pusch M, Gschnait F (1989) Marked increase of liver transaminases after khellin and UVA therapy. J Am Acad Dermatol 21:592–594
24. El Mofty (1948) A preliminary clinical report on the treatment leukoderma with Ammi majus Linn. J Royal Egypt Med Assoc 31:651–655
25. Falabella F (1988) Treatment of localized vitiligo by autologous minigrafting. Arch Dermatol 124:1649–1655
26. Falabella R, Barona M, Escobar C, Borrero I, Arrunategui A (1995) Surgical combination therapy for vitiligo and piebaldism. Dermatol Surg 21:852–857
27. Frenk E (1986) Behandlung der Vitiligo. Hautarzt 37:1–5
28. Gokhale BB, Parakh AP (1983) Cyclophosphamide in vitiligo. Indian J Dermatol 28:7–10
29. Pathak MA, Fitzpatrick TB, Gonzalez S (1998) Use of 5-Methoxypsoralen (5-MOP) and Polypodium leucotomos extract (PLE) in PUVA photochemotherapy of vitiligo. In: Hönigsmann H, Knobler RM, Trautinger F, Jori G (eds.) Proceedings of the 12th International Congress on Photobiology. Landmarks in Photobiology. OEMFspa Publishers, Milan, pp 443–447
30. Grimes PE, Minus HR, Chakrabarti SG, Enteerline J, Halder R, Grough JE, Kenney JA Jr (1982) Determination of optimal topical photochemotherapy for vitiligo. J Am Acad Dermatol 7:771–778
31. Gupta AK, Haberman HF, Pawlowski D, Shulman G, Menon IA (1985) Canthaxanthin. Int J Dermatol 24:528–532
32. Halder RM, Grimes PE, Cowan CA, Enterline JA, Chakrabarti SG, Kenney JA Jr (1987) Childhood vitiligo. J Am Acad Dermatol 16:948–954
33. Halder RM, Battle EF, Smith EM (1995) Cutaneous malignancies in patients treated with psoralen photochemotherapy (PUVA) for vitiligo. Arch Dermatol 131:734–735
34. Hann SK, Lee HJ (1996) Segmental vitiligo: clinical findings in 208 patients. J Am Acad Dermatol 35:671–674
35. Hann SK, Cho MY, Im S, Park YK (1991) Treatment of vitiligo with oral 5-methoxypsoralen. J Dermatol 18:324–329
36. Handa S, Kaur I (1999) Vitiligo: clinical findings in 1436 patients. J Dermatol 26:653–657
37. Hann SK, Kim YS, Yoo JH, Chun YS (2000) Clinical and histopathological characteristics of trichome vitiligo. J Am Acad Dermatol 42:589–596
38. Harrist TJ, Pathak MA, Mosher DB, Fitzpatrick TB (1984) Chronic cutaneous effects of long-term psoralen and ultraviolet radiation therapy in patients with vitiligo. Natl Cancer Inst Monogr 66:191–196
39. Kenney JA (1971) Vitiligo treated by psoralens. A long-term follow-up study of the permanency of repigmentation. Arch Dermatol 103:475–480
40. Khalid M, Mujtaba G, Haroon TS (1995) Comparison of 0.05 % clobetasol propionate cream and topical Puvasol in childhood vitiligo. Int J Dermatol 34:203–205
41. Knoell KA, Schreiber AJ, Milgraum S (1997) Treatment of vitiligo with the ultrapulse carbon dioxide laser in patients concomitantly receiving oral psoralen plus UV-A therapy. Arch Dermatol 133:1605–1606
42. Koga M (1977) Vitiligo: a new classification and therapy. Br J Dermatol 97:255–261
43. Koster W, Wiskemann A (1990) Phototherapie mit UV-B bei Vitiligo. Z Hautkr 65:1022–1024
44. Kovacs SO (1998) Vitiligo. J Am Acad Dermatol 38:647–668
45. Kuiters GR, Hup JM, Siddiqui AH, Cormane RH (1986) Oral phenylalanine loading and sunlight as source of UVA irradiation in vitiligo on the Caribbean island of Curacao NA. J Trop Med Hyg 89:149–155
46. Le Poole IC, Das PK, van den Wijngaard RM, Bos JD, Westerhof W (1993) Review of the etiopathomechanism of vitiligo: a convergence theory (review; 97 refs). Exp Dermatol 2:145–153

47. Le Poole IC, van den Wijngaard RM, Westerhof W, Das PK (1996) Presence of T cells and macrophages in inflammatory vitiligo skin parallels melanocyte disappearance. Am J Pathol 148:1219–1228
48. Lerner AB, Nordlund JJ (1978) Vitiligo. What is it? Is it important? JAMA 239:1183–1187
49. Lerner AB, Halaban R, Klaus SN, Moellmann GE (1987) Transplantation of human melanocytes. J Invest Dermatol 89:219–224
50. Lotti TM, Menchini G, Andreassi L (1999) UV-B radiation microphototherapy. An elective treatment for segmental vitiligo. J Eur Acad Dermatol Venereol 113:102–108
51. Miescher G (1930) Das Problem des Lichtschutzes und der Lichtgewöhnung. Strahlentherapie 35:403
52. Morliere P, Honigsmann H, Averbeck D, Dardalhon M, Huppe G, Ortel B, Santus R, Dubertret L (1988) Phototherapeutic, photobiologic, and photosensitizing properties of khellin. J Invest Dermatol 90:720–724
53. Na GY, Seo SK, Choi SK (1998) Single hair grafting for the treatment of vitiligo. J Am Acad Dermatol 38:580–584
54. Nath SK, Majumder PP, Nordlund JJ (1994) Genetic epidemiology of vitiligo: multilocus recessivity cross-validated. Am J Hum Genet 55:981–990
55. Naughton GK, Reggiardo D, Bystryn JC (1986) Correlation between vitiligo antibodies and extent of depigmentation in vitiligo. J Am Acad Dermatol 15:978–981
56. Njoo MD, Das PK, Bos JD, Westerhof W (1999) Association of the Koebner phenomenon with disease activity and therapeutic responsiveness in vitiligo vulgaris. Arch Dermatol 135:407–413
57. Njoo MD, Bos JD, Westerhof W (2000) Treatment of generalized vitiligo in children with narrow-band (TL-01) UVB radiation therapy. J Am Acad Dermatol 42:245–253
58. Nordlund JJ, Halder R (1990) Melagenina. An analysis of published and other available data. Dermatologica 181:1–4
59. Nordlund JJ, Lerner AB (1982) Vitiligo. It is important. Arch Dermatol 118:5–8
60. Nordlund JJ, Majumder PP (1997) Recent investigations on vitiligo vulgaris. Dermatol Clin 15:69–78
61. Nordlund JJ, Ortonne JP (1992) Vitiligo and depigmentation. Curr Probl Dermatol 21:3–29
62. Nordlund JJ, Taylor NT, Albert DM, Wagoner MD, Lerner AB (1981) The prevalence of vitiligo and poliosis in patients with uveitis. J Am Acad Dermatol 4:528–536
63. Oakley AM (1996) Rapid repigmentation after depigmentation therapy: vitiligo treated with monobenzyl ether of hydroquinone. Austr J Dermatol 37:96–98
64. Orecchia G, Perfetti L (1992) Photochemotherapy with topical khellin and sunlight in vitiligo. Dermatology 184:120–123
65. Ortel B (1993) Die Photochemotherapie der Vitiligo-PUVA und KUVA. Aktuel Dermatol 19:90–94
66. Ortel B, Gonzalez S (1997) Phototherapie und Photochemotherapie der Vitiligo. In: Krutmann J, Hönigsmann H (eds) Handbuch der dermatologischen dermatologischen Phototherapie und Photodiagnostik. Springer, Berlin Heidelberg New York, pp 111–135
67. Ortel B, Tanew A, Honigsmann H (1986) Vitiligo treatment. Curr Probl Dermatol 15:265–271
68. Ortel B, Tanew A, Honigsmann H (1988) Treatment of vitiligo with khellin and ultraviolet A. J Am Acad Dermatol 18:693–701
69. Papadopoulos L, Bor R, Legg C (1999) Coping with the disfiguring effects of vitiligo: a preliminary investigation into the effects of cognitive-behavioural therapy. Br J Med Psychol 72:385–396
70. Parsad D, Saini R, Verma N (1998) Combination of PUVAsol and topical calcipotriol in vitiligo. Dermatology 197:167–170

71. Pasricha JS, Khaitan BK (1993) Oral mini-pulse therapy with betamethasone in viti-ligo patients having extensive or fast-spreading disease. Int J Dermatol 32:753–757
72. Pasricha JS, Khera V (1994) Effect of prolonged treatment with levamisole on viti-ligo with limited and slow-spreading disease. Int J Dermatol 33:584–587
73. Pathak MA, Fitzpatrick TB (1992) The evolution of photochemotherapy with psora-lens and UVA (PUVA): 2000 BC to 1992 AD (review). J Photochem Photobiol B Biol 14:3–22
74. Pathak MA, Mosher DB, Fitzpatrick TB, Parrish JA (1980) Relative effectiveness of three psoralens and sunlight in repigmentation of 365 Vitiligo patients. J Invest Der-matol 74:252
75. Pietzcker F, Kuner-Beck V (1979) "Pigment balance" through oral beta carotene. A new therapeutic principle in cosmetic dermatology. Hautarzt 30:308–311
76. Porter JR, Beuf AH, Lerner A, Nordlund J (1986) Psychosocial effect of vitiligo: a comparison of vitiligo patients with "normal" control subjects, with psoriasis patients, and with patients with other pigmentary disorders. J Am Acad Dermatol 15:220–224
77. Ronnerfalt L, Lydahl E, Wennersten G, Jahnberg P, Thyresson-Hok M (1982) Oph-thalmological study of patients undergoing long-term PUVA therapy. Acta Derm Venereol 62:501–505
78. Rosenbach T, Wellenreuther U, Nurnberger F, Czarnetzki BM (1993) Behandlung der Vitiligo mit Phenylalanine und UV-A. Hautarzt 44:208–209
79. Schallreuter KU, Wood JM, Ziegler I, Lemke KR, Pittelkow MR, Lindsey NJ, Gutlich M (1994a) Defective tetrahydrobiopterin and catecholamine biosynthesis in the depigmentation disorder vitiligo. Biochim Biophys Acta 1226:181–192
80. Schallreuter KU, Wood JM, Pittelkow MR, Gutlich M, Lemke KR, Rodl W, Swanson NN, Hitzemann K, Ziegler I (1994b) Regulation of melanin biosynthesis in the human epidermis by tetrahydrobiopterin. Science 263(5152):1444–1446
81. Schallreuter KU, Wood JM, Lemke KR, Levenig C (1995) Treatment of vitiligo with a topical application of pseudocatalase and calcium in combination with short-term UVB exposure: a case study on 33 patients (see comments). Dermatology 190:223–229
82. Schulpis CH, Antoniou C, Michas T, Strarigos J (1989) Phenylalanine plus ultraviolet light: preliminary report of a promising treatment for childhood vitiligo. Pediatr Dermatol 6:332–335
83. Sehgal VN (1971) Oral trimethylpsoralen in vitiligo in children: a preliminary report. Br J Dermatol 85:454–456
84. Siddiqui AH, Stolk LM, Bhaggoe R, Hu R, Schutgens RB, Westerhof W (1994) L-phenylalanine and UVA irradiation in the treatment of vitiligo. Dermatology 188:215–218
85. Siddiqui AH, Stolk L, Korthals Altes-Levij van Vinninghe HR, Kammeijer A, Cor-mane RH (1982) Microenema of 8-methoxypsoralen in photochemotherapy of pso-riasis. Arch Dermatol Res 273:219–223
86. Skouge J, Morison WL (1995) Vitiligo treatment with a combination of PUVA ther-apy and epidermal autografts. Arch Dermatol 131:1257–1258
87. Srinivas CR, Shenoi SD, Balachandran C (1990) Acceleration of repigmentation in vitiligo by topical minoxidil in patients on photochemotherapy (letter). Int J Der-matol 29:154–155
88. Stern RS, Laird N (1994) The carcinogenic risk of treatments for severe psoriasis. Cancer 73:2759–2764
89. Studniberg HM, Weller P (1993) PUVA, UVB, psoriasis, and nonmelanoma skin cancer. J Am Acad Dermatol 29:1013–1022
90. Suite M, Quamina DB (1991) Treatment of vitiligo with topical melagenine–a human placental extract. J Am Acad Dermatol 24:1018–1019

91. Szekeres E, Morvay M (1985) Repigmentation of vitiligo macules treated topically with Efudix cream. Dermatologica 171:55–59
92. Takeda H, Mitsuhashi Y, Kondo S (1998) Multiple squamous cell carcinomas in situ in vitiligo lesions after long-term PUVA therapy. J Am Acad Dermatol 38:268–270
93. Tham SN, Gange RW, Parrish JA (1987) Ultraviolet-B treatment of psoriasis in patients with concomitant vitiligo (letter). Arch Dermatol 123:26–27
94. Thiele B, Steigleder GK (1987) Repigmentierungsbehandlung der Vitiligo mit L-Phenylalanine und UVA Bestrahlung. Z Hautkr 62:519–523
95. Thissen M, Westerhof W (1997) Laser treatment for further depigmentation in vitiligo. Int J Dermatol 36:386–388
96. Tsuji T, Hamada T (1983) Topically administered fluorouracil in vitiligo. Arch Dermatol 119:722–727
97. Westerhof W (1993) Differentialdiagnose bei Vitiligo – ein Bldbericht. Aktuel Dermatol 19:80–86
98. Westerhof W, Nieuweboer-Krobotova L (1997) Treatment of vitiligo with UV-B radiation vs topical psoralen plus UV-A. Arch Dermatol 133:1525–1528
99. Westerhof W, Nieuweboer-Krobotova L, Mulder PG, Glazenburg EJ (1999) Left-right comparison study of the combination of fluticasone propionate and UV-A vs. either fluticasone propionate or UV-A alone for the long-term treatment of vitiligo. Arch Dermatol 135:1061–1066
100. Wildfang IL, Jacobsen FK, Thestrup-Pedersen K (1992) PUVA treatment of vitiligo: a retrospective study of 59 patients. Acta Derm Venereol 72:305–306
101. Yagi S, Hanawa S, Morishima T (1983) Bowen disease and bowenoid lesion arising on vitiliginous skin during long-term phototherapy (in Japanese). Nippon Hifuka Gakkai Zasshi 93:741–745

8 Photo(chemo)therapy of Graft-Vs-Host Disease

Beatrix Volc-Platzer

Contents

Introduction

Allogeneic stem cell transplantation (SCT) – i.e., bone marrow (BM) or peripheral blood stem cells (PBSC) – from human leukocyte antigen (HLA)-matched related donors is increasingly used to cure otherwise lethal hematological malignancies, hematological and immunological disorders, and certain errors of metabolism [1, 2]. Although remarkable progress has been achieved in the past 25 years [3, 4] based on improved supportive-care techniques, molecular determination of matching for histocompatibility antigens, prevention and development of standard treatment modalities, and adverse graft-vs-host reactions (GVHR) are a major complication affecting approximately 50 % of the patients and impairing the overall prognosis after SCT [1, 2]. Moreover, the use of unrelated donors and HLA-disparate stem cells has resulted in increased frequencies of severe graft-vs-host disease (GVHD) [5, 6]. Several other risk factors add to the development of GVHD, among them the age of donor and recipient, the number of T lymphocytes included in the graft, and the sex of donor and recipient (female donor, male recipient).

The severe, life-threatening symptoms of steroid-resistant acute GVHD, i.e., toxic epidermal necrolysis, liver failure, and severe gut involvement, and high-dose immunosuppression significantly enhance the risk of developing bacterial, fungal, and viral infections [7] or of relapse of the underlying disease. The immunosuppression associated with chronic GVHD per se, and the standard immunosuppression based on cyclosporine A (CSA) and corticosteroids used for prophylaxis and treatment of GVHD, respectively, do not only bear the risk of infectious complications [8] but also lead to the development of secondary malignancies [9].

Therefore, the use and further development of adjunct or alternative treatment modalities based on the immunomodulating effects of UV irradiation, which allow the reduction of, or maybe even replacement of, standard immunosuppression with corticosteroids is highly desirable for the treatment of acute and chronic GVHD. In addition, immune manipulation of grafts by ultraviolet (UV) irradiation may also be considered to prevent GVHD.

Graft-Vs-Host Disease

Definition and Immunopathological Concepts

In 1966, Billingham defined the three prerequisites for the development of GVHD:
1. immunologically competent T lymphocytes within the graft from a
2. HLA-disparate donor recognize tissues or cells of an
3. immunologically incompetent host as foreign [10].

The immunological event leading to injury of the main target organs – skin, gut, and liver – involves the activation and the clonal expansion of effector T cells in response to the recipient's disparate major or minor histocompatibility antigens (miHA) within the severely immunosuppressed host. Current evidence suggests that dysregulated cytokine production during sequential monocyte and T-lymphocyte activation is responsible – at least in part – for characteristic features of acute and chronic GVHD. Damage of host tissues by the conditioning regimen results in the release of inflammatory cytokines interleukins-1 and -6 (IL-1, IL-6) and tumor necrosis factor alpha (TNF-α), which increase the constitutive and the aberrant expression of class II alloantigen and adhesion molecules and contribute to an increased activation of donor T lymphocytes [11]. The T lymphocytes secrete predominantly IL-2 and IFN-γ, induce cytotoxic T-cell (CTL) and natural killer (NK)-cell responses, and prime monocytes to produce TNF-α and IL-1 [12]. Hallmarks of cutaneous and intestinal GVHD, such as dyskeratosis and apoptosis of epithelial cells [13], may be cytokine-induced via TNF-α [4], may occur via activation of the Fas/FasL system [15], and may be mediated by CTL and NK-cell effector molecules [15].

Clinical Symptoms, Histological Signs, and Immunopathological Findings

Acute GVHD develops around the time when the first peripheral leukocytes are detected within the peripheral blood ("graft take"), which usually occurs between days +14 and +21. Occasionally, acute GVHD may be detected as early as within few days after SCT in recipients who are not HLA-matched with the donor or in patients not given any prophylaxis. Acute GVHD is observed in up to 50 % of patients, the target organs being skin, liver, and gut. The skin lesions are characterized by a maculopapular rash, closely resembling, and sometimes essentially indistinguishable from a drug-induced or viral skin rash. The intensity of the skin rash may increase involving the entire integument (erythroderma) with blister formation and sloughing of the entire epidermis ("toxic epidermal necrolysis-like"). Staging of acute cutaneous, as well as liver and gut, GVHD and the overall grading, which take into account the symptoms of all three organ systems, are performed according to Glucksberg et al. [16] and are confirmed by histopathology [17]. Despite recent attempts to modify this grading and staging system in order to make it more suitable for biostatistical evaluations and analyses, it is most important that the original Glucksberg grading and staging system [16] is used by all transplantation centers for comparison of the outcome of patients and responses to new treatments such as UV-based therapies in clinical studies. Symptoms of acute GVHD may be seen as late as 2 to 3 months after transplantation, due to reduction or withdrawal of CSA around day +100. This "late" appearing form of acute cutaneous GVHD may already display features of lichen planus, clinically as well as histologically GVHD [18] and appears to be associated with higher morbidity.

Chronic cutaneous GVHD may present as a lichen-planus-like skin eruption, observed as early as around day +60 in up to 55 % of transplant recipients [19]. In addition, lichen sclerosis-like or morphea-like (i.e., localized scleroderma-like) eruptions of the skin and of the oral and/or genital mucosa are observed and predominate manifestations of chronic GVHD in other organs [20]. The skin and the mucosal sites are involved in more than 90 % [20] of cases, but also other organs such as the eyes, the gut, the liver, the musculoskeletal system, the central nervous system, the spleen, the pancreas, and the lungs may be involved, resembling – in part – the manifestations of autoimmune diseases (Sjögren's syndrome, autoimmune hepatitis, lupus erythematosus, dermatomyositis, scleroderma, etc.).

Mild GVHD of the skin, i.e., a maculopapular rash involving less than 25 % of the skin in the virtual absence of an inflammatory infiltrate body surface, histologically confirmed by a vacuolization of basal epidermal keratinocytes, is considered as not endangering the outcome of the patient. It is considered as an indicator of an ongoing graft-vs-leukemia (GVL) reaction closely associated with the GVHR. The GVL reaction is mediated by donor T lymphocytes, at minimum $1 \cdot 10^7$ CD3$^+$ T cells. At present, no phenotypic marker(s) are known to determine, and, in consequence, to isolate the GVL-effector cell population, although experimental data point to an important role of in vivo activated NK cells [21, 22, 22a]. Nevertheless, even after autologous BMT, e.g., following the treatment with ultra-high-dose chemotherapy, CSA and its withdrawal, respectively, is used to induce mild GVHD, hopefully associated with the desired GVL or graft-vs-tumor effect [23]. However, the risk of the subsequent development of lichen-planus-like GVHD and other symptoms of chronic cutaneous GVHD is also increased.

Whereas in numerous clinical trials different prophylactic protocols have been evaluated, only a few studies about the treatment of established GVHD have been reported. Standard immunosuppression with CSA and increasing the dose of corticosteroids [24], and – in case of steroid resistance – with antithymocyte globulin (ATG) is used for acute cutaneous GVHD stage II and more [25]. Essentially the same basic treatment is used for chronic GVHD. If CSA is not tolerated because of its side effects on the kidney or the central nervous system, it is replaced by FK 506 [26] or mycophenolate mofetil [27], respectively. In addition, thalidomide is used in selected cases of chronic GVHD [28]. Most importantly, UV radiation-based treatments [29], i.e., UVB, psoralen with UVA radiation (PUVA) – orally and as PUVA bath – and extracorporeal photochemotherapy ECP, have been evaluated for the treatment of steroid resistant, chronic, and – to a lesser extent – acute GVHD [30–38] within the last 15 years.

Photo(chemo)therapies with UVA

PUVA (8-Methoxypsoralen plus UVA)

Treatment of Chronic GVHD

The successful introduction and widespread use of PUVA in the management of psoriasis was the stimulus for evaluation of the therapeutic use of this non-ionizing radiation in other dermatoses. Due to clinical and histological similarities of idiopathic lichen planus and lichenoid GVHD, we and others treated this latter type of GVHD with PUVA [30, 31]. Between 1985 and 1999 the number of reports on the successful use of PUVA, in addition to standard immunosuppression of lichenoid GVHD, increased steadily (Table 1 [30–38]).

Reports on the results of PUVA treatment of scleroderma-like variants of cutaneous GVHD are controversial. According to our own experience, the more circumscribed, localized forms appear to respond to PUVA most readily, concomitantly softening the fibrotic, sclerotic connective tissue. However, more widespread, disseminated lesions hardly respond to PUVA therapy (B. Volc-Platzer, A. Tanew, H. Hönigsmann, unpublished observation).

It has been reported that PUVA may exert not only local but also systemic effects. We observed an initial improvement of mucosal erosions followed by healing upon treatment of chronic lichenoid GVHD with PUVA. Apparently, there is no improvement of GVHD of other organs, e.g., liver. Nevertheless, it is equally important that – on the other hand – deterioration of liver GVHD has never been reported since psoralens are metabolized by the liver.

The therapeutic regimen used for the treatment of chronic GVHD is essentially the same as for psoriasis or mycosis fungoides. One or 2 h after the ingestion of 5- or 8-methoxypsoralen (5-MOP, 8-MOP), respectively, patients are submitted to UVA radiation. Prior, during, and after the treatment the patients' eyes are shielded by protective sunglasses. Initial UVA doses vary between 0.5 and 2.0 J/cm^2 [30–38]. However, it appears difficult to establish the individual minimal erythema dose (MED) for each patient, due to unknown reasons. But UVA

Table 1. Treatment of acute and chronic GVHD with PUVA

Reference	Number of patients	Type of GVHD	Outcome
Hymes et al. 1985 [30]	1	Progressive lichenoid ccGVHD	CR
Atkinson et al. 1986 [32]	4	3 patients recalcitrant ccGVHD 1 patient acGVHD	4 CR after whole body and intraoral PUVA
Volc-Platzer et al. 1990 [31]	4	Extensive cGVHD (skin, oral mucosa, liver)	2 CR; 1 NR; 1 NE
Eppinger et al. 1990 [33]	11	7 extensive cGVHD, 4 aGVHD (III-IV)	3/7 CR and 2/4 CR; 6 PR
Jampel et al. 1991 [34]	6	Chronic limited GVHD	3 CR; 1 PR; 1 improved; 1 NR
Kapoor et al. 1992 [35]	15	Extensive chronic GVHD	12/15 patients evaluable: 4 CR; 4 PR; 2 improved; 2 stable disease
Reinauer et al. 1993 [36]	6	Acute cutaneous GVHD II–III	4/6 CR; 2/4 cGVHD
Aubin et al. 1995 [37]	11	7 chronic extensive GVHD, 4 acute GVHD III–IV	6 CR (3 acute and 3 chronic); 2 PR (chronic); 3 NE
Vogelsang et al. 1996 [38]	40	35 refractory chronic GVHD, 5 high-risk chronic GVHD	31 patients improved; 16/31 CR; 15/31 PR

CR, complete responder; PR, partial responder.

radiation doses should not be increased too much, in order to avoid erythema and possible (re)activation of GVHD. In general, increase of the UVA dose by 0.5 J/cm^2 at maximum after every second to fourth exposure can be recommended. Patients are exposed to UVA radiations 3–4 times weekly. After skin lesions have resolved, exposures are reduced to 2 times weekly for approximately one month, and, finally, to once per week for the last month ("maintenance").

One of the concerns is that UV-based treatments of cutaneous GVHD may lead to the development of skin tumors. Kelly et al. have investigated the effect of immunosuppressive drugs on UV-induced carcinogenesis in the animal model [39]. Altman and Adler [40] have reported on the development of multiple cutaneous squamous cell carcinomas during PUVA treatment for chronic cutaneous GVHD, but definitive proof is lacking that carcinogenesis has been triggered by the UV treatment. Their particular patient developed intermediately differentiated squamous cell carcinomas while being on the PUVA treatment regimen. Although PUVA cannot be definitively excluded as one cause of the tumor development, the influence of other risk factors has to be considered as well: conditioning with ionizing total-body irradiation and high-dose intravenous cyclophosphamide, transplantation during blast crisis of chronic myeloid leukemia (CML), an unrelated donor, preceding acute cutaneous GVHD of the skin, liver, and gut, treatment of acute GVHD with steroids, and ATG, and progressive onset chronic scleroderma-like GVHD treated with corticosteroids, CSA, azathioprine, and thalidomide. However, using the recommended doses for PUVA and limiting the treatment to a span of 3 months, it is highly unlikely that secondary malignancies are triggered by this UVA-based photochemotherapy. However, all bone marrow/peripheral stem cell recipients, no matter whether they had experienced cutaneous GVHD and whether or not they have been treated with photo(chemo)therapy, have to be examined on a regular basis by experienced dermatologists because of the overall increased risk of secondary malignancies, particularly of the skin and the mucous membranes [9].

Treatment of Acute GVHD

Within the last years, PUVA has been increasingly investigated as adjunct treatment in steroid-resistant acute GVHD. Aschan [41] could not demonstrate any benefit from PUVA, neither as monotherapy nor in combination with steroids, steroids plus CSA or methotrexate (MTX). Reinauer et al. [36] administered PUVA to 6 patients with acute cutaneous GVHD stage II to III, who remained on a basic standard immunosuppression with CSA. In all patients the authors noted an improvement after 5 – 12 exposures, and healing after 8–12 exposures. However, 2/6 patients developed chronic cutaneous GVHD with symptoms of lichen planus, poikiloderma, and Sicca syndrome. Eppinger et al. [33] reported 4 patients who had acute cutaneous GVHD. Interestingly only 2/4 patients who had developed "late onset" acute cutaneous GVHD, i.e., around day +70, experienced an improvement of their skin lesions 28 – 40 days after initiation of PUVA treatment. These patients were observed for 4 and 20 months, respectively, and did not develop any relapses of acute cutaneous or symptoms of chronic cutaneous GVHD.

The therapeutic regimen is the same as for the chronic forms of GVHD. Nevertheless, care has to be taken that the initial dose of UV radiation is not too high, although Reinauer et al. report initial doses of 2.5 J/cm^2 without any adverse effects [36].

PUVA "Bath"

Reports on the successful treatment of selected patients with localized scleroderma [42] and lichen planus [43], respectively, prompted us as well as others to investigate the therapeutic effect in selected patients with lichen planus-like and scleroderma-like GVHD. In the meantime, we have treated two children and one adolescent with chronic GVHD of different degrees. 8-MOP was applied in the concentration of 0.001%. The patients stayed in the water for 20 min, and the initial UV dose was 0.5 J/cm^2. Whereas we could notice a partial remission in one patient with a disseminated form of morphea-like and one patient with lichen planus-like GVHD, we could not achieve any improvement in the patient with a linear form of morphea-like GVHD on a lower limb. However, significant improvement has been observed in patients with lichenoid and patients with morphea-like GVHD by Lüftl et al. [44].

Extracorporeal Photopheresis

Initially, extracorporeal photopheresis (ECP) has been reported as successful treatment of cutaneous T-cell lymphoma (CTCL) [45] and selected patients with autoimmune diseases such as pemphigus vulgaris [46] and systemic sclero-derma [47]. Currently, it is approved by the FDA only for the treatment of CTCL. The mechanism of action of ECP is thought to be due to immunomodulatory effects, based on clinical and experimental observations, but many aspects thereof still need to be elucidated. The following possibilities are briefly discussed:

1. Psoralens bind to leukocyte DNA after photoactivation in vitro, thereby inhibiting DNA replication [48]. However, since during one ECP treatment only 2 % – 5 % of the patient's mononuclear cell population is affected [49], this direct action cannot fully explain the immunomodulatory effects of ECP.
2. Photopheresis-treated lymphocytes secrete cytokines such as IL-1, IL-6, and TNF-α [50], which affect the entire immune system with various molecular and biological effects.
3. Apoptosis has been observed in lymphocytes undergoing the ECP procedure [51], which may lead to deletion of graft-reactive T-cells.
4. Another possibility is that photoactivated 8-MOP may alter the idiotypes (e.g., HLA-class I-associated peptides of the T-cell receptor) expressed by clones of autoreactive T cells of known or unknown specificity by upregulation of class I expression [52]. The increased amounts of class I molecules might trigger the induction of specific anti-idiotypic autoregulatory T cells, most likely CD8$^+$ T lymphocytes with suppressive or cytotoxic capabilities [53]. The enhancement of a presumably already existent anti-idiotypic T-cell response may thus be boosted, permitting cytolysis of non-irradiated autoreactive cells expressing smaller amounts of the respective antigen. Findings in the animal model support this concept [55, 56].

Recently, we and others have reported on the successful adjunct treatment of steroid-refractory acute and chronic GVHD with ECP (Table 2 [57–67]). However, double-blind, controlled studies using standardized parameters to evaluate the effect of ECP on the various organ systems are awaited to unequivocally prove the benefit of this adjunct treatment. According to our own experiences, favorable responses are observed primarily in patients with early onset, lichenoid cutaneous GVHD [58, 61], whereas patients with scleroderma-like GVHD respond less well [61]. Patients with steroid-refractory acute cutaneous GVHD also respond well to ECP [61].

ECP treatments have been performed at our institution with the UVAR Photopheresis system (Therakos, West Chester, Pa.). Whereas the technical details are discussed elsewhere in this book, it should be noted that the mean treatment time for each photopheresis session was 3.5 h, and that two treatments on two

Table 2. Treatment of steroid refractory acute and chronic GVHD with ECP

Reference	Number of patients	Type of GVHD	Outcome
Besnier et al. 1997 [57]	7	2: Acute GVHD (Glucksberg IV); 5: Chronic extensive GVHD	2 deaths; 4/5 improved
Richter et al. 1997 [59]	1	Acute GVHD (Glucksberg III)	CR
Dall'Amico et al. 1998 [85]	13	4: Acute GVHD (no grading); 9: Chronic GVHD (no details)	Response in 3/4 patients; improvement in 6/9
Greinix et al. 1998 [61]	21	6: Acute GVHD (Glucksberg II-III); 15: Chronic extensive GVHD	5/6 CR; 12/15: skin CR, contractures PR; 15/15: oral CR; 7/10: liver CR
Owsianowski et al. 1994 [62]	1	Chronic extensive GVHD	Skin CR; Sicca PR
Rossetti et al. 1995 [63]	1	Chronic extensive GVHD	Improved
Balda et al. 1996 [64]	1	Chronic extensive GVHD	PR
Gerber et al. 1997 [58]	1	Chronic extensive cutaneous GVHD	CR
Dall'Amico et al. 1997 [65]	4	Chronic extensive GVHD	3 of 4 improved
Abhyankar and Bishop 1998 [66]	53	Chronic extensive GVHD	81 %: skin improved; 77 %: oral improvement
Sniecinski et al. 1998 [60]	48	11: acute GVHD; 37: chronic extensive GVHD	1/11 PR; 80 % skin CR or PR; 36 % liver CR or PR
Bishop et al. 1998 [67]	14	Chronic GVHD (no details)	4 CR, 2 PR

CR, complete responder; PR, partial responder.

consecutive days have been performed. ECP has been applied at 1- to 4-week intervals for various lengths of time.

However, despite the first promising results, controlled studies with larger numbers of patients are required to establish a treatment schedule with defined intervals between ECP treatments to identify a time frame in which ECP therapy should be applied. Moreover, it is of outmost importance to assess properly – based on controlled randomized studies – the benefits of the treatment for GVHD vs the effect on relapse of the underlying disease.

Phototherapy with UVB

The effect of UVB radiation on prolongation of graft survival has been investigated in various experimental situations [68–70]. Additional data point to an important role of UVB in the prevention of graft rejection and GVHD, respectively [71]. The mechanism of action of UVB, at least on human peripheral blood lymphocytes, appears to be based on the induction of apoptosis [72], whereas normal bone marrow stem cells are preserved at comparable doses [73].

Experience with UVB treatments of cutaneous GVHD is very limited. So far, UVB radiation has been used for treatment of cutaneous GVHD only in selected patients [74, 75]. Based on one study [75] it remains unclear whether irradiation of the skin shortly after transplantation is of benefit in the prevention of human cutaneous GVHD.

UV Radiation for the Prevention of GVHD and Graft Rejection After SCT

GVHD and graft rejection remain major problems in allograft recipients and result from allo-interactions between graft and recipient. Both radioresistant T cells of the host (CD8+ cytotoxic T lymphocytes equal CTL and major histocompatibility complex [MHC]-restricted) [76–79] that are capable of surviving the conditioning regimens, as well as donor lymphocytes, may function as effector cells in graft rejection. In addition, donor-derived dendritic cells contribute to graft rejection by initiating T-cell allorecognition and graft rejection [80]. However – at least in mice – selected donor lymphocyte subpopulations, i.e., activated killer cells [81], facilitate engraftment without increasing GVHD.

Most of the studies on modulation of allo-interactions have been performed with UVB in animal models [82]. Further investigations have been performed with human peripheral blood mononuclear cells irradiated with UVB and UVC [83]. Murine dendritic cells (DCs) viability is extremely sensitive to UVB and UVC radiation. Moreover, UVB irradiation of human DC prevents the normal upregulation of costimulatory cell-surface ligands such as ICAM-1 and B7/BB1 during clustering with allogeneic T lymphocytes, the critical event in primary stimulation of naive or non-sensitized T cells. HLA class II expression on mononuclear cells is reduced following UVB exposure with HLA-DQ and -DP expression on lymphocytes being more sensitive than that of HLA-DR and class I expression. In addition, cytokines involved in DC/T-cell interactions are affected by UV irradiation. UVB irradiation of human peripheral blood DC does not prevent cluster formation with alloantigen specific T lymphocytes but subsequent T lymphocyte proliferation and IL-2 secretion is impaired. Data from experiments with other APC populations point to a UV-induced antigen processing defect.

Apart from the experimental and in vitro data, possible clinical implications have emerged:

Most recently, the potency of immunomodulation by ECP and its benefit in preventing on graft rejection has been shown for heart transplant recipients in a preliminary, controlled, double-blind clinical study [84].

Summary and Outlook

Despite the use of steroids in addition to CSA and other immunosuppressants such as ATG, a certain percentage of patients with acute GVHD subsequent to hematopoietic stem cell transplantation does not respond even to high doses of corticosteroids. Patients with chronic GVHD, particularly those with extensive involvement of mucosal sites, may also require high doses of standard corticosteroid and CSA treatment or even require the addition or switch to other standard drugs such as azathioprine (Imurek) or less-well-investigated drugs such as FK506 (Prograf), mycophenolate mofetil (Cellcept), thalidomide, etc. Most of these treatments applied either as single agents or in combination bear the risks of life-threatening infections or – over the long term – of the development of secondary malignancies. Therefore, the search for alternative or at least adjunct treatment modalities has led to the exploration of the immunosuppressive potential of UV radiation applied as photo- or photochemotherapy. Whereas the value of the shorter wavelength UVB radiation (311 or 312 nm) still has to be evaluated, the potency of phototreatments based on UVA radiation has been – and still is – extensively investigated.

The currently available data suggest

1. the "lichen planus-like" skin manifestations of progressive onset and quiescent onset limited chronic cutaneous GVHD as well as of "late-occurring" acute GVHD after reduction or withdrawal of CSA respond best to photochemotherapies, and
2. that standard PUVA and ECP are probably equally effective in this particular clinical situation.
3. A beneficial systemic effect has been postulated based on the response of mucosal lesions, which are not directly exposed to the photochemotherapy.
4. Organ manifestations other than those of the skin, in particular liver involvement, appear to respond only to ECP, including GVHD of the gastrointestinal tract.
5. PUVA bath may be the phototherapy of choice for disseminated morphea-like lesions of limited, de novo onset chronic GVHD.
6. The effect of PUVA and ECP on acute GVHD has to be investigated in larger clinical trials. Although improvement of acute cutaneous GVHD has been reported – as we have shown in a preliminary study, standard immunosuppression can be reduced or terminated earlier in patients treated with ECP when compared to historical controls without ECP – the long-term effects on the prevention of chronic GVHD as well as of relapse of the underlying disease are still not entirely clear.

Whereas most studies performed by or in cooperation with dermatologists focus on the treatment of already ongoing GVHD, it should be kept in mind that

UV irradiation may well be effective in the prevention of rejection of solid organ as well as of hematopoietic stem cell grafts. Further investigation is needed to explore the possibilities to prevent GVHD in human bone marrow and peripheral stem cell recipients, and, perhaps, either to inactivate selectively those cell populations mediating GVHD or to selectively enhance the peripheral blood cells mediating the GVL effect.

References

1. Thomas ED, Storb R, Clift RA, Fefer A, Buckner CD, Neimann PE, Lerner KC (1975) Bone marrow transplantation. N Engl J Med 292:832–843, 895–902
2. Armitage JO (1994) Bone marrow transplantation. N Engl J Med 330:827–838
3. Clift RA, Buckner CD, Thomas ED, Bensinger WI, Bowden R, Bryant E, Deeg HJ, Doney KC, Fisher LD, Hansen JA, Martin P, McDonald GB, Sanders JE, Schoch G, Singer J, Storb R, Sullivan KM, Witherspoon RP, Appelbaum FR (1994) Marrow transplantation for chronic myeloid leukemia: a randomized study comparing cyclophosphamide and total body with busulfan and cyclophosphamide. Blood 84:2036–2043
4. Greinix HAT, Reiter E, Keil F, Fischer G, Lechner K, Dieckmann K, Leitner G, Schulenburg A, Höcker P, Haas OA, Knöbl P, Mannhalter C, Fonatsch C, Hinterberger W, Kalhs P (1998) Leukemia-free survival and mortality inpatients with refractory or relapsed acute leukemia given marrow transplants from sibling and unrelated donors. Bone Marrow Transplant 21:673–678
5. Hansen JA, Gooley TA, Martin PJ, Appelbaum F, Chauncey TR, Clift RA, Petersdorf EW, Radich J, Sanders JE, Storb RF, Sullivan KM, Anasetti C (1998) Bone marrow transplants from unrelated donors for patients with chronic myeloid leukemia. N Engl J Med 338:962–968
6. Lee SJ, Kuntz KM, Horowitz MM, McGlave PB, Goldman JM, Sobocinski KA, Hegland J, Kollmann C, Parsons SK, Weinstein MC, Weeks JC, Antin JH (1997) Unrelated donor bone marrow transplantation for chronic myeloid leukemia: a decision analysis. Ann Intern Med 127:1080–1088
7. Bowden RA (1990) Infections in patients with graft-vs.-host disease. In: Burakoff SJ, Deeg HJ, Ferrara J, Atkinson K (eds) Graft-vs.-host disease. Dekker, New York, pp 525–538
8. Socie G, Stone JV, Wingard JR, Weisdorf D, Henslee-Downey PJ, Bredeson C, Cahn JY, Passweg JR, Rowlings PA, Schouten HC, Kolb HJ, Klein JP (1999) Long-term survival and late deaths after allogeneic bone marrow transplantation. N Engl J Med 341:14–21
9. Curtis RE, Rowlings PA, Deeg HJ, Shriner DA, Socie G, Travis LB, Horowitz MM, Witherspoon RP, Hoover RN, Sobocinski KA, Fraumeni JF Jr, Boice JD Jr (1997) Solid cancer after bone marrow transplantation. N Engl J Med 336:897–904
10. Billingham RE (1966) The biology of graft-versus-host reactions. Harvey Lect 62:21–72
11. Ferrara JLM, Deeg HJ (1991) Graft-versus-host disease. N Engl J Med 324:828–834
12. Ferrara JL (1998) The cytokine modulation of acute graft-versus-host disease. Bone Marrow Transplant 21:S13–15
13. Gilliam AC, Whitaker-Menezes D, Korngold R, Murphy GF (1996) Apoptosis is the predominant form of epithelial target cell injury in acute experimental graft-versus-host disease. J Invest Dermatol 107:377–383
14. Piguet PF, Grau GE, Allet B, Vassalli P (1987) Tumor necrosis factor/cachectin is an effector of skin and gut lesions of the acute phase of the graft-vs-host disease. J Exp Med 166:1280–1289

15. Kagi D, Vignaux F, Ledermann B, Burki K, Depraetere V, Nagata S, Hengartner H, Golstein P (1994) Fas and perforin pathways as major mechanisms of T cell-mediated cytotoxicity. Science 265:528–530

16. Braun MY, Lowin B, French L, Acha-Orbea H, Tschopp J (1996) Cytotoxic T cells deficient in both functional Fas ligand and perforin show residual cytolytic activity yet lose their capacity to induce lethal acute graft-versus-host disease. J Exp Med 183:67–661

17. Glucksberg H, Storb R, Fefer A, Buckner CD, Neiman PE, Clift RA, Lerner KG, Thomas ED (1974) Clinical manifestations of graft-versus-host disease in human recipients of marrow from HLA-matched siblings. Transplantation 18:295–304

18. Lerner KG, Kao GF, Storb R, Buckner CD, Clift RA, Thomas ED (1974) Histopathology of graft-versus-host reaction (GVHR) in human recipients of marrow from HLA-matched siblings. Transplant Proc 6:367–371

19. Horn TD, Zahurak ML, Atkins D, Solomon AR, Vogelsang GB (1997) Lichen planus-like histopathologic characterisitics in the cutaneous graft-vs-host reaction. Arch Dermatol 133:961–965

20. Shulman HM, Sale GE, Lerner KG, Barker EA, Weiden PL, Sullivan K, Gallucci B, Thomas ED, Storb R (1980) Chronic cutaneous graft-versus-host disease. Am J Pathol 91:545–570

21. Sullivan KM, Shulman HM, Storb R, Weiden PL, Witherspoon RP, McDonald GB, Schubert MM, Atkinson K, Thomas ED (1981) Chronic graft-versus-host disease in 52 patients: adverse natural course and successful treatment with combination immunosuppression. Blood 57:267–276

22. Sullivan KM, Storb R, Buckner CD, Fefer A, Fisher L, Weiden PL, Witherspoon RP, Appelbaum FR, Banaji M, Hansen J et al (1989) Graft-versus-host disease as adoptive immunotherapy in patients advanced hematologic neoplasms. N Engl J Med 320:828–834

22a. Xun CQ, Thompson JS, Jennings CD, Brown SA (1995) The effect of human IL-2-activated natural killer and T cells on graft-versus-host disease and graft-versus-leukemia in SCID mice bearing human leukemic cells. Transplantation 60:821–827

23. Elmaagacli AH, Beelen DW, Trenn G, Schmidt O, Nahler M, Schaefer UW (1999) Induction of graft-versus-leukemia reaction by by cyclosporin A withdrawal as immunotherapy for leukemia relapsing after allogeneic bone marrow transplantation. Bone Marrow Transplant 23:771–777

24. Martin PJ, Schoch G, Fisher L, Byers V, Anasetti C, Appelbaum FR, Beatty PG, Doney K, McDonald GB, Sanders JE, Sullivan KM, Storb R, Thomas ED, Witherspoon RP, Lomen P, Hannigan J, Hansen JA (1990) A retrospective analysis of therapy for acute graft-versus-host disease: initial treatment. Blood 76:1464–1472

25. Doney KC, Weiden PL, Storb R, Thomas ED (1981) Treatment of graft-versus-host disease in human allogeneic marrow graft recipients: a randomized trial comparing antithymocyte globulin and corticosteroids. Am J Hematol 11:1–8

26. Ratanatharathorn V, Nash RA, Przepiorka D, Devine SM, Klein JL, Weisdorf D, Fay JW, Nademanee A, Antin JH, Christiansen NP, Van der Jagt R, Herzig RH, Litzow MR, Wolff SN, Longo WL, Petersen FB, Karanes C, Avalos B, Storb R, Buell DN, Maher RM, Fitzsimmons WE, Wingard JR (1998) Phase III study comparing methotrexate and tacrolimus (Prograf, FK 506) with methotrexate and cyclosporine for graft-versus-host disease prophylaxis after HLA-identical sibling bone marrow transplantation. Blood 92:2303–2314

27. Bornhauser M, Schuler U, Porksen G, Naumann R, Geissler G, Thiede C, Schwerdtfeger R, Ehninger G, Thiede HM (1998) Mycophenolate mofetil and cyclosporine as graft-versus-host disease prophylaxis after allogeneic blood stem cell transplantation. Transplantation 67:499–504

28. Vogelsang GB, Farmer ER, Hess AD, Altamonte V, Beschorner WE, Jabs DA, Corio RL, Levin LS, Colvin OM, Wingard JR et al (1992) Thalidomide for the treatment of chronic graft-versus-host disease. N Engl J Med 326:1055–1058

29. Hönigsmann H, Fitzpatrick TB, Pathak MA, Wolff K (1993) Oral photochemotherapy with psoralens and UVA (PUVA): principles and practice. In: Fitzpatrick TB, Eisen K, Wolff K, Freedberg IM, Austen KF (eds) Dermatology in General Medicine. McGraw-Hill, New York, pp 1728–1775

30. Hymes SR, Morison WL, Farmer ER, Walters LL, Tutschka PJ, Santos GW (1985) Methoxypsoralen and ultraviolet A radiation in treatment of chronic graft-versus-host reaction. J Am Acad Dermatol 12:30–37

31. Volc-Platzer B, Hönigsmann H, Hinterberger W, Wolff K (1990) Photochemotherapy improves chronic cutaneous graft-versus-host disease. J Am Acad Dermatol 23:220–228

32. Atkinson K, Weller P, Ryman W, Biggs J (1986) PUVA therapy for drug-resistant graft-versus-host disease. Bone Marrow Transplant 1:227–236

33. Eppinger T, Ehninger G, Steinert M, Niethammer D, Dopfer R (1990) 8-methoxypsoralen and ultraviolet A therapy for cutaneous manifestations of graft-versus-host disease. Transplantation 50:807–811

34. Jampel RM, Farmer ER, Vogelsang GB, Wingard J, Santos GW, Morison WL (1991) PUVA therapy for chronic cutaneous graft-vs-host disease. Arch Dermatol 127:1673–1678

35. Kapoor N, Pelligrini AE, Copelan EA, Cunningham I, Avalos BR, Klein JL, Tutschka PJ (1992) Psoralen plus ultraviolet A (PUVA) in the treatment of chronic graft versus host disease: preliminary experience in standard treatment resistant patients. Semin Hematol 29:108–112

36. Reinauer S, Lehmann P, Plewig G, Heyll A, Söhngen D, Hölzle E (1993) Photochemotherapie (PUVA) der akuten Graft-versus-Host Erkrankung. Hautarzt 44:708–712

37. Aubin F, Brion A, Deconinck E, Plouvier E, Herve P, Humbert P, Cahn JY (1995) Phototherapy in the treatment of cutaneous graft-versus-host disease. Transplantation 59:151–155

38. Vogelsang GB, Wolff D, Altomonte V, Farmer E, Morison WL, Corio R, Horn T (1996) Treatment of chronic graft-versus-host disease with ultraviolet irradiation and psoralen (PUVA). Bone Marrow Transplant 17:1061–1067

39. Kelly GE, Meikle W, Sheil AG (1987) Effects of immunosuppressive therapy on the induction of skin tumors by ultraviolet irradiation in hairless mice. Transplantation 44:429–433

40. Altman JS, Adler SS (1994) Development of multiple cutaneous squamous cell carcinomas during PUVA treatment for chronic graft-versus-host disease. J Am Acad Dermatol 31:505–507

41. Aschan J (1994) Treatment of moderate to severe acute graft-versus-host disease: a retrospective analysis. Bone Marrow Transplant 14:601–607

42. Kerscher M, Volkenandt M, Meurer M, Lehmann P, Plewig G, Röcken M (1994) Treatment of localized scleroderma with PUVA bath photochemotherapy. Lancet i:1233

43. Kerscher M, Volkenandt M, Meurer M, Lehmann P, Plewig G, Röcken M (1995) PUVA-bath photochemotherapy of lichen planus. Arch Dermatol 131:1210–1211

44. Lüftl M, Degitz K, Plewig G, Röcken M (1997) Psoralen bath plus UV-A therapy. Possibilities and limitations. Arch Dermatol 1597–1603

45. Edelson R, Berger C, Gasparro F, Jegasothy B, Heald P, Wintroub B, Vonderheid V, Knobler R, Wolff K, Plewig G, McKiernan G, Christiansen I, Oster M, Hönigsmann H, Wilfert H, Kokoschka E, Rehle T, Perez M, Stingl G, Laroche L (1987) Treatment of leukemic cutaneous T cell lymphoma with extracorporeally-photoactivated 8-methoxypsoralen. N Engl J Med 316:297–303

46. Rook AH, Heald PW, Nahass GT, Macey W, Witmer WK, Lazarus GS, Jegasothy BV (1989) Treatment of autoimmune disease with extracorporeal photochemotherapy: pemphigus vulgaris – preliminary report. Yale J Biol Med 62:647–652

47. Rook AH, Freundlich B, Nahass GT, Washko R, Macelis B, Skolnicki M, Bromley P, Witmer WK, Jegasothy BV (1989) Treatment of autoimmune disease with extracorporeal photochemotherapy: progressive systemic sclerosis. Yale J Biol Med 62:639–645

48. Lüftl M, Röcken M, Plewig G, Degitz K (1998) PUVA inhibits DNA replication, but not gene transcription at nonlethal dosages. J Invest Dermatol 111:399–405
49. Lee KH, Garro J Jr (1989) Engineering aspects of extracorporeal photochemotherapy. Yale J Biol Med 62:621
50. Vowels BR, Cassin M, Boufal MH, Walsh L, Rook AH (1992) Extracorporeal photochemotherapy induces the production of tumor necrosis factor-α by monocytes: implications for the treatment of cutaneous T-cell lymphoma and systemic sclerosis. J Invest Dermatol 98:686–692
51. Yoo EK, Rook AH, Elenitsas R, Gasparro FP, Vowels BR (1996) Apoptosis induction by ultraviolet light A and photochemotherapy in cutaneous T-cell lymphoma: relevance to mechanism of therapeutic action. J Invest Dermatol 107:235–242
52. Lambert M, Ronai Z, Weinstein IB et al (1989) Enhancement of major histocompatibility class I protein synthesis by DNA damage in cultured human fibroblasts and keratinocytes. Mol Cell Biol 9:847–850
53. Ware R, Jiang H, Braunstein N, Kent J, Wiener E, Pernis B, Chess L (1995) Human CD8$^+$ T lymphocyte clones specific for T cell receptor V beta families expressed on autologous CD4$^+$ T cells. Immunity 2:177–184
54. Jiang H, Zhang S-I, Pernis B (1992) Role of CD8$^+$ T cells in murine experimental allergic encephalomyelitis. Science 256:1213–1215
55. Berger CL, Perez M, Laroche L, Edelson R (1990) Inhibition of autoimmune disease in a murine model of systemic lupus erythematosus induced by exposure to syngeneic photoinactivated lymphocytes. J Invest Dermatol 94:52–97
56. Girardi M, Herreid P, Tigelaar RE (1995) Specific suppression of lupus-like graft-versus-host disease using extracorporeal photochemical attenuation of effector lymphocytes. J Invest Dermatol 104:177–182
57. Besnier DP, Chabannes D, Mahe B, Mussini JMG, Baranger TAR, Muller JY, Milpied N, Esnault VLM (1997) Treatment of graft-versus-host disease by extracorporeal photochemotherapy. Transplantation 64:49–54
58. Gerber M, Gmeinhart B, Volc-Platzer B, Kalhs P, Greinix H, Knobler R (1997) Complete remission of lichen-planus-like graft-versus-host disease (GVHD) with extracorporeal photochemotherapy (ECP). Bone Marrow Transplant 19:517–519
59. Richter HI, Stege H, Ruzicka T, Söhngen D, Heyll A, Krutmann J (1997) Extracorporeal photopheresis in the treatment of acute graft-versus-host disease. J Am Acad Dermatol 36:787–789
60. Sniecinski I, Parker P, Dagis A, Collier T, Wang S, Rickard K, Snyder D, Nademanee A, Spielberger R, Rodriguez R, Krishnan A, Fung H, Stein A, O'Donnell M, Rosenthal J, Sahebi F, Kogut N, Falk P, Molina A, Loui W, Planas I, Niland J, Forman S (1998) Extracorporeal photopheresis (ECP) is an effective treatment of chronic refractory graft-versus-host disease (GVHD). Blood 92S:454a
61. Greinix HT, Volc-Platzer B, Rabitsch W, Gmeinhart B, Guevara-Pineda C, Kalhs P, Krutmann J, Hönigsmann H, Ciovica M, Knobler RM (1998)Successful use of extracorporeal photochemotherapy in the treatment of severe acute and chronic graft-versus-host disease. Blood 92:3098–3104
62. Owsianowski M, Gollnick H, Siegert W, Schwerdtfeger R, Orfanos CE (1994) Successful treatment of chronic graft-versus-host disease with extracorporeal photopheresis. Bone Marrow Transplant 14: 845–848
63. Rossetti F, Zulian F, Dall'Amico R, Messina C, Montini G, Zacchello F (1995) Extracorporeal photochemotherapy as single therapy for extensive, cutaneous, chronic graft-versus-host disease. Transplantation 59:149–151
64. Balda BR, Konstantinow A, Starz H, Gnekow A, Heidemann P (1996) Extracorporeal photochemotherapy as an effective treatment modality in chronic graft-versus-host disease. J Eur Acad Dermatol Venereol 7:155
65. Dall'Amico R, Rossetti R, Zulian F, Montini G, Murer L, Andreetta B, Messina C, Baraldi E, Montesco MC, Dini G, Locatelli F, Argiolu F, Zaccello G (1997) Photophere-

sis in paediatric patients with drug-resistant chronic graft-versus-host disease. Br J Haematol 97:848 – 854

66. Abhyankar S, Bishop M (1998) Adjunctive treatment of resistant chronic graft versus host disease with extracorporeal photopheresis using UVADEX sterile solution. Blood 92(S1):454a

67. Bishop MR, Ketcham M, Lynch J, Tarantolo SR, Pavletic ZS, Oria N, Morris M, Reddy RL, Armitage JO, Kessinger A (1998) Extracorporeal photopheresis permits steroid withdrawal in steroid-resistant chronic graft-versus-host disease. Blood 92(S1):455a

68. Hill JC, Sarvan J, Maske R, Els WJ (1994) Evidence that UV-B irradiation decreases corneal Langerhans cells and improves corneal graft survival in the rabbit. Transplantation 57:1281 – 1284

69. De Fazio SR, Gozzo J (1994) Prolongation of skin allograft survival by cotransplantation of ultraviolet B-irradiated skin. Transplantation 58:1044 – 1057

70. Habibullah CM, Ayesha Q, Khan AA, Naithani R, Lahiri S (1995) Xenotransplantation of UV-B-irradiated hepatocytes . Survival and immune response. Transplantation 59:1495 – 1497

71. Ohajewke OA, Hardy MA, Oluwole SF (1995) Prevention of graft-versus-host disease and the induction of transplant tolerance by low-dose UV-B irradiation of BM cells combined with cyclosporine immunosuppression. Transplantation 60:1510 – 1516

72. Yaron I, Yaron R, Oluwole SF, Hardy MA (1996) UVB irradiation of human-derived peripheral blood lymphocytes induces apoptosis but not T-cell anergy: additive effects with various immunosuppressive agents. Cell Immunol 168:258 – 266

73. Gowing H, Lawler M, Hagenbeek A, McCann SR, Pamphilon DH, Hudson J, van Weelden H, Braakman E, Martens ACM (1996) Effect of ultraviolet-B light on lymphocyte activity at doses at which normal bone marrow stem cells are preserved. Blood 87:1635 – 1643

74. Van Dooren-Greebe RJ, Schattenberg A, Koopman RJJ (1991) Chronic cutaneous graft-versus-host disease: successful treatment with UVB. Br J Dermatol 125:498 – 499

75. Torinuki W, Mauduit G, Guyotat, Archimbaud E, Fiere D, Thivolet J (1987) Effect of UVB radiation on the skin after allogeneic bone-marrow transplantation in man. Arch Dermatol Res 279:424 – 426

76. Butturini A, Seeger RC, Gale RP (1986) Recipient immune-competent T lymphocytes can survive intensive conditioning for bone marrow transplantation. Blood 68:954 – 958

77. Bierer BE, Emerson SG, Antin J et al (1988) Regulation of cytotoxic T lymphocyte-mediated graft rejection following bone marrow transplantation. Transplantation 46:835 – 839

78. Kernan NA, Flomenberg N, Dupont B, O'Reilly RJ (1987) Graft rejection in recipients of T cell depleted HLA-nonidentical marrow transplants for leukemia. Transplantation 43:842 – 847

79. Fleischhauer K, Kernan NA, O'Reilly RJ, Dupont B, Yang SY (1990) Bone marrow allograft rejection by T lymphocytes recognising a single amino acid difference in HLA-B44. N Engl J Med 323:1818 – 1822

80. Oluwole SF, Engelstad K, James T (1993) Prevention of graft-versus-host disease and bone marrow rejection: kinetics of induction of tolerance by UVB modulation of accessory cells and T cells in the bone marrow inoculum. Blood 81:1658 – 1665

81. Azuma E, Hatsumi Y, Kaplan J (1989) Use of lymphokine-activated killer cells to prevent bone marrow graft rejection and lethal graft-vs-host disease. J Immunol 143:1524 – 1529

82. Ohajewke OA, Hardy MA, Oluwole SF (1995) Prevention of graft-versus-host disease and the induction of transplant tolerance by low-dose UV-B irradiation of BM cells combined with cyclosporine immunosuppression. Transplantation 60:1510 – 1516

83. Deeg HJ (1988) Ultraviolet irradiation in transplantation biology. Transplantation 45:845 – 851

84. Barr ML, Meiser BM, Eisen HJ, Roberts RF, Livi U, Dall'Amico R, Dorent R, Rogers JG, Radovancevic B, Taylor DO, Jeevanadam V, Marboe CC (1998) Photopheresis for the prevention of rejection in cardiac transplantation. N Engl J Med 339:1744–1751
85. Dall'Amico R, Zacchello G (1998) Treatment of graft-versus-host disease with photopheresis. Transplantation 65:1283–1284

9 Phototherapy and Photochemotherapy: Less Common Indications for Its Use

Thomas Schwarz, Anita Rütter, John Hawk

Contents

The use of ultraviolet (UV) phototherapy and photochemotherapy for the treatment of skin disease has steadily expanded over recent decades. During that time, in addition to its confirmed efficacy for classical indications such as psoriasis vulgaris, atopic dermatitis, mycosis fungoides, polymorphic light eruption, and vitiligo, the treatment modality has also shown promise in the therapy of a variety of other dermatoses; however, since these conditions have been treated mostly on a tentative or trial basis, success rates have been poorly defined. Nevertheless, there has unquestionably been a steady increase in the number of dermatoses for which phototherapy can now be regarded as a standard therapeutic option, and such disorders include in particular scleroderma, urticaria pigmentosa, and lichen planus. In addition, a large number of case reports also suggest the efficacy of the treatment in a variety of other dermatoses; however, in these last instances, the reports are based mostly on single cases and no definite positive conclusions can be drawn. The true value of phototherapy in these disorders will therefore only become clear should controlled studies eventually become possible. This chapter now briefly reviews the evidence for the likely efficacy of phototherapy in all these rarer disorders; precise technical details from the various reports have not always been included, however, and in these instances the reader is strongly recommended to consult the original literature if the treatment is definitely being considered.

Lichen Planus

The apparent beneficial effect of PUVA in lichen planus was first reported shortly after the introduction of the technique as a treatment modality. In that study [8], remission was achieved in 15 patients with exanthematic lichen planus during the course of six systemic PUVA exposures. Ortonne et al. [83] confirmed these reports, demonstrating that six of seven patients with generalized forms of the disease also responded to systemic PUVA with remission. Subsequent studies then indicated an overall likely response rate of between 50 and 90 %, suggesting lichen planus to be less responsive to PUVA than psoriasis; in addition, more treatment sessions were generally necessary for complete clearance, while marked post-inflammatory hyperpigmentation sometimes led to significant long-lasting cosmetic disability. Further, by exposure of just half the body, Gonzalez et al. [23] also observed improvements in the unirradiated skin of 50 % of patients, thus suggesting PUVA might, in addition, exert a systemic effect, while the beneficial effect as well of bath PUVA was described in 1980 by Väätainen et al. [114], as apparently being even better than oral PUVA [33]. However, early relapses occurred with both regimens. In most of the Scandinavian bath studies, trioxsalen was used, although Kerscher et al. [50] have also recently demonstrated a successful outcome with 8-methoxypsoralen (8-MOP) in four patients with only lowish cumulative UVA doses ($7.2 - 11.2$ J/cm^2), while an improvement in the non-treated mucosal lesions of three patients again suggested that the PUVA may also act systemically; however, the complete remission of mucosal lesions purely by treatment of the skin appears unlikely. The same group has now confirmed the beneficial effect of bath PUVA in 12 further patients (53), all except one responding completely within 6 weeks, although with slightly higher cumulative doses ($10.1 - 23.9$ J/cm^2) than previously used.

Since mucosal lichen planus is a particularly difficult therapeutic problem, intraoral photochemotherapy has been tried for this aspect of the disease, Jansén et al. [41] having used a filtered irradiation device normally reserved for the hardening of dental fillings, with the psoralen administered systemically. In seven of eight patients marked improvements were observed. But although this advantageous effect was later confirmed in other studies [61, 64, 79], homogeneous irradiation of the oral cavity for an appropriate length of time has frequently presented major technical problems, being both difficult for the patient and potentially associated with severe thermal burning from the device if great care is not taken. Use of the technique has not, therefore, become widespread.

Disseminated and particularly hyperkeratotic forms of lichen planus can also be successfully treated by combined therapy with PUVA and retinoids, the latter generally being started some $2 - 3$ weeks before the former, as also recommended for psoriasis [21].

Thus, overall, PUVA is an effective therapeutic option for extensive lichen planus; however, this disease is usually much more resistant than psoriasis, for example, longer treatment periods and higher cumulative doses generally being necessary. In addition, early relapse is possible, while lichen planus can also sometimes be actinically induced [117]; in such cases, PUVA may also conceivably aggravate the condition [23].

Pityriasis Lichenoides and Lymphomatoid Papulosis

Both pityriasis lichenoides acuta (PLA) and chronica (PLC) can have prolonged courses and be markedly resistant to therapy. However, the well-accepted useful effect of sunlight on the latter was noted by LeVine [63], who also successfully administered UVB phototherapy for the condition; similar beneficial effects have been observed for PUVA [7, 36, 90], although UVB should probably be used first and PUVA reserved for resistant cases [37]. Brenner et al. [8] also demonstrated the effectiveness of PUVA in PLA, a finding later confirmed by Powell et al.; in fact, since PLA lesions are often more indurated and erosive than those of PLC, thus generally responding relatively poorly to UVB, Honig et al. [37] recommend PUVA as the treatment of choice for the former, although relapse may still occur.

In the study by Brenner et al. [8], a patient with the probably related lymphomatoid papulosis was also successfully treated with PUVA, the therapy then being tapered off over 3 1/2 months; however, relapse occurred 4 months after the treatment was finally stopped. Lange-Wantzin and Thomsen [55] also demonstrated the beneficial effect of PUVA in five lymphomatoid papulosis patients, although this study in addition clearly indicated limitations of the therapy. Thus, complete remission was achieved in only one patient, with only a partial response in the other four, while in most cases too, relapse occurred when the PUVA was stopped, thus leading to a requirement for continuous therapy; because of its potential long-term side effects, however, this cannot safely be recommended, and Willemze and Beljaards [125], therefore, regard lymphomatoid papulosis as only a relative indication for PUVA. Nevertheless, bath PUVA has recently been used successfully in a 6-year-old child with the condition [119], complete clearance of the disorder being noted within 30 sessions (cumulative dose: 28.5 J/cm^2). Whether or not such treatment is undertaken, however, the regular follow-up of all patients with the condition is recommended to ensure early detection of any possible progression towards malignant lymphoma.

Pityriasis Rosea

Pityriasis rosea is a benign, relatively self-limiting dermatosis not generally requiring specific therapy. However, Arndt et al. [4] did evaluate the effect of UVB in a controlled study, 20 patients being treated over just half their bodies with five exposures starting at 80 % of the initial minimal erythema dose; 50 %

reported a significant improvement in pruritus on the treated side. Further, since these patients suffered their pityriasis rosea for an average of only 9 days as a result, the authors recommended the early initiation of phototherapy for the condition. A further bilateral comparison study undertaken elsewhere on 17 patients then apparently confirmed this beneficial effect [59], the placebo side however not being left untreated on this occasion but exposed to 1 J/cm^2 of UVA 5 times weekly over 2 weeks; improvement just on the UVB side was noted after only three exposures. Later evaluation, however, failed to confirm any advantage of the UVB, while any pruritus present was also apparently unaffected by the therapy. Taken together, therefore, these studies suggest pityriasis rosea to be a questionable indication for UVB therapy, particularly because of its self-limiting benign course; furthermore, inflammatory irritated pityriasis rosea should probably not be treated in this way because of its potential to deteriorate with the treatment.

Seborrheic Dermatitis

UV radiation appears to exert a relatively beneficial effect on seborrheic dermatitis, the condition generally improving in summer and on sunny holidays; however, deterioration too may occur in some subjects. Nevertheless, useful effects can often be achieved with artificial UVB, while PUVA has also been used in three cases of erythrodermic disease [15], the patients having suffered disease deterioration after the cessation of long-term topical steroid therapy; however, 8 % of psoriatic patients undergoing PUVA therapy in one study demonstrated a worsening of their facial seborrheic features [112].

Palmoplantar Dermatoses

Chronic allergic contact dermatitis of the hands may, on occasion, present a severe therapeutic problem, particularly if the causative contact agent cannot be identified or avoided; in such instances, the regular application of topical corticosteroid preparations has been the major therapeutic option, although their occasional potential to induce side effects has led to a search as well for other effective treatments. Thus, Mørk and Austad [76] attempted to treat the condition with UVB in 1983, their rationale being the presumed immunosuppressive activity of the radiation [5, 52]; although seven of their ten patients responded excellently, the exposure sessions had to be continued at least weekly to achieve long-term remissions. Sjövall and Christensen [99] then compared the local and systemic effects of UVB and UVA on the allergic patch test reactions of patients sensitive to nickel, UVA not having any effect while UVB caused significant reductions in the responses. Reduced patch test activity was also observed when the patch areas were spared but the rest of the body exposed, again suggesting a systemic effect for UVB and that patch tests should perhaps best not be performed in recently UVB-exposed patients. The authors also further evaluated the local and systemic effects of UVB on chronic palmar eczema [100]. Eighteen patients with contact dermatitis to a variety of allergens were subjected variously to placebo irradiation, UVB exposure of the hands, and UVB exposure of the hands and the body. No change was observed in the placebo group, but a marked improvement after irradiation of the hands was even greater after total body irradiation as well. However, relapse then generally occurred after cessation of the treatment, as also in Mørk and Austad's study [76].

Bruynzeel et al. [10] also successfully treated six of nine allergic contact dermatitis patients with systemic PUVA, complete remissions being observed after a mean 23 exposures; however, recurrent exposure courses were necessary to maintain the remissions. Hawk and LeGrice [31] further reported the beneficial effect of topical as well as systemic PUVA in chronic palmoplantar eczema, although some treatment failures occurred in severe cases, and relapses were usual; palmoplantar psoriasis also responded, but the pustular form less well. The beneficial effect of local as well as systemic PUVA for palmoplantar pustulosis has also been noted by other groups [74, 77, 88], while LeVine et al. [62] reported the successful use of systemic PUVA in dyshidrotic eczema.

Bath PUVA of the palms and soles is also of value in the management of chronic palmoplantar eczema, and is better than the previously used topical paint PUVA, having as advantages the usual absence of photosensitivity and hyperpigmentation reactions; thus Schemp et al. [95] achieved an excellent or good response in 93 % of patients with dyshidrotic and 86 % of patients with hyperkeratotic eczema. Cream PUVA therapy may also represent an interesting alternative in clinical practice [106], the 8-MOP being applied some 2 h before UVA exposure in a cream containing 0.0006 % 8-MOP in a 30 % water-in-oil emulsion. Phototherapy and photochemotherapy thus appear valuable therapeutic options in the treatment of palmoplantar eczemas, an efficacy confirmed by our own experience, which also suggests, however, that the treatment failure rate may be higher than reported, perhaps because of an investigator tendency to report successes rather than failures, except in rare instances [40].

Keratosis Lichenoides Chronica

Keratosis lichenoides chronica is a non-life-threatening but generally extremely disabling dermatosis characterized by extensive areas of linear, reticulate hyperkeratosis affecting particularly the face and by swollen, often hyperkeratotic, periungual areas. Optimistically, however, Lang [54] has reported the successful use of PUVA in one patient resistant to all other therapies; this efficacy was also noted by Ryatt et al. [93], while the combination of PUVA with systemic retinoids may be even more effective [16, 18].

Purpura Pigmentosa

Purpura pigmentosa is a harmless but often cosmetically unpleasant disorder frequently resistant to conventional treatment. Simon and Hunyadi [98], however, have reported the successful use of PUVA in the condition, a response also achieved in a side-by-side study by Wong and Ratnam in a further patient [127]; another of their patients too, initially resistant to UVB, was successfully treated with PUVA, while Krisza et al. [53] confirmed the efficacy of PUVA in seven other patients. Thus, PUVA appears to be the treatment of choice for purpura pigmentosa, once underlying causes such as its possible induction by drugs have been excluded.

Scleroderma

Localized scleroderma (morphea) is a not uncommon disorder generally resistant to therapy. Young adults are most often affected, females more than males; widely disseminated morphea may also be associated with restricted joint and chest wall mobility. Pathogenesis is uncertain, genetic, immunological, toxic, viral, hormonal, and vascular factors having all been invoked; at least in some cases, however, Borrelia burgdorferi infection appears implicated, which may explain the occasional therapeutic success of antibiotics such as penicillin in some inflammatory forms.

In other variants, a selection of other treatments, particularly phenytoin, chloroquine, griseofulvin, penicillamine, and retinoids have also been used with very limited success. A major breakthrough, however, was claimed with the use of bath PUVA therapy, Kerscher et al. [51] in 1994 having described two patients treated in this way. A 20-min immersion of the patient in 8-MOP solution followed by UVA irradiation of the affected skin starting with a dose of 0.2 J/cm^2 was undertaken, 20 sessions 4 times weekly being used initially and gradually reduced to twice weekly over 5 weeks. After 30 sessions, complete or almost complete remission of the sclerotic patches was noted in both patients, all the lesions softening clinically and improving histologically. The efficacy of bath PUVA has since been confirmed [48], although a minimum treatment duration of 6–8 weeks is needed and relapse rates have yet to be evaluated. Bath PUVA has also been reported as useful in scleroderma adultorum [28]. Further, in our hands, although in relatively few patients, oral PUVA too has been effective, as it has also in the treatment of a child with severely disabling pansclerotic morphea [94]. Thus, this 8-year-old girl had rapidly developed progressive morphea with joint contractures, systemic corticosteroids, and interferon-γ either as monotherapies or in combination with pentoxifylline being initially unsuccessful. Systemic PUVA was therefore initiated with oral 8-MOP at a dose of 15 mg and a UVA commencement dose of 0.5 J/cm^2, four exposures per week being given over 2 months increasing up to a maximum irradiation dose of 1.8 J/cm^2, after which maintenance therapy at that dose was undertaken twice weekly for 6 months. A marked reduction in dermatosclerosis, the complete healing of all ulceration-ions, and an improvement in joint mobility were observed, although relapse then occurred over a further 14 months. Recently, the successful administration of UVA-1 phototherapy in localized morphea has also been reported by Kerscher et al. [47] in ten patients suffering from extensive disease. Thus over 6 weeks, the patients were subjected to exposures of 20 J/cm^2 4 times weekly, leading in all cases to complete remission of the dermatosclerotic lesions within, at most, 15 exposures; by 24 treatments, over 80 % of the lesions were in regression. Histopathological and sonographic studies (20 MHz ultrasound) confirmed the clinical impressions. Successful outcomes were also reported in 30 further patients irradiated with 20 J/cm² UVA-1 over 12 weeks (total number of treatments: 30; cumulative dose: 600 J/cm²) [49]; this regimen was also incidentally effective in a 16-year-old male with disabling pansclerotic morphea [27]. Stege et al. then also used high-dose UVA-1-therapy for localized morphea, 17 patients being irradiated over 30 visits with either 130 J/cm² or 20 J/cm² [105], the high-dose regimen appearing superior.

The mode of action of PUVA and UVA-1 therapy in scleroderma remains to be determined. However, both in vitro and in vivo studies have demonstrated that UV irradiation induces the synthesis of collagenase, thus resulting in increased collagen degradation [105, 126]; since morphea is associated with increased collagen synthesis, phototherapy may well act through this mechanism in the disease. In addition, both UVA and PUVA bring about the release of cytokines, particularly tumor necrosis factor-α and interleukin-6, which also induce collagenase and inhibit collagen synthesis; this perhaps further contributes to the beneficial effect of phototherapy. Finally, the well-recognized immunosuppressive effect of phototherapy may contribute as well.

Granuloma Annulare

Granuloma annulare is a benign disorder of generally little significance apart from its, at times, unsightly appearance and rare associated pruritus; in addition, it usually has a self-limiting course such that the need for major therapy is at most relative, particularly since topical treatments such as corticosteroids or occasionally cryotherapy are frequently sufficient in any case. On the other hand, the disorder is at times disseminated and may thus lead to requests for therapy for purely cosmetic reasons; in that the underlying cause of the disease remains unknown, however, many varying treatments such as, for example, sulfones, potassium iodide, chloroquine, niacinamide, gold, and oral or topical corticosteroids have been tried, usually without major success. In 1981, PUVA was added to this list [66], topical therapy with a 0.15 % 8-MOP solution proving effective. Since then, other studies have confirmed this efficacy, cumulative UVA doses varying from 10.5 to 110 to 400 J/cm² [35, 46, 129]; a more recent report [56], however, and our own experience in three cases, suggest that bath and systemic PUVA are equally effective. The mode of action of PUVA in granuloma annulare nevertheless remains to be determined, while the numerous therapeutic variations tried also suggest there is no clear optimal regimen of administration. Therefore, the potential side-effect profile of the therapy must be considered before the treatment is offered, particularly as spontaneous regression of the disorder in children and young adults is relatively frequent; PUVA should thus only be used when all other reasonable approaches have failed and the patient remains insistent on treatment.

Mastocytosis

Mastocytosis is a spectrum of disorders characterized by the abnormal proliferation of mast cells within a variety of organs, especially the skin; since there are both benign and malignant forms, such as, for example, mastocytoma and mast cell leukemia, differing therapeutic approaches must be adopted. Thus, localized mastocytoma and diffuse mastocytosis in the very young generally regress spontaneously without treatment; on the other hand, systemic mastocytosis with its associated internal organ involvement may require systemic interferon-α or other chemotherapy such as chlorambucil, while in cases associated with systemic flushing, diarrhea, or tachycardia, H1 and H2 antihistamines may also be necessary. Finally, classical urticaria pigmentosa with its disseminated maculopapules may lead to patient requests for therapy for purely cosmetic reasons, even without subjective symptoms or internal organ involvement; on the other hand, pruritus may also be severe in the condition, often in association with whealing after mechanical trauma, the so-called Darier's sign.

Classical urticaria pigmentosa is generally resistant to conventional therapy, although corticosteroids topically under occlusion or by intralesional injection may sometimes improve localized lesions. With the introduction of PUVA, however, a new therapeutic regimen for the condition became available; thus, Christophers et al. [12] first reported the efficacy of the therapy, all ten of his patients showing marked improvements in their pruritus and Darier's signs, even if most of the hyperpigmented lesions did not regress. Vella Briffa et al. [118] then similarly treated eight patients, one with systemic involvement, all except the last again reporting significant improvements in pruritus and whealing, but now also in the typical macules, some even disappearing completely; initially, however, the patients complained of worse pruritus, which then gradually improved as the irradiation doses increased. In children too, PUVA is often helpful, seeming justified particularly in widespread, disabling mastocytosis [101]; thus, four children who had not responded to various other treatment modalities dramatically improved or remitted with systemic PUVA, no relapses occurring over a further 6 years.

To avoid the possible effects of sudden mediator release from treated mast cells in urticaria pigmentosa, a PUVA regimen of gradually increasing doses, especially initially, seems advisable, although the therapy should otherwise be undertaken according to usual guidelines with 0.6 mg/kg body weight of 8-MOP and 2, 3, or 4 times weekly treatment. Therapeutic responsiveness may also be evaluated during treatment by the scoring of any improvements in pruritus, flushing, or Darier's sign. Biopsies before and after PUVA, however, did not show any mast cell changes in one study, whether from involved or uninvolved skin; similarly, no changes in skin histamine concentrations occurred [118]. On the other hand, significant decreases in mast cell numbers and in the urinary histamine metabolite, 1-methyl-4-imidazoloacetic acid, after PUVA occurred in another, these findings correlating with similar reductions in pruritus and the typical maculopapules [26]. Väätäinen et al. [114] also used bath PUVA in urticaria pigmentosa, 5 patients responding successfully to trioxsalen baths followed by UVA irradiation; in contrast, however, Godt et al. found the bath method ineffective but systemic PUVA helpful [25], perhaps because topically applied 8-MOP may concentrate mostly in the epidermis but systemically more readily reach the dermis where the mast cells are located. Overall, therefore, cutaneous urticaria pigmentosa appears generally to respond moderately to PUVA, but usually only slowly, partially and with early relapse after treatment cessation. On the other hand, relatively prolonged remissions have been reported in four patients exposed to high-dose UVA-1 (111), 130 J/cm² being administered 5 times weekly for 2 weeks; their pruritus diminished after only three sessions, while any diarrhea and headache also improved, along with reductions in urinary histamine metabolites. Remissions then lasted 10–23 months; however, such prompt responses and long disease-free periods after only ten exposures are perhaps unexpected, and these encouraging observations now need confirmation in more extended studies.

Scleromyxedema

Scleromyxedema is a widespread, chronic, progressive, skin, and generally later systemic, disease, with unpredictable prognosis and poor response to treatment; in its advanced stages, internal organ involvement often requires chemotherapy with cyclophosphamide, the current treatment of choice. Early on, however, systemic PUVA may improve the cutaneous disease; Farr and Ive [19] first treated a patient who responded only somewhat to combined cyclophosphamide and steroid therapy, after which 2 months of PUVA markedly improved the infiltrative skin lesions. Schirren et al. [96] also reported a moderate cutaneous response in a patient with relatively advanced disease following the administration of melphalan and PUVA. From our own experience, the early use of PUVA appears appropriate; one 31-year-old female patient, for example, responded very satisfactorily to PUVA and systemic steroids [104].

These various reports thus clearly indicate that PUVA may often improve the cutaneous features of scleromyxedema without systemic effect, there generally being no change in circulating paraprotein levels; UVB phototherapy, however, does not appear effective and there has even been one report of its exacerbation of lichen myxedematosus [128]. Even after a satisfactory course of PUVA, however, regular patient follow-up is advisable to enable the early recognition of internal disease progression.

Histiocytosis X

Histiocytosis X behaves similarly to scleromyxedema as far as phototherapy is concerned. Thus while internal organ involvement is a clear indication for chemotherapy, PUVA may be recommended for the cutaneous lesions, especially in adults. Thus, Iwatsuki et al. [39] treated two patients with both UVB and PUVA, the latter being more effective. After the cessation of therapy, however, rapid relapse occurred, although the disease remained responsive to PUVA; these observations were then confirmed by Neumann et al. [80] and Kaudewitz et al. [45]. Further, since epidermal Langerhans' cells, the progenitors of histiocytosis X, are extremely UV-sensitive [1], such satisfactory responses are perhaps not unexpected.

Eosinophilic Dermatoses

Hypereosinophilic syndrome is characterized by a pronounced peripheral blood eosinophilia, disseminated eosinophilic organ involvement, and systemic symptoms; for firm diagnosis, however, other causes of eosinophilia, such as parasitic infection, must first be excluded. The syndrome apparently represents a spectrum of eosinophilic dermatoses, ranging from Nir-Westfried eosino-philic dermatitis on the one hand to eosinophilic leukemia [82] on the other; it is particularly characterized by severe generalized pruritus and very resistant to conventional therapy. Van den Hoogenband et al. [115], however, reported the successful treatment of its cutaneous lesions with PUVA when systemic steroids and sulfones had been ineffective; Wemmer et al. [124] also reported an excellent response in a patient with just skin involvement. Thus, PUVA appears to be the treatment of choice for the cutaneous features of hypereosinophilic syndrome, even in patients with the human immunodeficiency virus [67]; it may also be administered with steroids and cytostatic drugs if systemic involvement is present. Bath PUVA also appears effective [17]. In addition, the eosinophilic pustular folliculitis of Ofuji, perhaps a follicular variant of subcorneal pustular dermatosis and characterized by asymmetrically distributed circular papules and pustules of mainly the face and trunk, may also respond well to systemic PUVA [9].

Pruritus

UVB therapy can be beneficial in various forms of pruritus, particularly those associated with diabetes and hepatic disorders, and certain idiopathic types, while a number of controlled studies have also demonstrated its efficacy in uremic pruritus [22, 34]. Remissions in hepatic disease, however, are relatively short-lived [30], although Person [89] observed a remarkable improvement in one patient with cholestatic pruritus. Both bath and systemic PUVA have also been successfully used in aquagenic pruritus [69, 102], even in cases associated with polycythemia rubra vera, or the myelodysplastic syndrome [69]. The beneficial effect of PUVA on the pruritus of polycythemia rubra vera alone has also been reported by Swerlick [110] and Jeanmougin et al. [42], the pruritus of these hematological disorders often being so severe as to clearly justify this form of therapy [75], even with its usual need for maintenance treatment [42]. The mechanism of action of PUVA in the various forms of pruritus remains to be determined, although its effects on mast cell degranulation, cutaneous histamine reactivity, and neural sensitivity threshold may conceivably be responsible [75]; thus, Fjellner and Hägermark [20] demonstrated in 1982 that UVB, UVA, and PUVA can all significantly reduce cutaneous responsiveness to the histamine liberator 48/80, although UVB was effective only after the direct injection of histamine. It is worth noting, however, that dryness of the skin may result from long-term recurrent exposure to UV radiation, and the regular use of topical emollients by treated patients is therefore advised.

HIV-Associated Dermatoses

The safety or otherwise of phototherapy for human immunodeficiency virus (HIV)-infected patients remains uncertain [2]. Thus, many of the cutaneous problems able to occur during the disease, such as for example psoriasis, pruritus, pruritic papular eruption, and folliculitis, may respond favorably to such treatment; on the other hand, the therapy also tends to have an immunosuppressive effect [5, 52], while potentially inducing HIV replication as well [97, 122, 130]. Nevertheless, UVB phototherapy is in fact relatively effective in pruritic papular eruption, Pardo et al. [85] having treated eight patients with UVB 3 times weekly, the initial exposure dose being 60 % of that necessary for minimal erythema, followed by 10 % increments thereafter. Therapy was stopped a month later if the pruritus was clear, or continued if not; seven of the patients improved well, the inflammatory infiltrate of mainly CD4+, CD8+, and CD2+ cells also being reduced, although relapse always occurred by about 8 weeks. UVB has also been effective in HIV patients with eosinophilic pustular folliculitis [11, 72], while Weiss and Taylor [123] noted that the pruritus of HIV responds too, although once again there was rapid relapse after treatment stopped; Gorin et al. [24] then used PUVA for severe HIV pruritus, a marked improvement again being observed by 4 weeks, while any folliculitis present also responded. In four other patients, UVA therapy alone also helped HIV pruritus, while May et al. [67] reported almost complete remissions in the pruritus of HIV-associated hypereosinophilic syndrome in two patients. Overall, therefore, UVB phototherapy and PUVA both appear effective in the treatment of HIV-associated pruritus [38], although it remains unclear whether the treatments can also lead to progression of the HIV disease. Thus, Ranki et al. [91] treated five HIV-positive patients with systemic PUVA, their skin lesions of psoriasis, seborrheic dermatitis, folliculitis, or pruritus responding very well over a few weeks; in two patients, however, CD4+ lymphocyte numbers were also reduced, although their serum and urinary β_2-microglobulin and neopterin, and serum HIV antigen, levels were not affected. Further, interestingly, in two of the patients, the tuberculin recall reaction was negative before phototherapy and positive afterwards. Horn et al. [38], however, also treated a series of HIV-positive patients with PUVA, and noted no changes in CD4+ cell numbers or viral antigen concentrations, while Meola et al. [70] similarly treated six other patients, five with psoriasis, one with pruritus, with UVB for several weeks and again found no significant changes in serum CD4+ or CD8+ cell numbers or β_2-microglobulin concentrations; one of the patients, however, p24-antigen-negative at the start of therapy, did become positive later. Nevertheless, in none of the studies was an increase in patient opportunistic infections observed, and

UVB and PUVA thus appear at least relatively safe in HIV-positive patients. Notwithstanding these observations, however, one survey of interviews and literature searches has clearly suggested that HIV-positive patients are much more likely to be offered UVB than PUVA as compared with normal subjects, and also more likely to be treated for pruritic conditions than for psoriasis [108]. Thus, particularly in view of the various in vitro studies on the matter [97, 122, 130], it remains clear that decisions concerning the treatment of any given HIV-positive patient must be made on an individual basis by the supervising physician until larger scale, longer term, and better controlled clinical studies are available [2]; the possible risk of increased photosensitivity in such patients should also be taken into account before any phototherapy is commenced [84]. Finally, HIV patients should still generally be advised to protect themselves as much as reasonably possible from ambient UV exposure.

Alopecia Areata

The treatment of resistant alopecia areata remains one of the most difficult therapeutic problems in dermatology; thus it is not surprising that in addition to the many other therapeutic trials undertaken in the condition, phototherapy and in particular photochemotherapy have also been investigated. Thus, Rollier and Warcewski [92] reported in 1974 that the systemic administration of 8-MOP to patients followed by their exposure shortly afterwards to natural sunlight could lead to some hair regrowth. Lassus et al. [57] in 1980 then compared the efficacy of local and systemic PUVA in 41 patients with various forms of the disease, the best responses occurring in patients with localized hair loss; the totalis and universalis forms had much poorer success rates. Patients with atopy also appeared to respond less well, as did those with longstanding disease, while no response at all occurred if the condition had been present for more than 8 years; overall, however, PUVA seemed a reasonable therapeutic option for alopecia patients resistant to other forms of treatment. In 1983, Claudy et al. [14] again claimed that PUVA was effective in 23 patients, 11 of 17 with multiple lesions, alopecia totalis or alopecia universalis undergoing either complete remission or improvements of around 90 % after systemic PUVA, with average cumulative UVA doses of 505 J/cm^2; three did, however, relapse after the cessation of therapy. On the other hand, these findings were in sharp contrast to those of van der Schar and Sillevis Smitt [116], who instead noted very poor PUVA treatment outcomes; thus of 30 patients treated with systemic total body PUVA, only nine demonstrated any hair regrowth, and six had relapsed within 7.7 months. These findings are in accordance too with those of Mitchell and Douglass [73], who treated 22 patients with topical PUVA; although 45 % initially showed some regrowth, no long-term response was noted. As a result, Mitchell and Douglass were unable in general to recommend PUVA for alopecia areata, although they did suggest it might be tried in patients with particularly severe involvement. Another study, the largest to date on the matter, was then undertaken in 1993 by Healy and Rogers [32], 102 patients receiving 8-MOP systemically or topically followed by scalp or total body by UVA exposure; although 90 % hair regrowth was observed in 53 % of subjects, high relapse rates over follow-up periods of up to 10 years led the authors to conclude that PUVA cannot be recommended for alopecia areata. These conclusions were also reached by Taylor and Hawk [111], who studied the efficacy of PUVA in 70 patients with alopecia areata partialis, totalis, or universalis; a useful long-term response was observed in only 6.3 % of the alopecia areata partialis patients, 12.5 % of those with alopecia areata totalis and 13.3 % of those with alopecia areata universalis. Finally, Alabdulkareem et al. in a study of a further 25 patients again reached a similar conclusion [3].

Acne Vulgaris

Because of the modern availability of effective therapeutic agents for acne such as antibiotics and retinoids, the use of phototherapy and photochemotherapy for the condition is essentially of only historical value. However, a summer-time improvement in the disorder is well recognized by many patients [71], while more specific studies have also suggested a positive effect for UVB selective ultraviolet phototherapy (SUP) [58] and UVA [68]. On the other hand, a relatively large study of 126 patients did not note any beneficial effect from either UVB or PUVA [71], a finding in accordance too with that of Parrish et al. [86]; Nielsen and Thormann [81] also even observed the induction of acne-like lesions during PUVA, while a comedogenic effect following long-term UVB-exposure has been claimed as well. UVB and PUVA do not therefore appear indicated for the regular treatment of acne, although they may perhaps be worth an occasional trial for the urgent short-term therapy of patients attending special events in the near future.

Lupus Erythematosus

Phototherapy and photochemotherapy have been considered absolutely contra-indicated in lupus erythematosus because of the potential severity of the disease and its frequent clear exacerbations following UV exposure, a fact confirmed by experimental evidence. However, because of contraindications to treatment with corticosteroids and other immunosuppressive therapies in one 71-year-old female patient with the subacute cutaneous form of the disease, UVA-1 (340–400 nm) phototherapy was very tentatively administered instead, a total dose of 186 J/cm^2 being administered in two series of exposures over 9 weeks [103]. Remarkably, the inflammatory cutaneous lesions had considerably improved by 6 weeks, the regression then persisting over several months. Thus, although lupus is indeed potentially UV-induced, the action spectrum for its induction is apparently mostly in the UVB range [60], and this interesting report now needs confirmation in larger patient numbers. Until such data are available, however, great caution should be exercised in the use of UVA-1 therapy for lupus.

Other Dermatoses

Transient acantholytic dermatosis (Grover's disease) is usually characterized by exacerbations following UV exposure; however, Paul and Arndt [87], observed a marked improvement in the condition of one patient following systemic PUVA, a coincidental spontaneous remission being excluded by the lack of response on unexposed areas. Interestingly, the condition initially worsened, before significantly improving as treatment continued.

Papular erythroderma (of Ofuji) is characterized by a persistent pruritus, a circulating eosinophilia and the presence of extensive brown-red flat papules sparing skin folds (the so-called deck chair sign); Wakeel et al. [121] interestinaly achieved a 9-month remission in one such patient with systemic PUVA.

Ichthyosis linearis circumflexa has also responded to systemic PUVA in two patients with the condition [65, 78].

Prurigo nodularis is well known for its intractable nature, including often in our experience following systemic PUVA and UVB; however, Väätäinen et al. [113] and Karvonen et al. [44] instead reported beneficial effects in the condition from bath PUVA with trioxsalen. Further studies are needed for confirmation.

Prurigo simplex subacuta may also respond moderately to bath PUVA [13, 109].

Persistent arthropod reactions too have been claimed to respond to systemic PUVA [6]; however, these lesions also usually respond to much simpler treatments such as topical or injected corticosteroids, and phototherapy is likely to be at most very rarely needed.

Halkier-Sørensen et al. [29] have further used topical PUVA successfully in the treatment of 20 nail dystrophy, a 0.15 % 8-MOP solution being applied to the digit eponychial areas 45 min before UVA exposure; improvements only occurred on the exposed areas. In view of the lack of other therapeutic measures, however, this approach may represent an interesting advance, although so far based on only one report.

Finally, Kalimo et al. [43] have used PUVA successfully in five patients with dermatitis herpetiformis not responding to a gluten-free diet; nevertheless, the condition does generally respond to this diet or dapsone, and PUVA is again likely to be needed on at most extremely rare occasions.

References

1. Aberer W, Schuler G, Stingl G, Hönigsmann H, Wolff K (1981) Ultraviolet light depletes surface markers of Langerhans cells. J Invest Dermatol 76:202–210
2. Adams ML, Houpt KR, Cruz PD (1996) Is phototherapy safe for HIV-infected individuals? Photochem Photobiol 64:234–237
3. Alabdulkareem AS, Abahussein AA, Okoro A (1996) Minimal benefit from photochemotherapy for alopecia areata. Int J Dermatol 35:890–891
4. Arndt KA, Paul BS, Stern RS, Parrish JA (1983) Treatment of pityriasis rosea with UV radiation. Arch Dermatol 119:381–382
5. Baadsgaard O (1991) In vivo ultraviolet irradiation of human skin results in profound perturbation of the immune system. Arch Dermatol 127:99–109

6. Beacham BE, Kurgansky D (1990) Persistent bite reactions responsive to photoche-motherapy. Br J Dermatol 123:693–694
7. Boelen RE, Faber WR, Lambers JCCA, Cormane RH (1982) Long-term follow-up of photochemotherapy in pityriasis lichenoides. Acta Derm Venereol 62:442–444
8. Brenner W, Gschnait F, Hönigsmann H, Fritsch P (1978) Erprobung von PUVA bei verschiedenen Dermatosen. Hautarzt 29:541–544
9. Breit R, Röcken M (1991) Klassische Form einer eosinophilen pustulösen Follikulitis – erfolgreiche Therapie mit PUVA. Hautarzt 42:247–250
10. Bruynzeel DP, Boonk WJ, van Ketel WG (1982) Oral psoralen photochemotherapy of allergic contact dermatitis of the hands. Dermatosen 30:16–20
11. Buchness MR, Lim HW, Hatcher VA, Sanchez M, Soter NA (1988) Eosinophilic pus-tular folliculitis in the acquired immunodeficiency syndrome. Treatment with ultra-violet B phototherapy. N Engl J Med 318:1183–1186
12. Christophers E, Hönigsmann H, Wolff K, Langner A (1978) PUVA-treatment of urti-caria pigmentosa. Br J Dermatol 98:701–702
13. Clark AR, Jorizzo JL, Fleischer AB (1998) Papular dermatitis (subacute prurigo, "itchy red bump" disease): pilot study of phototherapy. J Am Acad Dermatol 38:929–933
14. Claudy AL, Gagnaire D (1983) PUVA treatment of alopecia areata. Arch Dermatol 119:975–978
15. Dahl KB, Reymann F (1977) Photochemotherapy of erythrodermic seborrheic der-matitis. Arch Dermatol 113:1295–1296
16. Duschet P, Schwarz T, Gschnait F (1987) Keratosis lichenoides chronica. Hautarzt 38:678–682
17. Eberlein A, von Kobyletzki G, Gruss C, Dirschka T, Kerscher M, Altmeyer P (1997) Erfolgreiche Monotherapie der hypereosinophilen Dermatitis mit PUVA-Bad-Photochemotherapie. Hautarzt 48:820–823
18. Elbracht C, Wolf AF, Landes E (1983) Keratosis lichenoides chronica. Z Hautkr 58:701–708
19. Farr PM, Ive FA (1984) PUVA treatment of scleromyxoedema. Br J Dermatol 110:347–350
20. Fjellner B, Hägermark Ö (1982) Influence of ultraviolet light on itch and flare reac-tions in human skin induced by histamine and the histamine liberator compound 48/80. Acta Derm Venereol 62:137–140
21. Fritsch PO, Hönigsmann H, Jaschke E, Wolff K (1978) Augmentation of oral methoxysalen-photochemotherapy with an oral retinoic acid derivative. J Invest Dermatol 70:178–182
22. Gilchrest BA (1979) Ultraviolet phototherapy of uremic pruritus. Int J Dermatol 18:741–748
23. Gonzalez E, Momtaz K, Freedman ST (1984) Bilateral comparison of generalized lichen planus treated with psoralens and ultraviolet A. J Am Acad Dermatol 10:958–961
24. Gorin I, Lessana-Leibowitch M, Fortier P, Leibowitch J, Escande JP (1989) Successful treatment of the pruritus of human immunodeficiency virus infection and acquired immunodeficiency syndrome with psoralen plus ultraviolet A therapy. J Am Acad Dermatol 20:511–513
25. Godt O, Proksch E, Streit V, Christophers E (1997) Short- and long-term effective-ness of oral and bath PUVA therapy in urticaria pigmentosa and systemic mastocy-tosis. Dermatology 195:35–39
26. Granerus G, Roupe G, Swanbeck G (1981) Decreased urinary histamine metabolite after successful PUVA treatment of urticaria pigmentosa. J Invest Dermatol 76:1–3
27. Gruss C, Stücker M, von Kobyletzki G, Schreiber D, Altmeyer P, Kerscher M (1997) Low dose UVA1 photochemotherapy in disabling pansclerotic morphoea of child-hood. Br J Dermatol 136:293–294

28. Hager CM, Sobhi HA, Hunzelmann, N, Wickenhauser C, Scharenberg R, Krieg T, Scharffetter-Kochanek K (1998) Bath PUVA therapy in three patients with scleroderma adultorum. J Am Acad Dermatol 38:240–242
29. Halkier-Sørensen L, Cramers M, Kragballe K (1990) Twenty-nail dystrophy treated with topical PUVA. Acta Derm Venereol 70:510–511
30. Hanid MA, Levi AJ (1980) Phototherapy for pruritus in primary biliary cirrhosis. Lancet ii:530
31. Hawk JLM, Le Grice P (1994) The efficacy of localized PUVA therapy for chronic hand and foot dermatoses. Clin Exp Dermatol 19:479–482
32. Healy E, Rogers S (1993) PUVA treatment for alopecia areata – does it work? A retrospective review of 102 cases. Br J Dermatol 129:42–44
33. Helander I, Jansén CT, Meurman L (1987) Long-term efficacy of PUVA treatment in lichen planus: comparison of oral and external methoxsalen regimens. Photodermatology 4:265–268
34. Hindson C, Taylor A, Martin A, Downey A (1981) UVA light for relief of uraemic pruritus. Lancet i:215
35. Hindson TC, Spiro JG, Cochrane H (1987) PUVA therapy of diffuse granuloma annulare. Clin Exp Dermatol 13:26–27
36. Hofmann C, Weissmann I, Plewig G (1979) Pityriasis lichenoides chronica – eine neue Indikation zur PUVA-Therapie? Dermatologica 159:451–460
37. Honig B, Morison WL, Karp D (1994) Photochemotherapy beyond psoriasis. J Am Acad Dermatol 31:775–790
38. Horn TD, Morison WL, Frazadegan H, Zmudzka BZ, Beer JZ (1994) Effects of psoralen plus UVA radiation (PUVA) on HIV-1 in human beings: a pilot study. J Am Acad Dermatol 31:735–740
39. Iwatsuki K, Tsugiki M, Yoshizawa N, Takigawa M, Yamada M, Shamoto M (1985) The effect of phototherapies on cutaneous lesions of histiocytosis X in the elderly. Cancer 57:1931–1936
40. Jansén CT, Malmiharju (1981) Inefficacy of topical methoxsalen plus UVA for palmoplantar pustulosis. Acta Derm Venereol 61:354–356
41. Jansén CT, Lehtinen R, Happonen RP, Lehtinen A, Söderlund K (1987) Mouth PUVA: a new treatment for recalcitrant oral lichen planus. Photodermatology 4:165–166
42. Jeanmougin M, Rain D, Najean Y (1996) Efficacy of photochemotherapy on severe pruritus in polycythemia vera. Ann Hematol 73:91–93
43. Kalimo K, Lammintausta K, Viander M, Jansén CT (1986) PUVA treatment of dermatitis herpetiformis. Photodermatology 3:54–55
44. Karvonen J, Hannuksela M (1982) Long term results of topical trioxsalen PUVA in lichen planus and nodular prurigo. Acta Derm Venereol [Suppl] 120:53–55
45. Kaudewitz P, Przybilla B, Schmoeckel C, Gollhausen R (1986) Cutaneous lesions in histiocytosis X: Successful treatment with PUVA. J Invest Dermatol 86:324–325
46. Kerker B, Huang CP, Morison WL (1990) Photochemotherapy of generalized granuloma annulare. Arch Dermatol 126:359–361
47. Kerscher M, Dirschka T, Volkenandt M (1995) Treatment of localised scleroderma by UVA1 phototherapy. Lancet 346:1166
48. Kerscher M, Meurer M, Sander C, Volkenandt M, Lehmann P, Plewig G, Röcken M (1996) PUVA bath photochemotherapy for localized scleroderma. Arch Dermatol 132:1280–1282
49. Kerscher M, Volkenandt M, Gruss C, Reuther T, von Kobyletzki G, Freitag M, Dirschka T, Altmeyer P (1998) Low-dose UVA1 phototherapy for treatment of localized scleroderma. J Am Acad Dermatol 38:21–26
50. Kerscher M, Volkenandt M, Lehmann P, Plewig G, Röcken M (1995) PUVA-bath photochemotherapy of lichen planus. Arch Dermatol 131:1210–1211

51. Kerscher M, Volkenandt M, Meurer M, Lehmann P, Plewig G, Röcken M (1994) Treatment of localised scleroderma with PUVA bath photochemotherapy. Lancet 343:1233
52. Kripke ML (1990) Photoimmunology. Photochem Photobiol 52:919–924
53. Krizsa J, Hunyadi J, Dobozy A (1992) PUVA treatment of pigmented purpuric lichenoid dermatitis (Gougerot-Blum). J Am Acad Dermatol 27:778–780
54. Lang PG (1981) Keratosis lichenoides chronica. Successful treatment with psoralen-ultraviolet-A therapy. Arch Dermatol 117:105–108
55. Lange-Wantzin G, Thomsen K (1982) PUVA-treatment in lymphomatoid papulosis. Br J Dermatol 107:687–690
56. Langrock A, Weyers W, Schill WB (1998) Balneophotochemotherapie bei disseminiertem Granuloma anulare. Hautarzt 49:303–306
57. Lassus A, Kianto U, Johansson E, Juvakoski (1980) PUVA treatment for alopecia areata. Dermatologica 161:298–304
58. Lassus A, Salo O, Förström L, Lauharnta J, Kanerva L, Juvakoski T (1983) Behandlung der Akne mit selektiver Ultraviolettphototherapie (SUP). Dermatol Monatsschr 169:376–379
59. Leenutaphong V, Jiamton S (1995) UVB phototherapy for pityriasis rosea: a bilateral comparison study. Arch Dermatol 33:996–999
60. Lehmann P, Hölzle E, Kind P, Goerz G, Plewig G (1990) Experimental reproduction of skin lesions in lupus erythematosus by UVA and UVB radiation. J Am Acad Dermatol 22:181–187
61. Lehtinen R, Happonen RP, Kuusilehto A, Jansén CT (1989) A clinical trial of PUVA treatment in oral lichen planus. Proc Finn Dent Soc 85:29–33
62. LeVine MJ, Parrish JA, Fitzpatrick TB (1981) Oral methoxsalen photochemotherapy (PUVA) of dyshidrotic eczema. Acta Derm Venereol 61:570–571
63. LeVine MJ (1983) Phototherapy of pityriasis lichenoides. Arch Dermatol 119:378–380
64. Lundquist G, Forsgren H, Gajecki M, Emtestam L (1995) Photochemotherapy of oral lichen planus. Oral Surg Oral Med Oral Pathol Oral Radiol Endod 79:554–558
65. Manabe M, Yoshiike T, Negi M, Ogawa H (1983) Successful therapy of ichthyosis linearis circumflexa with PUVA. J Am Acad Dermatol 8:905–906
66. Marsch WCH, Stüttgen G (1981) Granuloma anulare – eine Indikation für die Photochemotherapie? Z Hautkr 56:44–49
67. May LP, Kelly J, Sanchez M (1990) Hypereosinophilic syndrome with unusual cutaneous manifestations in two men with HIV infection. J Am Acad Dermatol 23:202–204
68. Meffert H, Kölzsch J, Laubstein B, Sönnichsen N (1986) Phototherapie bei Akne vulgaris mit dem Teilkörperbestrahlungsgerät "TuR" UV10. Dermatol Monatsschr 172:9–13
69. Menagé HduP, Norris PG, Hawk JLM, Greaves MW (1993) The efficacy of psoralen photochemotherapy in the treatment of aquagenic pruritus. Br J Dermatol 129:163–165
70. Meola T, Soter NA, Ostreicher R, Sanchez M, Moy JA (1993) The safety of UVB phototherapy in patients with HIV infection. J Am Acad Dermatol 29:216–220
71. Mills OH, Kligman AM (1978) Ultraviolet phototherapy and photochemotherapy of acne vulgaris. Arch Dermatol 114:221–223
72. Misago N, Narisawa Y, Matsubara S, Hayashi S (1998) HIV-associated eosinophilic pustular folliculitis: successful treatment of a Japanese patient with UVB phototherapy. J Dermatol 25:178–184
73. Mitchell AJ, Douglass MC (1985) Topical photochemotherapy for alopecia areata. J Am Acad Dermatol 12:644–649
74. Morison WL, Parrish JA, Fitzpatrick TB (1978) Oral methoxsalen photochemotherapy of recalcitrant dermatoses of the palms and soles. Br J Dermatol 99:297–302

75. Morison WL, Nesbitt JA (1983) Oral psoralen photochemotherapy (PUVA) for pruritus associated with polycythemia vera and myelofibrosis. Am J Hematol 42:409 – 410

76. Mørk NJ, Austad J (1983) Short-wave ultraviolet light (UVB) treatment of allergic contact dermatitis of the hands. Acta Derm Venereol 63:87 – 89

77. Murray D, Corbett MF, Warin AP (1980) A controlled trial of photochemotherapy for persistent palmoplantar pustulosis. Br J Dermatol 102:659 – 663

78. Nagata T (1980) Netherton's syndrome which responded to photochemotherapy. Dermatologica 161:51 – 56

79. Narwutsch M, Narwutsch M, Dietz H (1990) Erste Ergebnisse zum Langzeiteffekt des PUVA-therapierten Lichen ruber oralis. Dermatol Monatsschr 176:349 – 355

80. Neumann C, Kolde G, Bonsmann G (1988) Histiocytosis X in an elderly patient. Ultrastructure and immunocytochemistry after PUVA photochemotherapy. Br J Dermatol 119:385 – 391

81. Nielsen EB, Thormann J (1978) Acne-like eruptions induced by PUVA-treatment. Acta Derm Venereol 58:374 – 375

82. Oppolzer G, Duschet P, Schwarz T, Hutterer J, Gschnait F (1988) Die Hypereosinophile Dermatitis (Nir-Westfried). Eine Variante im Spektrum des Hypereosinophiliesyndroms. Z Hautkr 63:123 – 125

83. Ortonne JP, Thivolet J, Sannwald C (1978) Oral photochemotherapy in the treatment of lichen planus (LP). Br J Dermatol 99:77 – 87

84. Pappert A, Grossman M, DeLeo V (1994) Photosensitivity as the presenting illness in four patients with human immunodeficiency viral infection. Arch Dermatol 130:618 – 623

85. Pardo RJ, Bogaert MA, Penneys NS, Byrne GE, Ruiz P (1992) UVB phototherapy of the pruritic papular eruption of the acquired immunodeficiency syndrome. J Am Acad Dermatol 26:423 – 428

86. Parrish JA, Strauss JS, Fleming TS, Fitzpatrick TB (1978) Oral methoxsalen photochemotherapy for acne vulgaris. Arch Dermatol 114:1241 – 1242

87. Paul BS, Arndt KA (1984) Response of transient acantholytic dermatosis to photochemotherapy. Arch Dermatol 120:121 – 122

88. Paul R, Jansén CT (1983) Suppression of palmoplantar pustulosis symptoms with oral 8-methoxypsoralen and high-intensity UVA irradiation. Dermatologica 167:283 – 285

89. Person JR (1981) Ultraviolet A (UV-A) and cholestatic pruritus. Arch Dermatol 117:684

90. Powell FC, Muller SA (1984) Psoralens and ultraviolet A therapy of pityriasis lichenoides. J Am Acad Dermatol 10:59 – 64

91. Ranki A, Puska P, Mattinen S, Lagerstedt A, Krohn K (1991) Effect of PUVA on immunologic and virologic findings in HIV-infected patients. J Am Acad Dermatol 24:404 – 410

92. Rollier R, Warcewski Z (1974) Le traitement de la pelade par la méladinine. Bull Soc Fr Dermatol Syph 81:97

93. Ryatt KS, Greenwood R, Cotterill JA (1982) Keratosis lichenoides chronica. Br J Dermatol 106:223 – 225

94. Scharffetter-Kochanek K, Goldermann R, Lehmann P, Hölzle E, Goerz G (1995) PUVA therapy in disabling pansclerotic morphoea of children. Br J Dermatol 132:830 – 831

95. Schempp CM, Müller H, Czech W, Schöpf E, Simon JC (1997) Treatment of chronic palmoplantar eczema with local bath PUVA therapy. J Am Acad Dermatol 36:733 – 737

96. Schirren, CG, Bethe M, Eckert F, Przybilla B (1992) Skleromyxödem Arndt-Gottron. Fallbericht und Übersicht über die therapeutischen Möglichkeiten. Hautarzt 43:152 – 157

97. Schreck S, Panozzo J, Milton J, Libertin CR, Woloschak GE (1995) The effects of multiple UV exposures on HIV-LTR expression. Photochem Photobiol 61:378–382
98. Simon M Jr, Hunyadi J (1986) PUVA-Therapie der Ekzematid-artigen Purpura. Aktuel Dermatol 12:100–102
99. Sjövall P, Christensen OB (1986) Local and systemic effect of ultraviolet irradiation (UVB and UVA) on human allergic contact dermatitis. Acta Derm Venereol 66:290–294
100. Sjövall P, Christensen OB (1987) Local and systemic effect of UVB irradiation in patients with chronic hand eczema. Acta Derm Venereol 67:538–541
101. Smith ML, Orton PW, Chu H, Weston WL (1990) Photochemotherapy of dominant, diffuse, cutaneous mastocytosis. Pediatr Dermatol 7:251–255
102. Smith RA, Ross JS, Staughton RCD (1994) Bath PUVA as a treatment for aquagenic pruritus. Br J Dermatol 131:584
103. Sönnichsen N, Meffert H, Kunzelmann V, Audring H (1993) UV-A-1-Therapie bei subakut-kutanem Lupus erythematodes. Hautarzt 44:723–725
104. Ständer H, Nashan D, Schwarz T (1996) Skleromyxödem Arndt-Gottron: erfolgreiche Behandlung mit einer kombinierten Steroid-PUVA-Therapie. Z Hautkr (unpublished data)
105. Stege H, Berneburg M, Humke S, Klammer M, Grewe M, Grether-Beck S, Boedeker R, Diepgen T, Dierks K, Goerz G, Ruzicka T, Krutmann J (1997) High-dose UVA1 radiation therapy for localized scleroderma. J Am Acad Dermatol 36:938–944
106. Stege H, Berneburg M, Ruzicka T, Krutmann J (1997) Creme-PUVA-Photochemotherapie. Hautarzt 48:89–93
107. Stege H, Schöpf E, Ruzicka T, Krutmann J (1996) High dose UVA1 for urticaria pigmentosa. Lancet 347:64
108. Stern RS, Mills DK, Krell K, Zmudzka BZ, Beer JZ (1998) HIV-positive patients differ from HIV-negative patients in indications for and type of UV therapy used. J Am Acad Dermatol 39:48–55
109. Streit V, Thiede R, Wiedow O, Christophers E (1996) Foil bath PUVA in the treatment of prurigo simplex subacuta. Acta Derm Venereol (Stockh) 76:319–320
110. Swerlick RA (1985) Photochemotherapy treatment of pruritus associated with polycythemia vera. J Am Acad Dermatol 4:675–677
111. Taylor CR, Hawk JLM (1995) PUVA treatment of alopecia areata partialis, totalis and universalis: Audit of 10 years' experience at St John's Institute of Dermatology. Br J Dermatol 133:914–918
112. Tegner E (1983) Seborrheic dermatitis of the face induced by PUVA treatment. Acta Derm Venereol 63:335–339
113. Väätäinen N, Hannuksela M, Karvonen J (1979) Local photochemotherapy in nodular prurigo. Acta Derm Venereol 59:544–547
114. Väätäinen N, Hannuksela M, Karvonen J (1981) Trioxsalen baths plus UV-A in the treatment of lichen planus and urticaria pigmentosa. Clin Exp Dermatol 6:133–138
115. van den Hoogenband HM, van den Berg WHHW, van Diggelen MW (1985) PUVA therapy in the treatment of skin lesions of the hypereosinophilic syndrome. Arch Dermatol 121:450
116. van der Schaar WW, Sillevis Smitt JH (1984) An evaluation of PUVA therapy for alopecia areata. Dermatologica 168:250–252
117. van der Schroeff JG, Schothorst AA, Kanaar P (1983) Induction of actinic lichen planus with artificial UV sources. Arch Dermatol 119:498–500
118. Vella Briffa D, Eady RAJ, James MP, Gatti S, Bleehen SS (1983) Photochemotherapy (PUVA) in the treatment of urticaria pigmentosa. Br J Dermatol 109:67–75
119. Volkenandt M, Kerscher M, Sander C, Meurer M, Röcken M (1995) PUVA-bath photochemotherapy resulting in rapid clearance of lymphomatoid papulosis in a child. Arch Dermatol 131:1094

120. von Kobyletzki G, Gruss C, Altmeyer P, Kerscher M (1997) Balneophotochemothera-pie des Lichen ruber. Hautarzt 48:323–327
121. Wakeel RA, Keefe M, Chapman RS (1991) Papuloerythroderma. Another case of a new disease. Arch Dermatol 127:96–98
122. Wallace BM, Lasker JS (1992) Awakenings... UV light and HIV gene activation. Science 257:1211–1212
123. Weiss DS, Taylor JR (1990) Treatment of generalized pruritus in an HIV-positive patient with UVB phototherapy. Clin Exp Dermatol 15:316–317
124. Wemmer U, Thiele B, Steigleder GK (1988) Hypereosinophilie-Syndrom (HES) – erfolgreiche PUVA-Therapie. Hautarzt 39:42–44
125. Willemze R, Beljaards RC (1993) Spectrum of primary cutaneous CD30 (Ki-1)-positive lymphoproliferative disorders. J Am Acad Dermatol 28:973–980
126. Wlaschek M, Heinen G, Poswig A, Schwarz A, Krieg T, Scharffetter-Kochanek K (1994) UVA-induced autocrine stimulation of fibroblast-derived collagenase/MMP-1 by interrelated loops of interleukin-1 and interleukin-6. Photochem Photobiol 59:550–556
127. Wong K, Ratnam KV (1990) A report of two cases of pigmented purpuric dermatoses treated with PUVA therapy. Acta Derm Venereol 71:68–70
128. Yamazaki S, Fujisawa T, Yanatori A, Yamakage A (1995) A case of lichen myxedematosus with clearly exacerbated skin eruptions after UVB irradiation. J Dermatol 22:590–593
129. Ziemer A, Göring HD (1989) Disseminiertes Granuloma anulare – Rückbildung unter PUVA-Therapie. Z Hautkr 64:1095–1097
130. Zmudzka BZ, Beer JZ (1990) Activation of human immunodeficiency virus by ultraviolet radiation. Photochem Photobiol 52:1153–1162

10 Phototherapy of HIV-Infected Patients: Evidence Questioning and Addressing Safety

Ponciano D. Cruz Jr.

Contents

Introduction

Because most forms of medical treatment interfere with biological events in the course of accomplishing their beneficial task, unintended adverse effects are almost inevitable. Recent concern about the use of phototherapy in patients infected with the human immunodeficiency virus (HIV) illustrate this double-edged situation. Whereas the efficacy of ultraviolet (UV)B or PUVA (psoralen plus UVA) for the treatment of HIV-related psoriasis, eosinophilic folliculitis, atopic dermatitis, or pruritus is unchallenged, questions regarding safety have not been fully resolved.

In this chapter, we have summarized information regarding the effects of UV radiation exposure on HIV infection and propose guidelines for phototherapy of HIV-infected patients.

Evidence Questioning the Safety of UV Radiation

In vitro studies were the first to raise the possibility that UV radiation may promote HIV infection (Table 1) [1–5]. HeLa cells were transfected with the long terminal repeat (LTR) component of HIV (a sequence that serves as an "on/off" switch for viral replication), which in turn was fused to a reporter gene that encodes for a protein with readily detectable activity, chloramphenicol acetyl transferase (CAT). With CAT activity as the read-out signal, HeLa cells were exposed to different UV wavelengths. UVC (< 290 nm) stimulated CAT activity by 50- to 150-fold [2]; PUVA, UVB+UVA2 (280–340 nm), or sunlight also enhanced CAT activity, although by lesser magnitudes [5]. By contrast, neither γ-radiation (< 100 nm) nor UVA-1 (340–400 nm) promoted CAT activity [5].

More definitive stimulatory effects of UV radiation on HIV activation were demonstrated by Valerie and colleagues [2] and by Stanley and colleagues [3].

Table 1. Effects of UV and other agents on HIV activation in vitro

Year First author	Agents	Cell lines	Results
1987 Folks [1]	Phorbol esters GM-CSF IL-1, IL-2, IFN-γ, TNF-α	Promonocytes (U1) infected with HIV	Phorbol esters and GM-CSF stimulated HIV replication; IL-1, IL-2 IFN-γ, and TNF-α did not
1988 Valerie [2]	Mitomycin UVC (254 nm) Sunlight	HeLa cells with CAT gene controlled by HIV LTR	Mitomycin, UVC and sunlight enhanced HIV-CAT expression
		T cells infected with HIV	UVC and sunlight stimulated HIV replication in T cells
1989 Stanley [3]	UVC (254 nm) UVB (312 nm) UVA (320–380 nm)	Promonocytes (U1) infected with HIV	UVC and UVB increased reverse transcriptase activity and p24; UVA did not
1993 Zmudzka [4]	PUVA	HeLa cells with CAT gene linked to HIV promoter	PUVA enhanced CAT activity
Beer [5]	UVC (254 nm) UVB+UVA2 (280–340 nm) UVA-1 (340–400 nm) γ-radiation	HeLa cells with CAT gene linked to HIV promoter	UVC and UVB+UVA2 enhanced CAT activity; UVA-1 and γ-radiation did not

Using cultured cells latently infected with HIV, they showed that UVC, UVB, or sunlight can activate HIV itself (not just a HIV LTR construct).

Similar results were demonstrated in genetically altered mice. Working independently, three groups of investigators utilized different transgenes in mice to test the effect of UV radiation on HIV gene expression (Table 2) [6–8]. Cavard and his associates used bacterial β-galactosidase linked to the HIV LTR [6]; Morrey and colleagues employed firefly luciferase linked to the HIV LTR [7]; and Vogel and associates utilized the HIV LTR and *tat* genes directly [8]. All three groups showed that in vivo exposure to various UV wavelengths led to cutaneous expression of the protein encoded by the respective transgenes. As with the previously described results from in vitro studies [2–5], UVC, UVB, sunlight, and particularly PUVA activated HIV [6–8], whereas UVA did not [7].

We have developed a quantitative polymerase chain reaction (PCR)-based assay for measuring HIV load in skin (unpublished). In HIV(+) patients with psoriasis or eosinophilic folliculitis, we detected HIV in lesional and non-lesional skin. We also showed that a single minimal erythemogenic dose of UVB delivered in vivo or in vitro can activate the virus at least sixfold, similar to

Table 2. Effects of UV on HIV activation in transgenic mice

Year First author	Agents	Transgenes	Results
1990 Cavard [6]	UVC (254 nm) UVB (280–300 nm)	Bacterial lac-2 (encodes for β- galactosidase) con- trolled by HIV LTR	UVC and UVB stimulated β-galactosidase expres- sion in skin
1991 Morrey [7]	UVB UVA PUVA Sunlight Psoralens+sunlight	Firefly luciferase gene controlled by HIV LTR	UVB, PUVA, sunlight, and psoralens+sunlight stimulated luciferase activity in skin; UVA did not
1992 Vogel [8]	UVC (254 nm) UVB (290–320 nm) Sunlight	LTR and tat HIV genes	UVC, UVB, and sunlight stimulated expression of transgenes in skin

increments observed in the previously cited cell culture and transgenic mice studies. By contrast, high-dose UVA-1 did not activate the virus.

Possible Mechanisms of UV-Induced HIV Activation

How might UV radiation activate HIV? UV causes DNA damage and normal cells try to repair such DNA damage. During repair, cells turn on genes that may include viral genes (including HIV) integrated into host DNA [9]. In this respect, it is interesting to note that the capacity of different agents and UV treatments to produce DNA damage correlates with their reported ability to activate HIV. For example, mitomycin C, cis-platinum, and anthracycline are well-known genotoxic agents; so are UVC, UVB, and PUVA. Each of these agents has been shown to activate HIV [2, 10, 11]. By contrast, UVA, a poor genotoxic agent, fails to activate the virus [3].

What happens during cell repair to turn on HIV genes? Repair involves unwinding of DNA from its naturally highly coiled state within the chromosome. In its uncoiled state, exposed components of DNA not only become accessible to repair enzymes that correct the DNA damage, but may also act as targets for activation via binding with transcription factors [12].

Potential Mechanisms for Adverse Effects of Phototherapy

From a theoretical standpoint, phototherapy can exert detrimental effects on HIV-infected individuals through two pathways. As described previously, a direct pathway is activation and proliferation of HIV in tissues such as skin exposed to UV radiation [1–8].

Because HIV can remain in latent form within infected cells for many years, agents that can trigger activation should be viewed with great alarm. On the other hand, the skin may not be a significant reservoir for HIV [13–19]. Thus, even if UV irradiation induces HIV replication in skin, the overall effect may be minimal if the viral load in skin is small or nil to begin with.

UV radiation may also produce adverse effects in an indirect manner. UVB and PUVA have been shown to suppress T-cell-mediated responses via several mechanisms including the induction of suppressor T cells, perturbation of antigen presentation, secretion by skin cells (especially keratinocytes) of immunosuppressive cytokines such as interleukin-10, and tumor necrosis factor-α, and altered migration of antigen-presenting cells and T cells in and out of sites of UV exposure [19–22]. UVB exposure has also been postulated to inhibit protective immune responses (Th1), while favoring tolerogenic immune responses (Th2) [23]. It is also interesting to note that, independent of UV exposure, a switch from Th1- to Th2-dominant responses has been shown in many HIV-infected subjects in their progression towards the AIDS-defining phase of the disease [24–26].

Clinical Studies Addressing the Safety of Phototherapy

Research employing cell lines and transgenic mice can not completely mimic what happens in natural HIV infection in humans. In this respect, the high prevalence of photo-treatable skin diseases in HIV-infected patients has served as an opportunity for assessing the in vivo effects of UV radiation on HIV infection (Table 3) [10–17].

Ranki et al. [11] and Horn et al. [14] analyzed the effects of PUVA treatment of HIV-infected patients with psoriasis, eosinophilic folliculitis, or pruritus. In both studies, PUVA was shown to be effective in alleviating the skin disorders. Neither study showed evidence of overt deterioration in the immunological or clinical status of patients, although Ranki et al. documented slight increases in viral replication after photochemotherapy in two of eight evaluable patients [11].

The effects of UVB treatment on HIV-infected patients with similar skin diseases have also been reported. Meola et al. observed improvement in the skin disease of all patients treated, with no deterioration in immunological and viral parameters, except for one patient whose HIV p24 antigenemia became positive after 42 treatments [13]. Fotiades et al. compared UVB effects in HIV-positive and -negative patients with psoriasis [15]. The skin disease improved in both groups of patients, and there was no deterioration in the immunological status of HIV-infected patients [15, 16]. Contrasting results were noted in a study by Duvic et al. who also compared UVB effects in HIV-positive and -negative patients with psoriasis [17]. Although CD4 counts were unchanged, a significant increase in p24 antigen levels was observed in HIV-infected patients [17].

The most recent clinical study was by Gelfand et al. who assessed HIV (+) patients treated with UVB (24 treatments) for various skin disorders. They observed no significant change in CD4 count. They also reported no significant

Table 3. Effects of UV treatment in HIV-infected patients

Year First author	Treatment (# of treatments)	Patients (# of patients)	Results
1988 Buchness [10]	UVB (6–9)	HIV (+) with eosinophilic folliculitis (6)	Pruritus cleared in all patients
1991 Ranki [11]	PUVA (12–24)	HIV (+) with psoriasis, seborrheic dermatitis, folliculitis, or chronic urticaria (5)	Psoriasis improved in all patients; plasma HIV titers did not increase; skin tests converted from anergic to positive in 3 patients
1992 Pardo [12]	UVB (8)	HIV (+) with pruritic papular eruption (8)	Pruritus reduced in 7 patients; skin biopsies showed less inflammation in 6 patients; no change in plasma immunoglobulins
1993 Meola [13]	UVB (21–57)	HIV (+) with psoriasis (5) HIV (+) with pruritus (1)	All patients improved clinically; no change in CBC, CD4 and CD8 counts, serum β_2-microglobulin, HIV-1, and p24 levels; no acquisition of opportunistic infection or malignancy
1994 Horn [14]	PUVA (24)	HIV (+) with psoriasis, eosinophilic folliculitis, or pruritus (10)	No change in CD4 count and viral load; no acquisition of opportunistic infection. Two of 8 patients with evaluable data at 2 months showed increased viral loads.
1995 Fotiades [15]	UVB (21)	HIV (+) with psoriasis (14) HIV (−) with psoriasis (14)	No change in CBC, CD4, and CD8 counts, and β_2 microglobulin level
1995 Fotiades [16]	UVB (42)	HIV (+) with psoriasis (28)	No change in lymphocyte counts; β_2 microglobulin level rose significantly in 12 patients; no acquisition of opportunistic infection or malignancy
1995 Duvic [17]	UVB (18)	HIV (+) with psoriasis (28) HIV (−) with psoriasis treated with AZT (10) or with UVB or PUVA (10)	No change in CD4 count, but p24 levels increased

Table 3. Continued

Year First author	Treatment (# of treatments)	Patients (# of patients)	Results
1998 Gelfand [18]	UVB (24)	HIV(+) eosinophilic folliculitis (3), pruritus (3), prurigo (3), atopic dermatitis (2)	No change in CD4 count; 4 patients showed increase in plasma HIV load

rise in plasma HIV load (defined as a threefold increment), although at least four patients displayed increased plasma HIV counts [18].

The clinical studies cited here offer no compelling proof, at least in the short term, that UVB or PUVA treatment leads to deleterious effects in HIV-infected subjects. On the other hand, there has been a suggestion of phototherapy-associated increases in viral replication, as shown by elevation in plasma p24 or HIV-RNA levels in several patients [11, 14, 17, 18]. These opposing observations underscore the need for larger, randomized, and controlled studies conducted over longer time periods, stratified prospectively for the early and later stages of HIV disease, and monitored concurrently for viral, immunological, and clinical parameters.

Guidelines

Pending more definitive information regarding the safety of phototherapy in HIV-infected individuals, we believe that UVB and PUVA should remain therapeutic options in HIV+ patients with UV-responsive skin diseases. The decision as to whether to employ phototherapy or not depends upon responses to the following questions:

1. *Is the skin disease UV-responsive?* If the answer is yes, consider phototherapy.
2. *Do alternative therapies offer less risk to the patient?* If yes, it may be judicious to first try alternative treatments.
3. *Is anticipated improvement in morbidity following phototherapy enough to justify potential risks?* If yes, proceed with phototherapy.
4. *Is the patient sufficiently reliable to show up for treatment visits?* If yes, proceed with phototherapy. If no, consider other treatments.
5. *Are there other contraindications to phototherapy (e.g., medication that confers photosensitivity)?* If yes, weigh the risk/benefit ratio.

Currently, we recommend HIV serology in patients with skin disorders (particularly psoriasis, eosinophilic folliculitis, or pruritus of undetermined cause) who are candidates for phototherapy. We also recommend that HIV-infected patients treated with UVB or PUVA be monitored for CD4 count and viral load before treatment, on monthly intervals during treatment, and 3 months after treatment.

References

1. Folks TM, Justement J, Kinter A, Dinarello CA, Fauci AS (1995) Cytokine-induced expression of HIV-1 in a chronically infected promonocyte cell line. Science 228:800–802
2. Valerie K, Delers A, Bruck C, Thiriart C, Rosenberg H, Debouck C, Rosenberg M (1988) Activation of human immunodeficiency virus type 1 by DNA damage in human cells. Nature 333:78–81
3. Stanley SK, Folks TM, Fauci AS (1989) Induction of expression of human immunodeficiency virus in a chronically infected promonocytic cell line by ultraviolet irradiation. AIDS Res Hum Retroviruses 5:375–384
4. Zmudzka BZ, Strickland AG, Miller SA, Valerie K, Dall'Acqua F, Beer JZ (1993) Activation of the human immunodeficiency virus promoter by UVA radiation in combination with psoralens or angelicins. Photochem Photobiol 58:226–232
5. Beer JZ, Olvey KM, Lee W, Zmudzka BZ (1994) Reassessment of the differential effects of ultraviolet and ionizing radiation on HIV promoter: the use of cell survival as the basis for comparisons. Photochem Photobiol 59:643–649
6. Cavard C, Zider A, Vernet M, Bennoun M, Saragosti S, Grimber G, Briand P (1990) In vivo activation by ultraviolet rays of the human immunodeficiency virus type 1 long terminal repeat. J Clin Invest 86:1369–1374
7. Morrey JD, Bourn SM, Bunch TD, Jackson MK, Sidwell RW, Barrows LR, Daynes RA, Rosen CA (1991) In vivo activation of human immunodeficiency virus type 1 long terminal repeat by UV type A (UV-A) light plus psoralen and UV-B light in the skin of transgenic mice. J Virol 65:5045–5051
8. Vogel J, Cepeda M, Tschachler E, Napolitano LA, Jay G (1992) UV activation of human immunodeficiency virus gene expression in transgenic mice. J Virol 66:1–5
9. Stern RS, Mills DK, Krell K, Zmudzka BZ (1998) HIV-positive patients differ from HIV-negative patients in indications for and type of UV therapy used. J Am Acad Dermatol 39:48–55
10. Buchness MR, Lim HW, Hatcher VA, Sanchez M, Soter NA (1988) Eosinophilic pustular folliculitis in the acquired immunodeficiency syndrome. N Engl J Med 318:1183–1186
11. Ranki A, Puska P, Mattinen S, Lagerstedt A, Krohn K (1991) Effect of PUVA on immunologic and virologic findings in HIV-infected patients. J Am Acad Dermatol 24:404
12. Pardo RJ, Bogaert MA, Penneys NS, Byrne GE, Ruiz P (1992) UVB phototherapy of the pruritic papular eruption of the acquired immunodeficiency syndrome. J Am Acad Dermatol 26:423–428
13. Meola T, Soter NA, Ostreicher R, Sanchez M, Moy JA (1993) The safety of UVB phototherapy in patients with HIV infection. J Am Acad Dermatol 29:216–220
14. Horn TD, Morison WL, Farzadegan H, Zmudzka BZ, Beer JZ (1994) Effects of psoralen plus UVA radiation (PUVA) on HIV-1 in human beings: a pilot study. J Am Acad Dermatol 31:735–740
15. Fotiades J, Lim HW, Jiang SB, Soter NA, Sanchez M, Moy J (1995) Efficacy of ultraviolet B phototherapy for psoriasis in patients infected with human immunodeficiency virus. Photodermatol Photoimmunol Photomed 11:107–111
16. Fotiades J, Soter NA, Sanchez MR, Moy JA (1995) A three-year follow-up evaluation on 28 HIV-positive patients treated with ultraviolet B (UVB) phototherapy. J Invest Dermatol 104:660a
17. Duvic M, Ulmer R, Crane M, Goller M, Adu-oppong A, Lewis DE (1995) Treatment of HIV+ patients with UVB is associated with a significant increase in p24 antigen levels. J Invest Dermatol 104:581
18. Gelfand JM, Rudikoff D, Lebwohl M, Klotman ME (1998) Effect of UV-B phototherapy on plasma HIV type 1 RNA viral level: a self-controlled prospective study. Arch Dermatol 134:940–945

19. Simpson E, Dawson B, Cruz PD Jr (1997) UVB radiation activates HIV in human skin. J Invest Dermatol 110:485

20. Cruz PD Jr, Dougherty I, Ellinger L, Gilchrest BA (1997) Thymidine dinucleotides inhibit the induction of contact hypersensitivity and activate the gene for TNFα. J Invest Dermatol 110:491a

21. Romerdahl CA, Okamoto H, Kripke ML (1989) Immune surveillance against cutaneous malignancies in experimental animals. In: Norris DA (eds) Immune mechanisms in cutaneous disease. Dekker, New York, pp 749–769

22. Kripke ML, Morison WL (1986) Studies on the mechanism of systemic suppression of contact hypersensitivity by UVB radiation. II. Differences in the suppression of delayed and contact hypersensitivity in mice. J Invest Dermatol 86:787–790

23. Ullrich SE (1996) Does exposure to UV radiation induce a shift to a Th-2-like immune reaction? Photochem Photobiol 64: 254–258

24. Clerici M, Stocks NI, Zajac RA, Boswell RN, Lucey DR, Via CS, Shearer GM (1989) Detection of three distinct patterns of T helper cell dysfunction in asymptomatic, human immunodeficiency virus-seropositive patients. J Clin Invest 84:1892–1899

25. Clerici M, Shearer GM (1993) A T_H1/T_H2 switch is a critical step in the etiology of HIV infection. Immunol Today 14:107–111

26. Mosmann TR (1994) Cytokine patterns during the progression to AIDS. Science 265:193–194

III Special Phototherapeutic Modalities

11 Photodynamic Therapy in Dermatology

Rolf-Markus Szeimies, Sigrid Karrer, Christoph Abels, Michael Landthaler,
Craig A. Elmets

Contents

Introduction

Photodynamic therapy refers to a new form of phototherapy in which non-psoralen photosensitizing drugs are administered systemically or topically to an individual. The drugs alone are inactive, but once activated by high-intensity light usually from a laser, they are exceptionally effective at inhibiting the growth of hyperproliferative tissues. PDT was originally designed for the treatment of malignancies because of the unique property of several photosensitizers to localize preferentially within tumors. Porfimer sodium (Photofrin), a first generation PDT photosensitizer, has already received regulatory approval in the USA, Canada, Japan, and Europe for the management of bladder, esophageal, and lung cancers. Although PDT has not been formally approved for dermatological malignancies, its efficacy in the treatment of superficial skin cancer has been demonstrated in several clinical studies [23, 38, 43, 85, 103, 125, 151, 163, 185]. Clinical trials are currently being conducted for this indication and approval is likely within the next few years. Because of the accessibility of the skin, there is increasing interest in using this novel form of therapy for psoriasis and other benign cutaneous disorders as well.

History of Photodynamic Therapy

The ability of photosensitizers and light to cause photosensitized destruction of cells was discovered about 100 years ago by Oscar Raab. As part of his doctoral thesis he found that paramecia could be killed by exposing them to rose bengal and light [131]. The first reported clinical application of photodynamic therapy (PDT) was performed on a 70-year-old woman with a squamous cell carcinoma of the face [73, 169]. The tumor was painted repeatedly with a 5 % eosin solution over 2 months immediately ofter painting was followed by exposure to sunlight or light from a carbon-arc lamp. The tumor healed rapidly with an excellent cosmetic result. In 1905 von Tappeiner and Jesionek reported of PDT on six patients with skin tumors on the face, primarily basal cell carcinomas. The treatment was performed daily for 2 – 8 weeks using the same procedure [73]. Four patients were cured (Fig. 1). In 1937 Silver reported on the successful application of PDT for the treatment of chronic inflammatory skin diseases [151]. He treated a 27-year-old patient with chronic psoriasis with intramuscular and oral application of hematoporphyrin followed by irradiation with ultraviolet light. This treatment resulted in partial remission of large psoriatic plaques and in complete remission of small ones. Despited of these encouraging results, little was done with PDT until the early 1960s when Lipson and Baldes performed tissue localization experiments with intravenous hematoporphyrin-derivative [101]. Their intention was to diagnose tumors by the detection of fluorescence

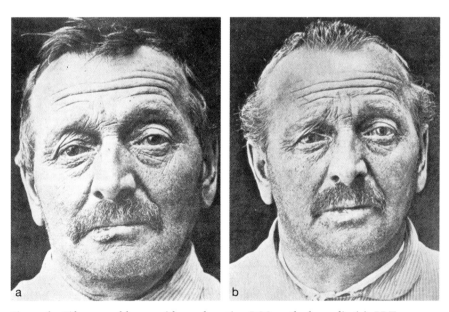

Fig. 1a, b. Fifty-year-old man with an ulcerating BCC on the lower lip (a). PDT was performed after application of an eosin solution (up to 5 %) and subsequent light exposure between March and May in 1904. A complete reepithelisation was observed at the end of the treatment (b), and there was a disease free interval of one year [73]

emitted by hematoporphyrin following exposure to light. In 1966 they treated an ulcerated, recurrent breast carcinoma by systemic PDT using hematoporphyrin. Although the tumor recurred after repeated treatments, a marked therapeutic effect was observed [102].

In the mid 1970s Thomas Dougherty showed that in animal models complete remissions and cures of several different types of tumors could be achieved after systemic PDT using hematoporphyrin derivative (HpD) and light from a xenon arc lamp [37]. HpD, which has improved activity compared to hematoporphyrin, is a mixture of oligomers from esterized and etherized hematoporphyrins. Three years later, he performed the first clinical trial treating 25 patients successfully with cutaneous and subcutaneous malignant tumors by systemic PDT with HpD. Of the 113 tumors, 111 showed complete or partial remissions [38]. Hematoporphyrin-derivative (porfimer sodium, also known by the trade name Photofrin or Photosan-3) PDT has been approved for clinical use in several countries throughout the world.

Aminolevulinic acid (ALA) is the newest PDT agent to receive regulatory approval. At this point the main indication for its use is the treatment of actinic keratoses. ALA itself is not a photosensitizer, but is metabolized to protoporphyrin IX (PpIX), which does have photosensitizing capabilities. The major advantage of ALA is that it can be given topically and thus is not associated with prolonged cutaneous photosensitivity.

Although porfimer sodium (Photofrin) is being used clinically to treat patients with malignancies, it is not a pure compound; the wavelengths of light used for therapy do not penetrate very deeply into tissues; and treatment is accompanied by severe cutaneous photosensitivity, which may last for up to 2 months. Because of these deficiencies, a number of second generation photosensitizers, which have fewer of these undesirable characteristics have been developed and are being evaluated.

Elements of Photodynamic Therapy

Photodynamic therapy requires the simultaneous presence of oxygen, a light-absorbing photosensitizer in the tissue, and light of the appropriate wavelength (Fig. 2).

Light Sources and Dosimetry

Although porfimer sodium (Photofrin), like other porphyrins, has stronger absorption peaks at shorter wavelengths, the absorption peak at 630 nm is employed for most Photofrin PDT protocols in order to achieve the greatest depth of penetration of light into tissue and thus to guarantee a sufficient absorption of photons by the photosensitizer. However, even at this wavelength, the depth of penetration into the skin is less than 4 mm. Currently, the light sources of choice are argon-ion pumped dye lasers ($\lambda = 630$ nm) and gold-vapor lasers ($\lambda = 628$ nm) [94], because they match the absorption band of Photofrin

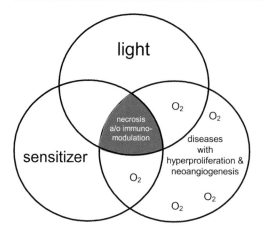

Fig. 2. Main requirements for a successful PDT is the simultaneous presence of a photosensitizer, oxygen and photoactivating light at the target site. If one factor is missing, PDT does not work

at 630 nm (Fig. 3). For the treatment of most non-cutaneous malignancies, e.g., the bladder, gastrointestinal tract, or bronchial tree, it is necessary to couple the light into fiber optic systems with high power density. The major drawbacks to the use of these laser systems are their high costs and the continuing need to replace and maintain optical parts. The development of diode lasers has become a promising field in the past few years, as these lasers are cheaper and more reliable. Moreover, they are much smaller compared with dye lasers.

Coupling light into endoscopic devices is not necessary in dermatology. Therefore, PDT in dermatology can be performed using incoherent light

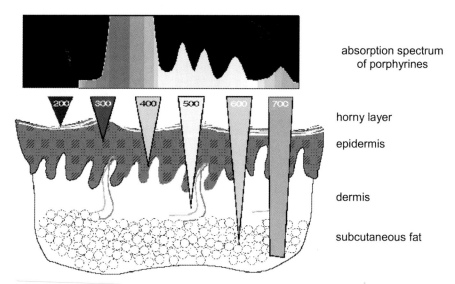

Fig. 3. At higher wavelengths (up to 1,100 nm) penetration of light into tissue increases. Therefore the last absorption band of the porphyrins at about 630 nm is used for PDT

Table 1. Comparison of different light sources for PDT

Light source	Advantages	Disadvantages
Sunlight	Free	Availability dosimetry
Lasers (metal vapor-, gas-, dye-laser)	Can be coupled to fibers Dosimetry	Expensive Requires maintenance Stationary systems Often limited to one wavelength
Diode lasers	Can be coupled to fibers Dosimetry Relatively inexpensive	Currently only available at higher wavelengths (630 nm and above) Limited to one wavelength
Broadband lamps	Inexpensive Can be used with several photosensitizers Large illumination fields	Only surface illumination possible Dosimetry

sources. Slide-projectors with special filters and high power density have been used for irradiation [50, 85, 182] and there are several high-powered lamps that are commercially available [159]. Another advantage of incoherent light sources are the low costs. Additionally, light sources with a broader emission spectrum permit the use of different photosensitizers with different absorption maxima (Table 1) [158].

To avoid nonspecific thermal effects, the light intensity should not exceed 200 mW/cm^2 in the treated area. Scars, crusts, scales, and melanin on the skin surface must be taken into account for selection of the most appropriate dose, since they can influence the amount of light that actually reaches the tissue. A standard light dose necessary for PDT must be determined for each of the different photosensitizers in order to establish standardized protocols with respect to the light intensity and light dose. With respect to Photofrin PDT, experimental and clinical experience has shown that a light dose of 100–150 J/cm^2 is necessary for the treatment of tumors. An irradiation procedure applying these parameters usually takes less than 30 min. For the treatment of chronic-inflammatory skin diseases such as psoriasis, less than half of the light dose is required [23, 100]. The reason for this relates to the fact that only sublethal damage or PDT-induced immunomodulation are responsible for the therapeutic response. Moreover, for these indications, fractionated treatments can be performed.

Photosensitizers

Photofrin is the only photosensitizer that has received regulatory approval for the treatment of tumors. Despite its proven efficacy, the drug has several characteristics that limit its therapeutic potential:

a) It cannot be synthesized as a pure compound.
b) Its selective accumulation in neoplastic versus normal tissue is poor.

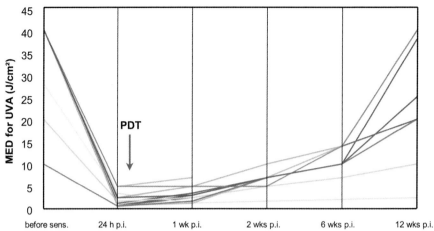

Fig. 4. Detection of the minimal erythema dose (MED) for UVA over time in patients ($n = 16$) undergoing systemic PDT with HpD for cancers of the urogenital- and GI-tract

c) Most Photofrin PDT protocols employ light sources in the 625–630 nm range. Light of these wavelengths penetrates tissue to a maximum depth of about 3 mm. Better photosensitizers are activated by light of longer wavelengths, since longer wavelengths of light have greater depth of penetration into tissue.

d) Photofrin is only active when delivered by intravenous injection.

e) After administration of Photofrin, there is a 24–72 h waiting period before the drug can be activated by light. This requires two visits for most treatment regimens.

f) Photofrin is associated with severe and persistent cutaneous photosensitivity, a problem that has been attributed to prolonged retention of this photosensitizer in the skin (Fig. 4).

The optimal photosensitizer for use in dermatology should have the following characteristics:

1. Chemically pure substance. Due to legal requirements regarding approval and patenting of drugs, only chemically pure, characterized substances are being evaluated.

2. High quantum yield of singlet oxygen. Most photosensitizers generate singlet oxygen with a quantum yield between 5 and 20% [144]. A high quantum yield of singlet oxygen indicates that, when compared to a substance with low quantum yield, less substance has to accumulate to induce a photodynamic reaction within the tissue. However, this consideration is only of theoretical interest, as the efficacy of a photosensitizer also depends on its chemical characteristics (e.g., lipophilicity or hydrophilicity), which influence subcellular distribution of the dye [87, 99, 187] (Table 2).

3. Deep penetration into the tissue. As already mentioned, the penetration depth of the light into tissue is quite limited. Most photosensitizers currently being evaluated have absorption peaks between 600 and 700 nm. With these

Table 2. Cellular uptake and localization of different photosensitizers

Photosensitizer	Cellular mechanism of uptake	Intracellular distribution
Hydrophilic (rhodamines, cyanines, chlorines, TPPS$_4$)	Pinocytosis	Endosomes Lysosomes
Lipophilic (porphyrins, phthalocyanines, porphycenes)	Diffusion Low-density lipoprotein-mediated endocytosis	Membranes (nucleus and plasma membrane and membranes of organelles)

wavelengths, lesions can only be 3–4 mm in thickness. The synthesis of substances which absorb in the near infrared region and that also produce a high quantum yield of singlet oxygen, could allow for the treatment of thicker tumors. For inflammatory skin diseases such as psoriasis, the penetration depth of the current photosensitizers seems to be sufficient.

4. Selective accumulation in target tissue. When photosensitizers have high selectivity for diseased tissue, there is less damage to surrounding normal tissue during PDT. Multiple lesions (e.g., actinic keratoses) can be treated with an excellent cosmetic result [83, 161] (Fig. 5). Although selectivity is a desirable feature, it should be noted that for most PDT photosensitizers the selectivity of the uptake is rather modest. The tumor to normal tissue in general ratio is about 3:1 for most PDT photosensitizers currently being evaluated. Restriction of the light and drug application to the affected area also contributes to the selectivity of PDT. Attempts have been made to enhance the selectivity of photosensitizers by incorporating them into liposomes, esterifying them, or coupling them to antibodies [100, 146]. In general, these procedures have met with limited success.

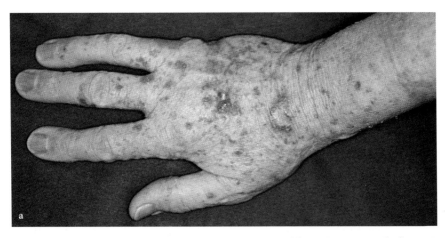

Fig. 5a–c. (a) Arsenic-induced skin cancers in a 62-year-old psoriatic patient before PDT. The right fifth finger had already been amputated due to an invasive Bowen's carcinoma

Of all of the photosensitizers currently being evaluated for clinical use, ALA shows the highest selectivity [2, 96]. The ratio between affected (tumor) and surrounding tissue after topical application of ALA is > 10:1 [93, 162]. The reason for this selectivity is not yet known.

5. Lack of cutaneous photosensitivity. Because generalized cutaneous photosensitivity, which may last for weeks, has a dramatic effect on the quality of life of patients after systemic PDT, the optimal photosensitizer should have little or none of this side effect. It should be rapidly metabolized and should not accumulate within the skin.

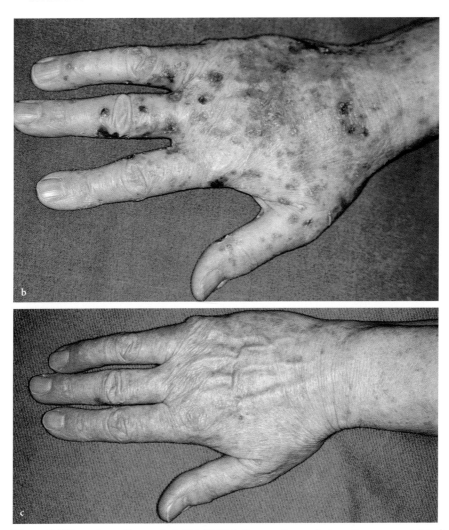

Fig. 5. (b) Three days after topical ALA-PDT: Inflammation and ulcerations are restricted to affected tissue (c) Six months after PDT: Biopsy-proven complete remission (Reprinted with permission from [160])

Table 3. Photosensitizers of potential interest in dermatology and current status of development

Company	Photosensitizer[a]	Wavelength	Indications	Route of administration	Status
QLT Photo-Therapeutics, Sanofi Winthrop, USA, Europe	Porfimer sodium (Photofrin)	630 nm	Approved for bladder, esophagus, lung cancers; BCC, cutaneous metastases under investigation	i.v.	Approved in Canada, USA, Japan, Europe; phase II/III for cutaneous tumors
DUSA, Berlex, USA	5-Aminolevulinic acid (ALA, Levulan)	635 nm	Actinic keratoses, BCC, cutaneous T-cell lymphoma, psoriasis, permanent hair removal	Topical	Approved in the USA for actinic keratoses (with blue light)
Medac, Germany	ALA Spectrila	635 nm	Diagnosis of bladder cancer	Intravesical	Approval expected in Germany in 2001
Photocure, Norway	ALA-methylester Metvix	635 nm	AK, BCC	Topical	Phase II/III
Miravant, USA	Tin ethyl etiopurpurin (SnET$_2$, Purlytin)	660–665 nm	Cutaneous metastases, Kaposi's sarcoma, macular degeneration	i.v., lipid emulsion	Phase II/III
Pharmacyclics, USA	Lutetium texaphyrin PCI-0123 (Lu-Tex)	720–760 nm	Skin cancer	i.v.	Phase II/III
Cytopharm Inc., USA	9-Acetoxy-2,7,12,17-tetrakis-(β-methoxyethyl)-porphycen (ATMPn)	640 nm	Psoriasis	Topical	Phase II
QLT Photo-Therapeutics, Canada	Benzoporphyrin derivative monoacid ring A (BPD-MA, Verteporfin)	690 nm	BCC, psoriasis, macular degeneration (MD)	i.v., liposomal formulation	Phase II, approval for MD
Scotia Pharmaceuticals, United Kingdom	meso-tetra-hydroxyphenyl-chlorin (mTHPC, Foscan)	650 nm	BCC, head and neck cancer	i.v., topical	Phase I/II
Nippon Petrochemical, Japan	Mono-L-aspartyl chlorin e6 (NPe6)	660–665 nm	Skin cancer	i.v.	Phase I/II

[a] The authors do not claim completeness of this table. The trade names were included because they were reported in published literature or electronic media (Internet).

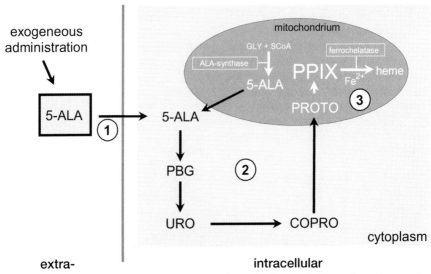

Fig. 6. Biosynthesis of heme: Accumulation of porphyrin metabolites when the negative feedback mechanism (ALA-synthesis) is bypassed. The tissue selectivity of synthesized porphyrins is now based on an enhanced uptake of ALA (1), an enhanced porphyrin synthesis (2), or a reduced activity of ferrochelatase (3). (*GLY*, glycine; *SCoA*, succinyl-CoA; *5-ALA*, 5-aminolevulinic acid; *PBG*, porphobilinogen; *URO*, uroporphyrinogen; *COPRO*, coproporphyrinogen; *PROTO*, protoporphyrinogen; *PpIX*, protoporphyrin IX)

A number of second generation photosensitizers are currently being evaluated as potential supplements or replacements for Photofrin. Table 3 shows the photosensitizers currently under clinical investigation, the potential indications, and their different properties.

ALA recently has been approved for the treatment of actinic keratoses in the US. Its mechanism of action is unique. ALA is not a photosensitizer, but is a metabolite in the biosynthetic pathway of heme, which induces the synthesis of porphyrins, particularly protoporphyrin IX [15, 158]. Increased uptake, enhanced synthesis of porphyrins or decreased turnover of heme due to decreased ferrochelatase activity in diseased cells may be some reasons for the selective accumulation of this agent [84] (Fig. 6).

Mechanisms of Action

Oxygen Dependence

PDT-induced effects are mediated by photooxidative reactions (Fig. 7). The term "photodynamic" is used for this type of reaction, to distinguish it from the process of sensitization without the need for oxygen. During irradiation the photosensitizer absorbs light, which results in its conversion to an energetically

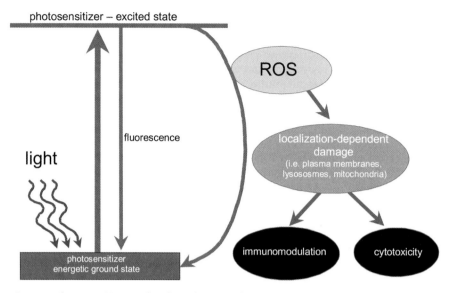

Fig. 7. A photosensitizer molecule in the excited state is able to form reactive oxygen species (*ROS*), mainly singlet oxygen (reaction type II) via photooxidation. Depending on the subcellular localization of the dye, organelle-specific damage occurs. The specific damage sites plus the extent of damage lead then to immunomodulation and/or cytotoxicity

higher status, the "singlet-status." After a short half-life (approx. 10^{-9} s) the activated photosensitizer returns to the ground state. This results either in emission of fluorescence or its internal conversion. Alternatively, the activated photosensitizer changes from the singlet state into a more stable triplet state with a longer half-life (10^{-3} s) ("intersystem crossing"). In the type I photooxidative reaction there is a direct hydrogen and electron transfer from the triplet state of the photosensitizer to a substrate. This reaction results in the generation of radicals of the substrate. These radicals are able to react directly with molecular oxygen and form peroxides, hydroxyl radicals and superoxide anions. This type I reaction is strongly concentration-dependent. Direct damage to cells by this reaction can occur, especially when the photosensitizer is bound to easily oxidizable molecules. In type II reactions, energy or electrons are directly transferred to molecular oxygen in the ground state (triplet) and singlet oxygen is formed. The highly reactive state of singlet oxygen results in a very effective method of oxidation of biological substrates. Both reaction types can occur in parallel. It is important to note that the extent to which one reaction occurs rather than the other depends on the photosensitizer, the subcellular localization of the dye, and the substrate and oxygen supply around the activated photosensitizer. Indirect experiments in vitro indicate that singlet oxygen is the main mediator of many PDT-induced biological effects [76, 176], although there is evidence from experimental systems that superoxide anion may be involved in the development of cutaneous photosensitivity [11, 12].

Biological Mechanisms

The biological effects of PDT can be divided into direct or indirect effects. Direct effects refer to direct actions on tumor cells. Indirect effects refer to actions of PDT on the immune and inflammatory response and on the tumor vasculature, which promotes tumor regression by restricting the blood supply to the tumor.

Direct Effects

Direct cellular damage can be detected following PDT [97]. This appears to be the major mechanism by which disulfonated and silicon phthalocyanine photosensitizers mediate tumor destruction [8, 48]. Besides the type of photosensitizer, the cell structures affected depend on the subcellular localization of the photosensitizer at the time of light treatment. The cell structures reported to be damaged by PDT include mitochondria [87], lysosomes [178] and the endoplasmatic reticulum [113]. Membrane damage initiates a cascade of events that result in apoptosis of cells that can be detected both in vivo and in vitro [3, 97, 191] and can affect cell cycle regulatory proteins [4]. On a molecular basis, PDT can also induce stress-proteins [57] (Fig. 8).

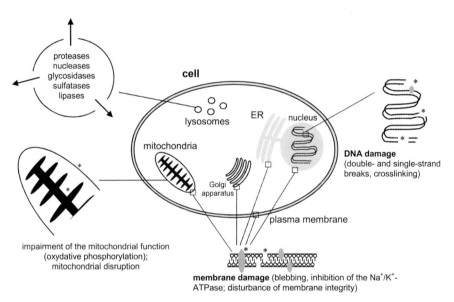

Fig. 8. PDT-related subcellular damages depend on the localization of the photosensitizer used. Significant damage occurs mostly at the plasma membranes, lysosomes, and mitochondria. This results in a disturbance of the membrane integrity, the release of lysosomal enzymes, and impairment of the respiratory chain. Damage to the DNA does not contribute significantly to cell death

Indirect Effects

When Photofrin is used in PDT protocols, indirect effects predominate with the most important biological effect for destruction of solid being the irreversible damage of pathologically altered tumor vasculature [47, 64] (Fig. 9). Photofrin PDT causes vasoconstriction of arterioles within the tumor, reduction of the erythrocyte flow velocity in venules of the surrounding tissue, stasis and thrombosis of tumor vessels, and perivascular edema [28, 31, 46, 153]. When enough photosensitizer and light is given, these effects are irreversible. Increase of the interstitial liquid pressure with compression of the tumor vessels [60, 98] is followed by tumor ischemia and accumulation of energetic phosphates within tumor cells [32]. The release of histamine [86], the induction of arachidonic-acid-metabolites, e.g., prostaglandin-E_2 [65] or thromboxane-B_2 [46], and other procoagulants, e.g., von-Willebrand-factor [51] participate in the vascular effects in the surrounding tissue and in the tumor.

In addition to the indirect effects on the tumor vasculature, there are a number of immunological and inflammatory effects that are at least in part responsible for PDT-induced tumor ablation. These effects are also being exploited for treatment of a number of benign conditions [35, 36, 90]. Profound inflammation is a consistent finding in PDT-treated tissues, and there is convincing evidence that inflammatory cells participate in PDT-induced tumor regression [29, 31, 47, 91]. For example, in animal models, neutropenia significantly reduced cure rates following Photofrin PDT [29, 89]. Moreover, the response to PDT could be significantly improved in experimental systems by co-administration of PDT with granulocyte colony-stimulating factor (G-CSF), a cytokine that increases neutrophil counts [92].

Cells of monocyte/macrophage lineage also contribute to PDT-induced tumor regression. In mice, low concentrations of porphyrins and light have an immunopotentiating effect [189, 190]. This may be because macrophages, which pref-

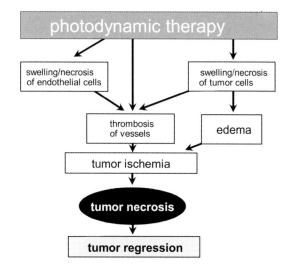

Fig. 9. On a cellular level PDT leads to swelling and/or necrosis of endothelial or tumor cells. The higher fragility of tumor cells leads to occlusion of vessels mostly due to thrombosis. The resulting tumor ischemia is further enhanced by compression of the vascular system due to an increased interstitial pressure based on cell swelling and perivascular edema

erentially target PDT treated cancer cells, release tumor necrosis factor-alpha (TNF-α) following Photofrin PDT [41, 88].

The development of T-cell mediated immunity also contributes significantly to PDT-induced tumor cures. Tumor specific T-cells can eliminate small foci of malignant cells, and this is likely to be the way in which tumor cells that have escaped the direct cytotoxicity and vascular effects of PDT are removed. Strong evidence that PDT, in fact, does lead to the induction of tumor-specific immunity comes from studies in animal models demonstrating that long-term tumor cures cannot be achieved in immunodeficient mice, but occur in immunocompetent animals [89, 90].

Inflammatory processes are often initiated by the synthesis and release of pro-inflammatory mediators [9, 41, 56, 119]. The production of several of these mediators is increased by PDT. Histamine and other vasoactive amines [9], cytokines such as TNF-α [9, 41, 119], interleukin (IL)-2 [119], IL-6 [56], IL-10 [56] IL-1β [30] and G-CSF [30], acute phase reactants [45, 122], and complement components have all been reported to increase following PDT.

In contrast to the treatment of superficial skin cancer or precancerous lesions, the aim in the treatment of chronic inflammatory dermatoses is not irreversible destruction of the tissue. There is evidence in the literature for immunosuppressive effects of PDT, e.g., decreased contact hypersensitivity, increased survival of skin transplants, and improvement in such experimental autoimmune diseases as collagen-induced arthritis and experimental allergic encephalomyelitis [21, 39, 66, 74, 100, 107, 121, 130, 132, 135, 139]. The investigation of PDT-induced immunological effects is an important goal of future research and will help to define new indications for PDT.

PDT in Dermatology

An overview of the clinical indications suitable for PDT in dermatology is given in Table 4. In contrast to other organs, the skin can be easily exposed to light after sensitization by either intravenous or direct topical or intralesional application of the photosensitizers.

Table 4. Indications for PDT in dermatology

Oncological	Mycosis fungoides
Actinic keratoses (also arsenical keratoses)	Cutaneous metastases
Bowen's disease	Non-oncological
Superficial basal cell carcinomas	Psoriasis vulgaris
Gorlin-Goltz syndrome	HPV-associated dermatoses
Keratoacanthoma	Epidermodysplasia verruciformis
Initial squamous cell carcinoma	Condylomata acuminata
Kaposi's sarcoma	

Systemic Photodynamic Therapy

The porphyrin mixture HpD and the partially purified and clinically approved form porfimer sodium are the only agents for which extensive clinical data are currently available. Systemic PDT has been used for the treatment of skin tumors, including Bowen's disease, basal cell carcinoma, squamous cell carcinoma, and recurrent metastatic breast cancer (Table 5). Although a large number of clinical studies on systemic PDT of non-melanoma skin cancer have been published, most are uncontrolled open trials with small numbers of patients using a wide variety of drug concentrations and light doses, and with differences in duration of follow-up, types of tumors, and patients.

Systemic PDT for Oncological Indications

Photofrin and HpD

Systemic PDT for Bowen's disease is very effective. Application of porfimer sodium (2 mg/kg of body weight [b.w.]) and light at $\lambda = 630$ nm (20–50 J/cm^2) induced complete remission in 98 %–100 % of the treated lesions [24, 140, 171]. A lower dose of porfimer sodium (1 mg/kg b.w.) was used to minimize cutaneous photosensitization. A complete remission of Bowen's disease ($n = 8$) was also achieved using higher light doses (630 nm, 185–250 J/cm^2) [75]. However, applying light doses of 50–100 J/cm^2 and 1 mg/kg b.w. porfimer sodium resulted in a complete remission in only 50 % of Bowen's disease patients [24, 140].

Squamous cell carcinomas (SCC) of the skin do not respond as well to systemic PDT as Bowen's disease. A 50 % recurrence rate was reported within 6 months after PDT of 32 SCCs treated with HpD (5.0 mg/kg b.w.) [128]. A possible explanation for the poor response rate could be the low light dose of light (30 J/cm^2) used in this study. Similar results were reported by McCaughan and co-workers for HpD (3 mg/kg b.w.) and porfimer sodium (2 mg/kg b.w.) also using low light doses of 20–30 J/cm^2 [109]. One year after PDT of 5 SCCs there was only a 40 % remission rate. There is only one case report showing the complete remission of a large squamous cell carcinoma of the lower lip during a follow-up 6 months after systemic PDT (porfimer sodium, 2 mg/kg b.w., 630 nm, 150 J/cm^2) [58].

More information is available for systemic PDT of basal cell carcinomas (BCC). In 1981, Dougherty [34] first used HpD (5 mg/kg b.w.) for curative PDT of three BCCs located in the face of a 72-year-old man. Irradiation was performed twice with a xenon-lamp (600–700 nm, 100 mW/cm^2, 120 J/cm^2) 4 days and 5 days after HpD administration. Feyh and co-workers treated 67 BCCs with HpD (2 mg/kg b.w.) and an argon-ion pumped dye laser (630 nm, 100 J/cm^2). Only three recurrences were reported in the 4.5 years of follow up [42]. Another study published by the same group showed poor response rates for BCCs located on the eyelid when treated with the same parameters [67]. Tse and co-workers treated 40 BCCs in three patients with nevoid BCC syndrome with HpD and light from a dye laser or a xenon-lamp [167]. All tumors resolved clinically within 4–6 weeks following therapy. However, histological examination of the treated tumors revealed nests of the tumor cells in 17.5 %. During the follow up period

Table 5. Results of systemic PDT for oncological indications in dermatology

Indication	Author	Lesions treated	Sensitizer, dose	Wavelength and lightdose	Complete remission
Bowen's disease	Waldow et al. 1987 [171]	3	Photofrin 2.0 mg/kg	630 nm 40–60 J/cm^2	100 %
	Robinson et al. 1988 [140]	>500 90	Photofrin 2.0 vs 1.0 mg/kg	628 nm 25 vs 50 J/cm^2	100 % 50 %
	Buchanan et al. 1989 [24]	50	Photofrin 2.0 mg/kg	630 nm 50 J/cm^2	98 %
	McCaughan et al. 1989 [109]	2	HpD/Photofrin 3.0/2.0 mg/kg	630 nm 20–30 J/cm^2	50 %
	Jones et al. 1992 [75]	8	Photofrin 1.0 mg/kg	630 nm 185–250 J/cm^2	100 %
Squamous cell carcinoma	Pennington et al. 1988 [128]	32	HpD 5.0 mg/kg	630 nm 30 J/cm^2	< 50 %
	McCaughan et al. 1989 [109]	5	HpD/Photofrin 3.0/2.0 mg/kg	630 nm 20–30 J/cm^2	40 %
	Gross et al. 1990 [58]	1	Photofrin 2.0 mg/kg	630 nm 150 J/cm^2	100 %
	Feyh et al. 1993 [42]	7	Photosan-3 2.0 mg/kg	630 nm 100 J/cm^2	86 %
Basal cell carcinoma	Tse et al. 1984 [167]	40	HpD 3.0 mg/kg	600–700 nm 38–180 J/cm^2	83 %
	Bandieramonte et al. 1984 [14]	42	HpD 3.0 mg/kg	480–515, 630 nm 60–120 J/cm^2	60 %
	Waldow et al. 1987 [171]	6	Photofrin 1.5–2.0 mg/kg	630 nm 40–60 J/cm^2	100 %
	Pennington et al. 1988 [128]	21	HpD 5.0 mg/kg	630 nm 30 J/cm^2	0 %
	Robinson et al. 1988 [140]	15	Photofrin 2.0 mg/kg	628 nm 50 J/cm^2	93 %
	Buchanan et al. 1989 [24]	13	Photofrin 1.5–2.0 mg/kg	630 nm 50–100 J/cm^2	39 %
	McCaughan et al. 1989 [109]	27	HpD/Photofrin 3.0/2.0 mg/kg	630 nm 20–30 J/cm^2	15 %
	Feyh et al. 1993 [42]	67	Photosan-3 2.0 mg/kg	630 nm 100 J/cm^2	97 %
	Calzavara et al. 1991 [26]	17	HpD/Photofrin 3.0/2.5–3.0 mg/kg	600–700 nm 25–225 J/cm^2	59 %
	Wilson et al. 1992 [180]	151	Photofrin 1.0 mg/kg	630 nm 72–288 J/cm^2	89 %
	Hintschich et al. 1993 [67]	27	Photosan-3 2.0 mg/kg	630 nm 100 J/cm^2	52 %
Cutaneous metastases of breast cancer (CR and PR in last row)	Dougherty 1981 [34]	35	HpD 2.5–5.0 mg/kg	? ?	97 %
	Schuh et al. 1987 [147]	30	Photofrin 1.0–2.0 mg/kg	630 nm 36–288 J/cm^2	80 %
	McCaughan et al. 1989 [109]	29	HpD/Photofrin 3.0/2.0 mg/kg	630 nm 20–30 J/cm^2	100 %
	Sperduto et al. 1991 [152]	20	Photofrin 1.5 mg/kg	630 nm 20–359 J/cm^2	65 %
	review Schlag et al. 1992 [145]	846	HpD/Photofrin 1.0–5.0 mg/kg	– 8–300 J/cm^2	83 %

of 12–14 months the recurrence rate was 10.8 %. Recurrences of large, ulcerative, or crusted tumors accounted for much of the poor response rate [167].

Another indication for systemic PDT is the palliative treatment of cutaneous metastases of breast cancer [145]. In all reported cases, PDT was performed after conventional therapies had failed (radiation, chemotherapy, hormone-therapy, conventional surgery). The aim of therapy was eradication of the tumor or the reduction of tumor bulk in order to avoid ulceration or uncontrollable bleeding (Table 5). Dougherty achieved partial remissions ($>$ 50 % reduction of tumor bulk) in 34 of 35 patients with cutaneous or subcutaneous metastases of breast cancer 4–6 weeks after PDT with HpD (2.5–5.0 mg/kg b.w.) [34]. McCaughan showed a partial or complete remission in all patients with cutaneous metastases of breast cancer after treatment with HpD (3 mg/kg b.w.) or porfimer sodium (2 mg/kg b.w.) and subsequent irradiation with 60–120 J/cm^2 [109]. Summarizing all patients (n = 118, total number of lesions=846) with cutaneous metastases of breast cancer treated by systemic PDT, Schlag et al. found a complete remission in 63 % of the treated lesions, a partial remission in 20 %, and no response in 16 % [145]. The best results were achieved in the treatment of tumors smaller than 2 cm.

Boehncke and co-workers showed in vitro that PDT was as effective as psoralen plus ultraviolet A (PUVA) in the treatment of cutaneous T-cell lymphoma using comparable photosensitizer concentrations and light doses (UVA 0.75 J/cm^2 vs laser 630 nm, 1 J/cm^2) [22]. In 1980, Forbes et al. succeeded in treating a patient with mycosis fungoides (plaque stage) with HpD (5 mg/kg b.w.) and repeated irradiations with an incoherent light source (λ = 620–640 nm, 40 mW/cm^2, 48–96 J/cm^2, irradiation 72 h and 96 h after sensitization) [50]. He also achieved a partial remission in a patient with metastatic Kaposi's sarcoma using the same treatment regimen [50]. Dougherty [34] and Calzavara [26] applied 2.5–3.0 mg/kg b.w. HpD and a light dose of 120 J/cm^2 vs 50–200 J/cm^2 in patients with classic Mediterranean Kaposi's sarcoma. All tumors (100 %) in three patients and 85 % of the tumors in four patients treated with PDT showed complete remission.

Schweitzer and Visscher treated five patients with AIDS-associated Kaposi's sarcoma with 2 mg/kg b.w. porfimer sodium and red light given both as surface illumination and interstitially (50–200 J/cm^2). Complete or partial remission of cutaneous or mucosal nodular lesions was observed 8 weeks after therapy in 54 of 92 lesions (58.7 %) [150]. Almost the same results were presented by Hebeda et al. for eight HIV-positive patients with a total of 83 Kaposi's sarcoma lesions treated with 2 mg/kg b.w. porfimer sodium and irradiation with a dye laser (630 nm, 70–120 J/cm^2). Although the remission rate was 60–70 %, the cosmetic results were unsatisfactory since long lasting hyperpigmentation and scar formation occurred [63].

Second Generation Photosensitizers

Benzoporphyrin derivative-monoacid ring A (verteporfin, BPD-MA) represents one of a number of alternatives to the first generation photosensitizers, Photofrin and HpD. It has a significantly shorter tissue half-life. It is a semisynthetic porphyrin synthesized from PpIX. A major advantage to BPD-MA is that both drug and the irradiation procedure can be administered on the same day. In contrast to HpD, BPD-MA is metabolized and excreted in an inactive form [16, 162]. The duration of potential susceptibility to cutaneous photosensitivity is therefore less than 72 h [103, 186]. Phase I/II studies with BPD-MA have confirmed the efficacy of this photosensitizer in the treatment of some epithelial skin tumors after intravenous administration of 0.375–0.50 mg/kg b.w. in a liposomal formulation followed by irradiation at 690 nm (50–150 J/cm^2) 2–6 h later. Remission rates of about 100 % were achieved [100].

Phase-I studies with lutetium texaphyrin, a compound with an expanded porphyrin macrocycle, have been completed in 19 patients with BCC, Kaposi's sarcoma, and metastatic melanoma. This agent has peak absorption at 732 nm, which allows for greater depth of penetration within tissues. Lutetium texaphyrin appears to be highly selective for tumors versus normal skin and shows no significant skin phototoxicity when given systemically [136].

SnET$_2$, a chlorin photosensitizer, is currently in phase II trials for the treatment of cutaneous metastatic breast cancer and Kaposi's sarcoma [36]. An overall 75 % complete response rate in 121 Kaposi's sarcoma lesions with a superb cosmetic result was described [5]. A complete response rate of 92 % was achieved in eight patients with advanced breast cancer metastases (total number of lesions = 86) after a single PDT with SnET$_2$ (1.2 mg/kg b.w.) and laser light (660 ± 3 nm, 150 mW/cm^2, 200 J/cm^2) [6].

Another chlorin photosensitizer tetra(m-hydroxyphenyl)chlorin (mTHPC), which is undergoing clinical trials for head and neck cancer in Europe and the United States, appears to be the most active of all photosensitizers requiring only very low drug and light doses [33].

The activity of another new photosensitizer, mono-L-aspartyl chlorin e$_6$ (Npe6) was evaluated in a phase I clinical study for 11 patients with a variety of solid skin tumors (BCC, SCC, recurrent breast cancer) [165]. Npe6 offers the advantage of being rapidly cleared from tissues resulting in a reduced duration of cutaneous photosensitivity. Using Npe6 doses of 2.5–3.5 mg/kg b.w. combined with 100 J/cm^2 of light energy resulted in 66 % of sites remaining tumor-free 12 weeks after therapy.

Systemic PDT for Non-Oncological Indications

Psoriasis

As early as 1937 Silver reported on the clinical application of hematoporphyrin and UV-light for the treatment of psoriasis. Six patients with psoriasis received HpD intramuscularly and orally on consecutive days followed by irradiation with UV-light. Two weeks after initiation of therapy, a significant reduction in psoriatic plaques was observed [151]. Low HPD doses given intravenously (1 mg/kg b.w.) and UVA irradiation for 15 days led to a 90 % remission of extensive plaque type psoriasis in 15 of 19 patients without significant side effects [18]. Emtestam and co-workers treated 10 patients with psoriasis with a single dose of tin-protoporphyrin (2.0 µmol/kg b.w.) and UVA for several days [40]. The cumulative UVA-dose necessary to induce a photodynamic reaction was 98.3 J/cm^2, which was fractionated over 21 days. In all patients psoriatic plaques improved significantly [40].

The successful use of HpD and UV-light by Berg and Emtestam demonstrates that the deeper penetration of red light into the skin is not necessary for an effective PDT of psoriasis. This would facilitate introduction of PDT into clinical practice, as UVA-light sources are widely available. Weinstein et al. treated 8 patients with psoriasis with a single dose of porfimer sodium (0.5 mg/kg b.w.) followed by irradiation with UVA-light vs light at 405 nm or at 630 nm [175]. The efficacy of UVA-light or light at 405 nm was significantly lower than that of light at 630 nm [175]. At present, systemic PDT with BPD-MA is being investigated for psoriasis. In a phase-I study (0.2 mg/kg b.w., irradiation 3 h later, 690 nm, 75 J/cm^2) complete remission of psoriatic plaques was achieved for 60 days after a single treatment [100].

Portwine stains

To evaluate the effect of systemic PDT on portwine stains, 15 patients were treated with porfimer sodium (0.75 and 1 mg/kg b.w.) and irradiated at different times thereafter (15, 30, 60 min, 2, 4, 8, 24 h) with different light doses (630 nm, 40–50 mW/cm^2, 25–100 J/cm^2). There was a marked improvement in those patients, who received a light dose of 75–100 J/cm^2 and were irradiated 30 min–2 h after photosensitizer administration. The lighting of portwine stains persisted up to 6 months after therapy. The treatment did not result in scarring or atrophy [117].

Xiao-xi et al. used PsD-007, a purified mixture of porphyrin molecules, for PDT of portwine stains. Compared to first-generation porphyrins, PsD-007 is activated at longer wavelengths and exhibits a lower degree of cutaneous photosensitivity after systemic administration. One-hundred thirty patients with portwine stains received intravenous injections of 4–7 mg/kg b.w. PsD-007. Less than half an hour later, the lesions were irradiated with a copper vapor laser (578 nm, 40–90 mW/m2). Of 118 patients reviewed retrospectively, 98.3% responded to PDT with varying degrees of success after one-time treatment. Side effects, such as hypertrophic scars and permanent hyper- or hypopigmentation did not occur. This positive effect on portwine stains is thought to be based on a PDT-mediated endothelial cell injury and death of abnormal capillaries beneath the overlying epidermis [188].

Topical Photodynamic Therapy

The most significant side effect of systemic PDT is prolonged cutaneous photosensitivity. For many dermatological diseases, this side effect can be avoided by topical application of photosensitizers. However, the molecular weight of porphyrins is too high (molecular weight approx. 900 g/mol) to allow for penetration into the skin in sufficient amounts [137]. In contrast, there is excellent percutaneous absorption of small hydrophilic molecules such as ALA, especially if parakeratotic horn is present as in epithelial tumors or psoriasis [84].

Because epithelial tumors show high and selective porphyrin accumulation they can be destroyed without damage to the surrounding tissue [2, 84, 158]. There are several potential reasons for the selective uptake of topical ALA into diseased tissue. Intact stratum corneum of normal skin is less permeable than skin in which the integrity is compromised. Additionally, the abnormal structure of tumor stroma with a large interstitial space and higher amounts of free water may allow for faster diffusion of the hydrophilic ALA [120]. Also, a selective accumulation of ALA-induced porphyrins occurs within cells [77]. Other factors contribute to the tissue selectivity of ALA-induced porphyrins: epidermal cells and the pilosebaceous units synthesize porphyrins in higher amounts than fibroblasts, myocytes, or endothelial cells [84, 124]. Fluorescence-microscopy of BCCs after incubation with ALA shows significantly higher fluorescence intensity within the tumor than the surrounding stroma due to a selective porphyrin accumulation in the tumor [106, 164].

Several studies in human volunteers and animals proved that ALA-induced PpIX is almost completely cleared from the body within 24 h after administration, either orally, topically, or intravenously [2, 19, 84]. This rapid clearance reduces the risk of PpIX accumulation leading to prolonged photosensitivity, even if a PDT treatment is repeated as often as every other day. Moreover, there is no significant systemic accumulation of porphyrins and porphyrin precursors after topical ALA application [54].

Possible improvements in topical ALA PDT to force accumulation of endogenously synthesized porphyrins have been proposed. These include adding inhibitors of ferrochelatase [133, 134], the addition of iron chelators [43, 61, 123] or the use of esterized ALA molecules (i.e., ALA-methylester). However, currently there is no clinical evidence of an increased effectiveness compared to ALA alone. Only for EDTA in patients suffering from basal cell carcinomas (tumor thickness < 2 mm) an improvement in the therapeutic response has been demonstrated [126].

The only relevant side effect of topical ALA PDT is a stinging pain that occurs during irradiation. When treating large areas, e.g., the whole scalp for actinic keratoses, some patients cannot tolerate the pain, making analgesics or even anesthesia necessary [157, 160, 161]. Recently an allergic contact dermatitis from ALA or its derivatives was reported [55].

There are few photosensitizers, other than ALA, that have been used topically. Tetrasodium-meso-tetraphenylporphinesulfonate (TPPS$_4$), a porphin isomer, has been tried for topical PDT. Thirty-three primary and recurrent neoplastic lesions (23 BCCs, 8 Bowen's disease, 1 SCC, 1 recurrent breast carcinoma) of the skin were treated. Complete remission was obtained in 25 of 27 lesions with histological tumor-thickness of less than 1 mm [143]. Sacchini and co-workers also treated 50 patients with 292 BCCs with a tumor thickness less than 2 mm with a 2 % TPPS$_4$ solution and a dye laser at 645 nm (120 – 150 J/cm^2). TPPS$_4$ was applied topically 24, 6, and 3 h before irradiation. In 93.5 %, a complete remission of the tumor was achieved. Recurrences were seen in 10.6 % of the treated tumors [143]. However, these initially promising studies were not continued due to possible neurotoxicity of the drug [181] and to extensive damage that occurred to the surrounding normal tissue as a consequence of a non-selective penetration of TPPS$_4$ into the subcutaneous fat [69].

A promising new group of compounds for topical PDT are the porphycenes [79, 137]. Chemically, porphycenes are synthetic porphin isomers that consist of four pyrrole rings [168]. They generate high yields of singlet oxygen [10] and show good tumor targeting properties [59]. The porphycene 9-acetoxy-2,7,12,17-tetrakis-(β-methoxyethyl)-porphycene (ATMPn) can be applied systemically within liposomes [1] as well as topically as an ethanolic gel-formulation [78]. Phase II clinical studies to investigate the efficacy, safety, and tolerability of topical PDT with ATMPn for the treatment of psoriasis and superficial basal cell carcinomas are currently being performed.

Topical PDT for Oncological Indications

The first clinical results with topical ALA PDT were reported by Kennedy and co-workers in 1990 [85]. After application of a 20 % ALA o/w formulation and an incubation time of 3–6 h, lesions were irradiated with a 500-W slide projector (150–300 mW/cm^2, 15–150 J/cm^2). Out of 80 BCCs 90 % showed a complete remission within 2–3 months after therapy (Table 6). Also each of 6 in situ or early invasive SCCs showed complete remission after PDT. Nine of 10 actinic

Table 6. Results of topical PDT with ALA for oncological indications in dermatology

Indication	Author	Lesions treated	ALA dose	Wavelength and light dose	Complete remission
Basal cell carcinoma	Kennedy et al. 1990 [85]	80[a]	20 % 3–6 h	150–300 mW/cm^2 15–150 J/cm^2	90 %
	Kennedy and Pottier 1992 [84]	300[a]	20 % 3–6 h	150–300 mW/cm^2 15–150 J/cm^2	79 %
	Warloe et al. 1992 [173]	96	20 % > 3 h	100–150 mW/cm^2 50–100 J/cm^2	96 %
	Wolf et al. 1993 [185]	37[a] 10[b]	20 % 4 h	50–100 mW/cm^2 –	97 %[a] 10 %[b]
	Hürlimann et al. 1994 [71]	72[a] 15[b]	20 % –	– –	94 %[a] 33 %[b]
	Cairnduff et al. 1994 [25]	16	20 % 3–6 h	150 mW/cm^2 125–250 J/cm^2	50 %
	Svanberg et al. 1994 [157]	55[a] 25[b]	20 % 4–6 h	110 mW/cm^2 60 J/cm^2	100 %[a] 64 %[b]
	Lang et al. 1995 [95]	12	10 % 6 h	– 100 J/cm^2	83 %
	Lui et al. 1995 [106]	8[a]	20 % 3 h	19–44 mW/cm^2 100 J/cm^2	50 %
	Calzavara-Pinton 1995 [27]	23[a] 30[b]	20 % 6–8 h	100 mW/cm^2 60–80 J/cm^2	87 %[a] 50 %[b]
	Fijan et al. 1995 [43]	34[a] 22[b]	20 %+3 % desferrioxamine 20 h	150–250 mW/cm^2 > 300 J/cm^2	88 %[a] 32 %[b]
	Fink-Puches et al. 1998 [49]	95[a]	20 % 4 h	– 18–131 J/cm^2	56 %
	Hürlimann et al. 1998 [70]	81[a]	10 % (nanocolloidal) 6 h	– 240 J/cm^2	84 %
	Szeimies et al., unpublished	149[a]	10–20 % 5–6 h	120–150 J/cm^2 120–180 J/cm^2	77 %

Table 6. (Continued)

Indication	Author	Lesions treated	ALA dose	Wavelength and light dose	Complete remission
Squamous cell carcinoma	Kennedy et al. 1990 [85]	6	20 % 3–6 h	150–300 mW/cm^2 15–150 J/cm^2	100 %
	Wolf et al. 1993 [185]	6[a]	20 % 4 h	50 mW/cm^2 –	83 %
	Hürlimann et al. 1994 [71]	4[a]	20 % –	–	100 % –
	Lui et al. 1995 [106]	3[a] 2[b]	20 % 3 h	19–44 mW/cm^2 100 J/cm^2	67 %[a] 0 %[b]
	Calzavara-Pinton 1995 [27]	12[a] 6[b]	20 % 6–8 h	100 mW/cm^2 60–80 J/cm^2	83 %[a] 33 %[b]
Actinic Keratoses	Kennedy et al. 1990 [85]	10	20 % 3–6 h	150–300 mW/cm^2 15–150 J/cm^2	90 %
	Wolf et al. 1993 [185]	9	20 % 4 h	50–100 mW/cm^2 –	100 %
	Calzavara-Pinton 1995 [27]	50	20 % 6–8 h	100 mW/cm^2 60–80 J/cm^2	84 %
	Fijan et al. 1995 [43]	43	20 % + 3 % desferrioxamine 20 h	150–250 mW/cm^2 > 300 J/cm^2	81 %
	Szeimies et al. 1996 [161]	17 head 19 hands and arms	10 % 5–6 h	160 mW/cm^2 150 J/cm^2	71 % head 0 % hands and arms
	Jeffes et al. 1997 [72]	55 head 112 hands and arms	10/20/30 % 3 h	– 10–150 J/cm^2	76 % head 38 % hands and arms
	Karrer et al. 1999 [80]	200 head	20 % 6 h	60–160 J/cm^2 (lamp) 16 J/cm^2 (laser 585 nm)	84 % (lamp) 79 % (laser)
Bowen's disease	Hürlimann et al. 1994 [71]	6	20 % –	– –	100 %
	Cairnduff et al. 1994 [25]	36	20 % 3–6 h	150 mW/cm^2 125–250 J/cm^2	89 %
	Svanberg et al. 1994 [157]	10	20 % 4–6 h	110 mW/cm^2 60 J/cm^2	90 %
	Calzavara-Pinton 1995 [27]	6	20 % 6–8 h	100 mW/cm^2 60–80 J/cm^2	100 %
	Fijan et al. 1995 [43]	10	20 %+3 % desferrioxamine 20 h	150–250 mW/cm^2 > 300 J/cm^2	30 %
	Morton et al. 1996 [116]	20	20 % 4 h	– 125 J/cm^2	100 %
	Wennberg et al. 1996 [177]	11	20 % 3 h	– 100 J/cm^2	100 %
	Szeimies et al., unpublished	10	10 % 6 h	150 mW/cm^2 150–180 J/cm^2	80 %

[a] Superficial tumors.
[b] Nodular tumors.

keratoses also responded well to a single treatment with ALA PDT. However, a remission could not be induced by ALA PDT in metastatic breast cancer [85]. Two years later the same group reported on ALA PDT of more than 300 superficial BCCs, showing complete remission in 79 % 3 months after therapy [84]. Warloe and co-workers treated 11 patients with 96 BCCs with a 20 % ALA emulsion. After 3 h of incubation, the lesions were irradiated. Most lesions received ALA PDT once, 11 lesions were treated twice and 2 lesions were treated 3 times. Three months after therapy 96 % of all lesions were cured, and the cosmetic results were considered excellent [173]. Hürlimann and co-workers had very good results after ALA PDT using an 20 % ALA formulation. A complete remission was achieved in 68 of 72 treated superficial BCCs, in all 6 Bowen's disease lesions and in all 4 treated SCCs. For nodular BCC the cure rate was only 33 %. Also, 9 cutaneous lymphomas treated with ALA PDT showed only minimal responsiveness [71]. Hürlimann et al. also treated 19 patients with 55 superficial BCCs using a novel nanocolloid lotion containing 10 % ALA followed by irradiation with light from a conventional slide projector [70]. This new ALA formulation was developed because of the chemical instability of ALA in aqueous solution at high pH levels. A complete response was found in 85 % of the carcinomas with a follow-up period of 6 months. Harth et al. used a modified topical formulation in which penetration enhancers (2 % EDTA and 2 % DMSO) were added to ALA 20 % in cream base. After 12 h of incubation with this formulation the tumors were exposed to a high output source emitting red and infrared light to utilize hyperthermia [62]. Complete responses were achieved after 1–3 ALA PDT treatments in 26 of 31 lesions of superficial or small nodular BCC (84 %) and in 4 of 5 lesions of superficial SCC (80 %). Wennberg and colleagues achieved a 92 % clearance of 157 superficial BCCs treated with a 20 % ALA emulsion and a filtered xenon lamp [177]. Wolf et al. treated 13 patients with 70 skin tumors with topical ALA PDT (20 % ALA emulsion, irradiation with a slide projector). Five of 6 initial SCCs, all 9 actinic keratoses, and 36 of 37 superficial BCCs showed a complete remission. Cutaneous metastases of malignant melanoma did not respond to therapy [185]. Pigmented BCCs ($n = 4$) also did not respond [27]. These and other pigmented tumors probably do not allow sufficient penetration of light into the neoplastic tissue due to their melanin content. Therefore, pigmented lesions are a contraindication for most forms of PDT. Very good results were reported from Svanberg et al., who showed a 100 % cure rate of 55 superficial BCCs and a 90 % cure rate of 10 Bowen's disease when treated with topical ALA PDT (630 nm light from a laser, 110 W/cm^2, 60 J/cm^2). Nodular BCCs ($n = 25$) did not respond as well to PDT (remission only in 64 %) [157]. Calzavara-Pinton achieved good results after repeated treatments with topical ALA PDT using a 20 % ALA emulsion and irradiation with an argon-ion-pumped dye laser (100 mW/cm^2, 60–80 J/cm^2) [27]. Treatments were performed every second day, until clinically detectable tumor was no longer apparent (usually 1–3 treatments). Forty-eight percent of 50 actinic keratoses, 87 % of 23 superficial BCCs, 100 % of 6 Bowen's disease, 84 % of 12 superficial SCCs, 50 % of 30 nodular BCCs and 33 % of 6 nodular SCCs showed a clinical complete remission [27]. In the only phase III study reported so far in the treatment of Bowen's disease, ALA PDT using a nonlaser light source appeared to be as effective as cryotherapy with fewer adverse effects [116].

In a phase II study, Szeimies and co-workers investigated the efficacy and tolerability of topical ALA PDT in the treatment of actinic keratoses according to GCP-guidelines [161]. Thirty-six actinic keratoses in ten patients were treated. A 10 % ALA emulsion was applied to the lesions for 5–6 h before irradiation with an incoherent light source (Waldmann PDT 1200, 160 mW/cm^2, 150 J/cm^2). Seventy-one percent of the actinic keratoses located on the head showed complete remission up to 3 months after therapy. For lesions located on the lower arms and hands, only partial remissions were seen, probably due to greater hyperkeratosis overlying the lesions [161]. Jeffes et al. treated 40 patients with actinic keratoses according to a similar treatment protocol (0 %, 10 %, 20 % or 30 % ALA, 3 h incubation, irradiation with an argon pumped dye laser, 630 nm, 10–150 J/cm^2). Eight weeks after a single treatment with 30 % ALA there was total clearing of 91 % of lesions on the face and scalp and 45 % of the lesions on the trunk and extremities. No significant differences were found in clinical responses for the different concentrations of ALA (10–30 %) [72]. Recently DUSA Pharmaceuticals (Toronto, Canada) reported the results of two phase III clinical trials using ALA for topical PDT of patients with actinic keratoses of the face and scalp. A total of 240 patients received either 20 % ALA or placebo overnight followed by irradiation with blue light at 10 J/cm^2. In the two studies, 86 % and 81 % of the treated lesions cleared after a single treatment. This was statistically significant compared with a clearance of 32 % and 20 % in the placebo group [36].

In order to further reduce irradiation time and lower the only side effect so far of ALA PDT which is pain during irradiation, Karrer et al. performed a comparative study in 24 patients [80]. Topical ALA PDT was performed on actinic keratoses on the head (n = 200) after application of a 20 % ALA emulsion for 6 h and irradiation by either an incoherent light source (160 mW/cm^2, 60–160 J/cm^2) or a long pulsed flash lamp pumped dye laser (LPDL) (t = 1.5 ms; λ = 585 nm; 16 J/cm^2). Twenty-eight days after PDT a complete remission was achieved in 79 % of 100 actinic keratoses treated by the LPDL and in 84 % of 100 actinic keratoses treated by the incoherent lamp. Pain during light treatment was significantly reduced by using the LPDL. Control lesions treated by the LPDL without ALA did not clear.

An important potential indication for topical ALA PDT is the Gorlin-Goltz syndrome (nevoid BCC syndrome) in which the multiple tumors can be clinically and cosmetically controlled in an effective way [83, 112]. Topical ALA PDT is also efficient in patients with arsenic-induced skin cancer or with epithelial skin cancer due to immunosuppression after kidney transplantation [44, 160, 172].

To investigate the influence of tumor thickness on the efficacy of PDT, Thiele and co-workers treated 19 BCCs in 11 patients with a 20 % ALA emulsion and a light dose of 50–100 J/cm^2. Histological investigation after therapy showed a destruction of superficial parts of the tumor. However, the deeper dermis of nodular lesions remained unchanged after therapy [166]. Fink-Puches and co-workers investigated the long-term effects and histological changes of superficial BCCs and superficial SCCs after ALA PDT with polychromatic light [49]. Their study revealed a poor long-term cure rate with a disease-free rate of only 50 % for BCC and 8 % for SCC 36 months after therapy. Histopathological studies after ALA PDT revealed fibrosis in the dermis, which reached deeper than the initial depth of invasiveness of the tumor, suggesting that the poor results of ALA PDT could not be explained by insufficient penetration of the therapy. As a possible factor for the poor response, an insufficient marking of tumors by PpIX was postulated [49]. Hoerauf reported an insufficient response of BCCs of the eye-lid after topical PDT with a 20 % ALA emulsion [68]. Four to 8 weeks after PDT, the former tumor bearing area was surgically removed in 10 patients. Histological examination showed residual tumor [67]. In a phase I study Cairnduff et al. achieved a complete remission in 89 % of 36 Bowen's disease lesions after treatment with a 20 % ALA ointment and irradiation with a dye laser at 630 nm. However, only 50 % of the 16 BCCs treated this way showed a complete remission. In this study, the lesions that were most likely to recur were ones that had been incubated for only 3 – 4 h with ALA [25]. Szeimies et al. performed fluorescence microscopy of BCCs that had been incubated with a 10 % ALA ointment before excision. After incubation with ALA for only 4 h prior to excision, porphyrin fluorescence could be detected solely within the pilosebaceous unit. Only after longer incubation times of at least 6 h could porphyrin fluorescence be detected in superficial or nodular BCCs [164]. However, morpheaform BCCs showed a very heterogeneous fluorescence even after longer incubation times of up to 12 h [164]. This is probably due to reduced porphyrin synthesis within this subtype of BCC [164, 179]. A penetration study using a 20 % ALA formulation in 16 patients with 18 BCCs (7 superficial, 10 nodular, 1 infiltrating) and an average incubation time of 6.9 h revealed PpIX fluorescence corresponding to full tumor thickness only in six of the superficial and four of the nodular tumors [108]. These results correlate with the experience of different working groups, that ALA PDT is not a reliable regimen for BCCs with a tumor thickness exceeding 3 – 4 mm thus making standard treatment modalities like excision, Moh's micrographic surgery, or cryotherapy necessary [27, 43, 71, 156, 157, 185].

According to the data discussed above, the only current indications for curative topical ALA PDT (occlusive application of 20 % ALA o/w emulsion for 4 – 6 h, irradiation with 100 – 150 mW/cm^2; 100 – 150 J/cm^2) of epithelial precancerous or cancerous lesions are actinic keratoses, Bowen's disease and superficial basal cell carcinomas (tumor thickness < 3 mm). For irradiation, an incoherent lamp is suitable without loss of efficacy [43, 161]. With respect to these indications and following these treatment parameters, PDT offers a good alternative to established treatments with the advantage of a better cosmetic result and the ability to treat many lesions simultaneously. However, a final judgment of topical ALA PDT is not possible until well-documented phase III studies with sufficiently long follow-up periods have been completed.

Besides epithelial skin tumors ALA PDT has also been used successfully for the treatment of mycosis fungoides. Two patients with plaque stage mycosis fungoides were treated with a 20 % ALA emulsion for 4 – 6 h and were then irradiated with a slide projector (44 mW/cm^2, 40 J/cm^2). After five treatment sessions within 18 weeks in one patient and after four treatments within 7 weeks in another patient, a complete clinical and histological remission could be achieved [182]. The same working group has now treated more than 60 mycosis fungoides lesions in another four patients. Treatment parameters, e.g., wavelength of the light source (UVA and visible light), light dose (0.5–60 J/cm^2) and number of treatments (up to three within 10–25 days) in this study varied significantly. Only repeated treatments led to a clinical remission of the lesions [183]. After a single treatment with ALA PDT, histological examination revealed persistence of atypical lymphocytes in the dermis, although clinically a remission was observed [7]. Oseroff and co-workers [124] from the Roswell Park Cancer Institute in Buffalo treated eight patients with different stages of mycosis fungoides with more than 50 solitary tumors, including ulcerated tumors with a tumor thickness up to 1.5 cm. A 2–20% ALA ointment was applied to the lesions for 12 h and then the lesions were irradiated with a dye laser (30–150 mW/cm^2, 50–150 J/cm^2). For comparison, two patients were treated with topical nitrogen mustard. PDT was performed every 2–4 weeks. Patches and thin plaques resolved after about two treatment cycles, thicker tumors needed five to seven therapy cycles until a histologically proven complete remission was achieved. Ulcerated tumors showed re-epithelization after a single treatment. In superinfected ulcerative CTCL lesions, bacterial concentrations in treated areas diminished leading to rapid granulation and better healing. Tumors treated with ALA PDT healed faster than those treated with nitrogen mustard. The result at the end of therapy was comparable for both treatment methods. Thus, there was a histologically proven remission in 61% of the treated lesions; in 39% a partial remission was achieved [13]. However, a randomized prospective clinical study with topical ALA PDT for mycosis fungoides has not been conducted yet.

Topical PDT for Non-Oncological Indications

A very promising indication for topical PDT is the treatment of benign skin diseases, e.g., psoriasis vulgaris. In contrast to tumor PDT, a single treatment probably will not be sufficient to achieve the desired clinical effect in most chronic disorders [23, 174]. Hürlimann et al. achieved a partial remission in 15 psoriatic plaques after 1–5 treatment sessions with ALA PDT [71]. Weinstein and co-workers treated plaques of psoriatic patients once a week for 4 weeks using either 10%, 20% or 30% ALA and irradiation by a dye laser (10–150 J/cm^2). He observed the best results for 30% ALA with repeated treatments [174]. McCullough and Weinstein undertook a pilot drug and light dose-ranging study using UVA and ALA PDT of psoriasis [110]. A total of 14 patients with plaque psoriasis were treated with topical ALA (2%, 10%, 20%) in an o/w emulsion for 3 h. They were then exposed to incremental dosages of UVA (2.5–30 J/cm^2). The result of this pilot study showed approximately 50% improvement after four weekly treatments with 10% (total UVA 80–120 J/cm^2) and 20% ALA (total UVA 1–39 J/cm^2). Treatment with 2% ALA was ineffective. To compare the effectiveness of ALA PDT with dithranol in three patients with chronic plaque-type psoriasis, Boehncke applied 10% ALA ointment for 5 h and irradiated the areas with an incoherent lamp (70 mW/cm^2, 25 J/cm^2) 3 times a week. In one patient, the PDT-treated areas cleared 1 week earlier than the side treated with dithranol [23]. An early phase II clinical study was conducted to evaluate the efficacy and tolerability of topical PDT with ATMPn in 29 patients with chronic plaque type psoriasis [78]. After a single treatment with a 0.1 % ethanol ATMPn formulation and irradiation with an incoherent light source, psoriasis plaques improved significantly. Further studies are under way to investigate whether repeated treatments using this new photosensitizer are able to induce a complete and prolonged remission of psoriatic plaques.

In contrast to PUVA or UVB radiation, which are known to be carcinogenic [142, 155], the target of cytotoxicity in PDT is not the DNA. There are no reports in the literature, which document an increased risk of the development of skin tumors in the long follow-up of patients with erythropoetic protoporphyria (Goerz, personal communication). Furthermore, it is likely that the total number of treatments necessary for therapeutic success is probably lower for PDT compared to PUVA. However, a better understanding of the basic mechanisms of PDT in psoriasis, which are distinctly different from that in cutaneous malignancies, is needed.

The ability of photosensitizers to inactivate viruses or bacteriophages has been known since the 1930s [141, 148]. This was demonstrated for herpes simplex viruses in vitro (for a review see [20]). As a consequence, this therapeutic approach was investigated in patients with genital herpes simplex infections. Neutral red (1.0 % aqueous solution) was used as a photosensitizer followed by irradiation with fluorescence light. In 30 patients a significant reduction of symptoms was observed and the frequency of recurrence was decreased [53]. Proflavine and methylene blue also showed therapeutic efficacy as photosensitizers for this disease (review see [20]). However, in four other studies, partly double-blind and placebo-controlled, PDT was found to be ineffective (review see [20]). Due to the potential carcinogenicity of proflavine and methylene blue and due to the introduction of antiviral chemotherapeutic treatments, PDT has been abandoned for this indication. PDT is being evaluated, however, for viral inactivation of blood products (e.g., HIV). [17, 118].

Another potential indication for topical PDT is human papilloma virus (HPV)-associated skin diseases. The benefits of PDT for these conditions are the lack of a virus-containing laser plume, which does occur with CO_2 and pulsed tunable dye lasers, and possibly a lower recurrence rate due to eradication of subclinical lesions. Frank and co-workers reported complete remission of anogenital condyloma acuminata in four of seven patients after topical ALA PDT (20 % ALA gel; 14 h incubation, argon dye laser 75–100 mW/cm^2, 100 J/cm^2) [52]. Recalcitrant hand and foot warts have also been shown to respond to ALA PDT. Stender et al. [154] treated 45 patients with verrucae vulgaris of the hands and feet with ALA PDT (20 % ALA cream; 4 h incubation; 70 J/cm^2 from a red light source) or placebo PDT. There was 100 % reduction in wart area in the ALA PDT treated group compared to a 71 % reduction in the placebo-treated wart group after six treatments over 18 weeks. However, some of the authors' own studies on six patients with verrucae vulgaris on hands or soles did not show any effect of ALA PDT, although a sufficient keratolysis was done before application of the 20 % ALA emulsion for 6 h and subsequent irradiation with an incoherent light source ($50-150$ mW/cm^2, 100 J/cm^2). HPV-associated warts in patients with epidermodysplasia verruciformis respond very well to ALA PDT [81, 184].

Photodynamic antimicrobial chemotherapy has been shown to be effective in vitro against bacteria, including drug-resistant strains, yeasts and parasites [82, 170]. Therefore, photodynamic antimicrobial chemotherapy is being proposed as a potential approach to the disinfection of blood products and to the treatment of locally occurring infections.

Few topical photosensitizers other than ALA have entered clinical evaluation for benign conditions. Monfrecola et al. treated two patients with alopecia areata with topical HPD-PDT. A 0.5% HPD-formulation was applied 3 times a week to the hairless areas followed by irradiation ($360-365$ nm). After $8-10$ weeks fine vellus hair grew in the treated areas, after further $4-8$ weeks it was replaced by terminal hairs [115]. In 1989 Meffert and Prěs performed topical PDT with HpD in 29 patients with psoriasis vulgaris, 17 of these patients suffered from palmoplantar psoriasis [111, 129]. Meffert treated 12 plaques with a 0.0001% HpD-ointment with 5% DMSO. On 3 consecutive days, PDT was performed with visible or UV-light (2, 4, 6 J/cm^2). The treated plaques responded well to therapy, some showing a complete remission [111]. Prěs treated the 17 patients with palmoplantar psoriasis using the same HPD-formulation in up to 20 treatment sessions. Irradiation was performed with visible light (17 J/cm^2). PDT resulted in nearly complete clearing of the lesions [129].

It has been proposed that topical ALA PDT may be effective for the management of acne, hirsutism, and alopecia areata since, after topical ALA, PpIX can be detected in adnexal structures [104, 127]. At this point, there is little clinical evidence to confirm or deny its efficacy for these diseases.

Perspectives

The evidence clearly demonstrates that PDT is effective in the treatment of superficial neoplastic tumors of the skin, especially actinic keratoses, Bowen's disease and superficial basal cell carcinomas as well as in the treatment of chronic inflammatory skin diseases like psoriasis.

For systemic PDT, treatment is currently restricted to subjects with multiple tumors or for large tumors in elderly people because of the prolonged cutaneous photosensitivity caused by porfimer sodium. However, systemic PDT shows great potential once second generation systemic photosensitizers that lack this side effect are approved. Currently, the clinically best-known topical photosensitizer is ALA, which recently has been approved in the United States for the treatment of actinic keratoses.

The advantages of topical PDT are that it is a non-invasive procedure which can be used repeatedly with excellent cosmetic results. Moreover, unlike many other forms of phototherapy, PDT mediates its effects by causing membrane damage and thus has a much lower potential for causing DNA damage, mutations, and carcinogenesis [114]. Nevertheless, the limitations of PDT must be considered. The depth of the penetration of light as well as the penetration of the photosensitizer into the skin is a crucial point and should be individualized for each patient. Moreover, for skin cancers with a potential risk of metastases, very careful should be patient selection considered. Histological confirmation and determination of tumor thickness are a prerequisite.

The goal of future studies will be to determine additional indications for this therapeutic approach and to standardize the treatment parameters as well as to compare PDT with surgery or radiation in long-term clinical trials of cutaneous oncological patients.

References

1. Abels C, Dellian M, Szeimies RM, Steinbach P, Richert C, Goetz AE (1996) Targeting of the tumor microcirculation with a new photosensitizer. In: Ehrenberg B, Jori G, Moan J (eds) Photochemotherapy: photodynamic therapy and other modalities. Proc SPIE 2625:164–169
2. Abels C, Heil P, Dellian M, Kuhnle GEH, Baumgartner R, Goetz AE (1994) In vivo kinetics and spectra of 5-aminolevulinic acid-induced fluorescence in an amelanotic melanoma of the hamster. Br J Cancer 70:826–833
3. Agarwal R, Korman NJ, Mohan RR, Feyes DK, Jawed S, Zaim MT, Mukhtar H (1996) Apoptosis is an early event during phthalocyanine photodynamic therapy-induced ablation of chemically induced squamous papillomas in mouse skin. Photochem Photobiol 63:547–552
4. Ahmad N, Feyes DK, Agarwal R, Mukhtar H (1998) Photodynamic therapy results in induction of WAF1/CIP1/P21 leading to cell cycle arrest and apoptosis. Proc Natl Acad Sci USA 95:6977–6982
5. Allison RR, Mang TS (1997) A phase II/III clinical study for the treatment of HIV-associated cutaneous Kaposi's sarcoma with tin ethyl etiopurpurin (SnET2)-induced photodynamic therapy. Presented at the European Cancer Conference (ECC09), Hamburg, Germany
6. Allison RR, Mang TS, Wilson BD (1998) Photodynamic therapy for the treatment of nonmelanomatous cutaneous malignancies. Semin Cut Med Surg 17:153–163
7. Ammann R, Hunziker T (1995) Photodynamic therapy for mycosis fungoides after topical photosensitization with 5-aminolevulinic acid. J Am Acad Dermatol 33:541
8. Anderson CY, Elmets CA (manuscript in preparation)
9. Anderson C, Hrabovsky S, McKinley Y, Tubesing K, Tang HP, Mukhtar H and Elmets CA (1997) Phthalocyanine (Pc) photodynamic therapy: disparate effects of pharmacologic inhibitors on cutaneous photosensitivity and on tumor regression. Photochem Photobiol 65:895–901
10. Aramendia PF, Redmond RW, Nonell S, Schuster W, Braslavsky SE, Schaffner K, Vogel E (1986) The photophysical properties of porphycenes: potential photodynamic therapy agents. Photochem Photobiol 44:555–559
11. Athar M, Mukhtar H, Elmets CA, Zaim MT, Lloyd JR, Bickers DR (1988) In situ evidence for the involvement of superoxide anions in cutaneous porphyrin photosensitization. Biochem Biophys Res Commun 151:1054–1059
12. Athar M, Elmets CA, Bickers DR, Mukhtar H (1989) A novel mechanism for the generation of superoxide anions in porphyrin mediated cutaneous photosensitization: Activation of the xanthine oxidase pathway. J Clin Invest 83:1137–1143
13. Babich D, Whitaker J, Conti C, Blaird-Wagner D, Stoll HL, Dozier S, Oseroff AR (1996) Treatment of all stages of cutaneous T-cell lymphomas with fractionated photodynamic therapy using topical δ-aminolevulinic acid. J Invest Dermatol 106:840

14. Bandieramonte G, Marchesini R, Melloni E, Andreoli C, Di pietro D, Spinelli P, Pava G, Zunino F, Emanuelli H (1984) Laser phototherapy following HpD administration in superficial neoplastic lesions. Tumori 70:327–334
15. Batlle AM del C (1993) Porphyrins, porphyrias, cancer and photodynamic therapy – a model for carcinogenesis. J Photochem Photobiol B: Biol 20:5–22
16. Bellnier DA, Ho YK, Pandey RK, Missert JR, Dougherty TJ (1989) Distribution and elimination of Photofrin II in mice. Photochem Photobiol 50:221–228
17. Ben-Hur E, Horowitz B (1995) Advances in photochemical approaches for blood sterilization. Photochem Photobiol 62:383–388
18. Berg H, Bauer E, Gollmick FA, Diezel W, Böhm F, Meffert H, Sönnichsen N (1985) Photodynamic hematoporphyrin therapy of psoriasis. In: Jori G, Perria C (eds) Photodynamic therapy of tumors and other diseases. Progetto Editore, Padova, pp 337–343
19. Berlin NI, Neuberger A, Scott JJ (1956) The metabolism of δ-aminolevulinic acid. 1. Normal pathways, studied with the aid of ^{15}N. Biochem J 64:80–90
20. Bockstahler LE, Coohill TP, Hellman KB, Lytle CD, Roberts JE (1979) Photodynamic therapy for herpes simplex: a critical review. Pharmacol Ther 4:473–499
21. Boehncke WH, König K, Kaufmann R, Scheffold W, Prümmer O, Sterry W (1994) Photodynamic therapy in psoriasis: suppression of cytokine production in vitro and recording of fluorescence modification during treatment in vivo. Arch Dermatol Res 286:300–303
22. Boehncke WH, König K, Rück A, Kaufmann R, Sterry W (1994) In vitro and in vivo effects of photodynamic therapy in cutaneous T cell lymphoma. Acta Derm Venereol (Stockh) 74:201–205
23. Boehncke WH, Sterry W, Kaufmann R (1994) Treatment of psoriasis by topical photodynamic therapy with polychromatic light. Lancet 343:801
24. Buchanan RB, Carruth JAS, McKenzie AL, Williams SR (1989) Photodynamic therapy in the treatment of malignant tumours of the skin and head and neck. Eur J Surg Oncol 15:400–406
25. Cairnduff F, Stringer MR, Hudson EJ, Ash DV, Brown SB (1994) Superficial photodynamic therapy with topical 5-aminolevulinic acid for superficial primary and secondary skin cancer. Br J Cancer 69:605–608
26. Calzavara F, Tomio L (1991) Photodynamic therapy: clinical experience at the department of radiotherapy at Padova general hospital. J Photochem Photobiol B Biol 11:91–95
27. Calzavara-Pinton PG (1995) Repetitive photodynamic therapy with topical δ-aminolevulinic acid as an appropriate approach to the routine treatment of superficial non-melanoma skin tumours. J Photochem Photobiol B Biol 29:53–57
28. Castellani A, Page GP, Concioli M (1963) Photodynamic effect of hematoporphyrin on blood microcirculation. J Pathol Bacteriol 86:99–102
29. de Vree WJ, Essers MC, de Bruijn HS, Star WM, Koster JF, Sluiter W (1996) Evidence for an important role of neutrophils in the efficacy of photodynamic therapy *in vivo*. Cancer Res 56:2908–2911
30. de Vree WJ, Essers MC, Koster JF, Sluiter W (1997) Role of interleukin 1 and granulocyte colony-stimulating factor in photofrin-based photodynamic therapy of rat rhabdomyosarcoma tumors. Cancer Res 57:2555–2558
31. Dellian M, Abels C, Kuhnle GE, Goetz AE (1995) Effects of photodynamic therapy on leukocyte-endothelium interaction: differences between normal and tumour tissue. Br J Cancer 72:1125–1130
32. Dellian M, Walenta S, Gamarra F, Kuhnle GE, Mueller-Klieser W, Goetz AE (1994) High-energy shock waves enhance hyperthermic response of tumors: effects on blood flow, energy metabolism, and tumor growth. J Natl Cancer Inst 86:287–293
33. Dilkes MG, De Jode ML, Rowntree-Taylor A (1997) m-THPC photodynamic therapy for head and neck cancer. Lasers Med Sci 11:23–30

34. Dougherty TJ (1981) Photoradiation therapy for cutaneous and subcutaneous malignancies. J Invest Dermatol 77:122–124
35. Dougherty TJ (1996) A brief history of clinical photodynamic therapy development at Roswell Park Cancer Institute. J Clin Laser Med Surg 14:219–221
36. Dougherty TJ, Gomer CJ, Henderson BW, Jori G, Kessel D, Korbelik M, Moan J, Peng Q (1998) Photodynamic therapy. J Natl Cancer Inst 90:889–905
37. Dougherty TJ, Grindey GB, Fiel R, Weishaupt KR, Boyle DG (1975) Photoradiation therapy. II. Cure of animal tumors with hematoporphyrin and light. J Natl Cancer Inst 55:115–121
38. Dougherty TJ, Kaufman JE, Goldfarb A, Weishaupt KR, Boyle D, Mittleman A (1978) Photoradiation therapy for the treatment of malignant tumors. Cancer Res 38:2628–2635
39. Elmets CA, Bowen KD (1986) Immunological suppression in mice treated with hematoporphyrin derivative photoradiation. Cancer Res 46:1608–1611
40. Emtestam L, Berglund L, Angelin B, Drummond GS, Kappas A (1989) Tin-protoporphyrin and long wavelength ultraviolet light in treatment of psoriasis. Lancet 1:1231–1233
41. Evans S, Matthews W, Perry R, Fraker D, Norton J, Pass HI (1990) Effect of photodynamic therapy on tumor necrosis factor production by murine macrophages. J Natl Cancer Inst 82:34–39
42. Feyh J, Gutmann R, Leunig A (1993) Die photodynamische Lasertherapie im Bereich der Hals-, Nasen-, Ohrenheilkunde. Laryngo Rhino Otol 72:273–278
43. Fijan S, Hönigsmann H, Ortel B (1995) Photodynamic therapy of epithelial skin tumours using delta-aminolevulinic acid and desferrioxamine. Br J Dermatol 133:282–288
44. Fijan S, Hönigsmann H, Tanew A (1996) Photodynamic therapy of keratoacanthoma using topical delta-aminolevulinic acid. J Invest Dermatol 106:945 (abstract)
45. Fingar VH (1996) Vascular effects of photodynamic therapy. J Clin Laser Med Surg 14:323–328
46. Fingar VH, Wieman TJ, Doak KW (1990) Role of thromboxane and prostacyclin release on photodynamic therapy-induced tumor destruction. Cancer Res 50:2599–2603
47. Fingar VH, Wieman TJ, Wiehle SA, Cerrito PB (1992) The role of microvascular damage in photodynamic therapy: the effect of treatment on vessel constriction, permeability, and leukocyte adhesion. Cancer Res 52:4914–4921
48. Fingar VH, Wieman TJ, Karavolos PS, Doak KW, Ouellet R, van Lier JE (1993) The effects of photodynamic therapy using differently substituted zinc phthalocyanines on vessel constriction, vessel leakage and tumor response. Photochem Photobiol 58:251–258
49. Fink-Puches R, Soyer HP, Hofer A, Kerl H, Wolf P (1998) Long-term follow-up and histological changes of superficial nonmelanoma skin cancers treated with topical δ-aminolevulinic acid photodynamic therapy. Arch Dermatol 134:821–826
50. Forbes IJ, Cowled PA, Leong ASY, Ward AD, Black RB, Blake AJ, Jacka FJ (1980) Phototherapy of human tumours using hematoporphyrin derivative. Med J Aust 2:489–493
51. Foster TH, Primavera MC, Marder VJ, Hilf R, Sporn LA (1991) Photosensitized release of von Willebrand factor from cultured human endothelial cells. Cancer Res 51:3261–3266
52. Frank RGJ, Bos JD, Vandermeulen FW, Sterenborg HJCM (1996) Photodynamic therapy for condylomata acuminata with local application of 5-aminolevulinic acid. Genitourin Med 72:70–71
53. Friedrich EG (1973) Relief for herpes vulvitis. Obstet Gynecol 41:74–77
54. Fritsch C, Verwohlt B, Bolsen K, Ruzicka T, Goerz G (1996) Influence of topical photodynamic therapy with 5-aminolevulinic acid on porphyrin metabolism. Arch Dermatol Res 288:517–521

55. Gniazdowska B, Rueff F, Hillemann P, Przybilla B (1998) Allergic contact dermatitis from δ-aminolevulinic acid used for photodynamic therapy. Contact Derm 38:348–349

56. Gollnick SO, Liu X, Owczarczak B, Musser DA, Henderson BW (1997) Altered expression of interleukin 6 and interleukin 10 as a result of photodynamic therapy in vivo. Cancer Res 57:3904–3909

57. Gomer CJ, Ferrario A, Rucker N, Wong S, Lee AS (1991) Glucose regulated protein induction and cellular resistance to oxidative stress mediated by porphyrin photosensitization. Cancer Res 51:6574–6579

58. Gross DJ, Waner M, Schosser RH, Dinehart SM (1990) Squamous cell carcinoma of the lower lip involving a large cutaneous surface. Photodynamic therapy as an alternative therapy. Arch Dermatol 126:1148–1150

59. Guardiano M, Biolo R, Jori G, Schaffner K (1989) Tetra-n-propylporphycene as a tumour localizer: pharmacokinetic and phototherapeutic studies in mice. Cancer Lett 44:1–6

60. Gutmann R, Leunig M, Feyh J, Goetz AE, Messmer K, Kastenbauer E, Jain RK (1992) Interstitial hypertension in head and neck tumors in patients: correlation with tumor size. Cancer Res 52:1993–1995

61. Hanania J, Malik Z (1992) The effect of EDTA and serum on endogenous porphyrin accumulation and photodynamic sensitization of human K562 leukemic cells. Cancer Lett 65:127–131

62. Harth Y, Hirshowitz B, Kaplan B (1998) Modified topical photodynamic therapy of superficial skin tumors, utilizing aminolevulinic acid, penetration enhancers, red light, and hyperthermia. Dermatol Surg 24:723–726

63. Hebeda KM, Huizing MT, Brouwer PA, van der Meulen FW, Hulsebosch HJ, Reiss P, Oosting JH, Veenhof CHN, Bakker PJM (1995) Photodynamic therapy in AIDS-related cutaneous Kaposi's sarcoma. J Acquir Immune Defic Syndr Hum Retrovirol 10:61–70

64. Henderson BW, Waldow SM, Mang TS, Potter WR, Malone PB, Dougherty TJ (1985) Tumor destruction and kinetics of tumor cell death in two experimental mouse tumors following photodynamic therapy. Cancer Res 45:572–576

65. Henderson BW, Donovan JM (1989) Release of prostaglandin E_2 from cells by photodynamic treatment in vitro. Cancer Res 49:6896–6900

66. Hendrich C, Hüttmann G, Diddens H, Seara J, Siebert WE (1996) Experimentelle Grundlagen einer photodynamischen Lasertherapie für die chronische Polyarthritis. Orthopäde 25:30–36

67. Hintschich C, Feyh J, Beyer-Machule C, Riedel K, Ludwig K (1993) Photodynamic laser therapy of basal-cell carcinoma of the lid. Ger J Ophthalmol 2:212–217

68. Hoerauf H, Hüttmann G, Diddens H, Thiele B, Laqua H (1994) Die Photodynamische Therapie (PDT) des Lidbasalioms nach topischer Applikation von δ-Aminolävulinsäure (ALA). Ophthalmologe 91:824–829

69. Hohenleutner U, Szeimies RM, Landthaler M (1993) Photodynamische Therapie zur Behandlung oberflächlicher Basaliome. In: Braun-Falco O, Plewig G, Meurer M (eds) Fortschritte der praktischen Dermatologie und Venerologie, vol 13. Springer, Berlin Heidelberg New York, pp 472–474

70. Hürlimann AF, Hänggi G, Panizzon RG (1998) Photodynamic therapy of superficial basal cell carcinomas using topical 5-aminolevulinic acid in a nanocolloid lotion. Dermatology 197:248–254

71. Hürlimann AF, Panizzon RA, Burg G (1994) Topical photodynamic treatment of skin tumors and dermatoses. Dermatology 3:327 (abstract)

72. Jeffes EW, McCullough JL, Weinstein GD, Fergin PD, Nelson JS, Shull TF, Simpson KR, Bukaly LM, Hoffmann WL, Fong NL (1997) Photodynamic therapy of actinic keratosis with topical 5-aminolevulinic acid. A pilot dose-ranging study. Arch Dermatol 133:727–732

73. Jesionek A, von Tappeiner H (1905) Zur Behandlung der Hautcarcinome mit fluorescierenden Stoffen. Dtsch Arch Klin Med 85:223–239
74. Jolles CJ, Ott MJ, Straight RC, Lynch DH (1988) Systemic immunosuppression induced by peritoneal photodynamic therapy. Am J Obstet Gynecol 158:1446–1453
75. Jones CM, Mang T, Cooper M, Wilson DB, Stoll HL (1992) Photodynamic therapy in the treatment of Bowen's disease. J Am Acad Dermatol 27:979–982
76. Jones LR, Grossweiner LI (1994) Singlet oxygen generation by Photofrin in homogeneous and light-scattering media. J Photochem Photobiol B Biol 26:249–256
77. Kappas A, Sassa S, Galbraith RA, Nordmann Y (1989) The porphyrias. In: Scriver CR, Beaudet AL, Sly WS, Valle D (eds) The metabolic basis of inherited disease, 6th edn. McGraw-Hill, New York, pp 1305–1366
78. Karrer S, Abels C, Bäumler W, Ebert A, Landthaler M, Szeimies RM (1996) Topical photodynamic therapy of psoriasis using a novel porphycene dye. J Invest Dermatol 107:466
79. Karrer S, Abels C, Szeimies RM, Bäumler W, Dellian M, Hohenleutner U, Goetz AE, Landthaler M (1997) Topical application of a first porphycene dye for photodynamic therapy – penetration studies in human perilesional skin and basal cell carcinoma. Arch Dermatol Res 289:132–137
80. Karrer S, Bäumler W, Abels C, Hohenleutner U, Landthaler M, Szeimies RM (1999) Long pulse dye laser for photodynamic therapy – investigations in vitro and in vivo. Lasers Surg Med 25(1):51–59
81. Karrer S, Szeimies RM, Abels C, Wlotzke U, Stolz W, Landthaler M (1999) Epidermodysplasia verruciformis: topical 5-aminolevulinic acid photodynamic therapy. Br J Dermatol 140:935–938
82. Karrer S, Szeimies RM, Ernst S, Abels C, Bäumler W, Landthaler M (1999) Photodynamic inactivation of staphylococci with 5-aminolevulinic acid or photofrin. Lasers Med Sci 14:54–61
83. Karrer S, Szeimies RM, Hohenleutner U, Heine A, Landthaler M (1995) Unilateral localized basaliomatosis: treatment with topical photodynamic therapy after application of 5-aminolevulinic acid. Dermatology 190:218–222
84. Kennedy JC, Pottier RH (1992) Endogenous protoporphyrin IX, a clinically useful photosensitizer for photodynamic therapy. J Photochem Photobiol B Biol 14:275–292
85. Kennedy JC, Pottier RH, Pross DC (1990) Photodynamic therapy with endogenous protoporphyrin IX: basic principles and present clinical experience. J Photochem Photobiol B Biol 6:143–148
86. Kerdel FA, Soter NA, Lim HW (1987) In vivo mediator release and degranulation of mast cells in hematoporphyrin derivative-induced phototoxicity in mice. J Invest Dermatol 88:277–280
87. Kessel D (1986) Sites of photosensitization by derivatives of hematoporphyrin. Photochem Photobiol 44:489–493
88. Korbelik M, Krosl G (1994) Enhanced macrophage cytotoxicity against tumor cells treated with photodynamic therapy. Photochem Photobiol 60:497–502
89. Korbelik MJ (1996) Induction of tumor immunity by photodynamic therapy. J Clin Laser Med Surg 14:329–334
90. Korbelik M, Krosl G, Krosl J, Dougherty GJ (1996) The role of host lymphoid populations in the response of mouse EMT6 tumor to photodynamic therapy. Cancer Res 56:5647–5652
91. Krosl G, Korbelik M, Dougherty GJ (1995) Induction of immune cell infiltration into murine SCCVII tumor by Photofrin-based photodynamic therapy. Br J Cancer 71:549–555
92. Krosl G; Korbelik M; Krosl J; Dougherty GJ (1996) Potentiation of photodynamic therapy-elicited antitumor response by localized treatment with granulocyte-macrophage colony-stimulating factor. Cancer Res 56:3281–3286

93. Korell M, Untch M, Abels C, Dellian M, Kirschstein M, Baumgartner R, Beyer W, Goetz AE (1995) Einsatz der photodynamischen Lasertherapie in der Gynäkologie. Gynäkol Geburtshilfl Rundsch 35:90–97
94. Landthaler M (1992) Premalignant and malignant skin lesions. In: Achauer BM, Vander Kam VM, Berns MW (eds) Lasers in plastic surgery and dermatology. Thieme, New York, pp 34–44
95. Lang S, Baumgartner R, Struck R, Leunig A, Gutmann R, Feyh J (1995) Photodynamische Diagnostik und Therapie von Neoplasien der Gesichtshaut nach topischer Applikation von 5-Aminolävulinsäure. Laryngo Rhino Otol 74:85–89
96. Langer S, Abels C, Szeimies RM, Goetz AE (1995) Photodynamic diagnosis and therapy of tumors with topically applied 5-aminolevulinic acid. J Invest Dermatol 105:511 (abstract)
97. Leunig A, Staub F, Peters J, Leiderer R, Feyh J, Goetz AE (1994) Die Schädigung von Tumorzellen durch die photodynamische Therapie. Laryngo Rhino Otol 73:102–107
98. Leunig M, Goetz AE, Gamarra F, Zetterer G, Messmer K, Jain RK (1994) Photodynamic therapy-induced alterations in interstitial fluid pressure, volume and water content of an amelanotic melanoma in the hamster. Br J Cancer 69:101–103
99. Leunig M, Richert C, Gamarra F, Lumper W, Vogel E, Jocham D, Goetz AE (1993) Tumour localisation kinetics of photofrin and three synthetic porphyrinoids in an amelanotic melanoma of the hamster. Br J Cancer 68:225–234
100. Levy JG, Jones CA, Pilson LA (1994) The preclinical and clinical development and potential application of benzoporphyrin derivative. Int Photodynam 1:3–5
101. Lipson RL, Baldes EJ (1960) The photodynamic properties of a particular haematoporphyrin derivative. Arch Dermatol 82:508–516
102. Lipson RL, Gray MJ, Baldes EJ (1966) Haematoporphyrin derivative for detection and management of cancer. Proc IX Internat Cancer Congr 393
103. Lui H, Anderson RR (1992) Photodynamic therapy in dermatology. Arch Dermatol 128:1631–1636
104. Lui H, Anderson RR (1993) Photodynamic therapy in dermatology: recent developments. Dermatol Clin 11:1–13
105. Lui H, Kollias N, Wimberly J, Anderson RR (1992) Photosensitizing potential of benzoporphyrin derivative-monoacid ring A (BPD-MA) in patients undergoing photodynamic therapy. Photochem Photobiol 55 [Suppl]:30S (abstract)
106. Lui H, Salasche S, Kollias N, Wimberly J, Flotte T, McLean D, Anderson RR (1995) Photodynamic therapy of nonmelanoma skin cancer with topical aminolevulinic acid: a clinical and histologic study. Arch Dermatol 131:737–738
107. Lynch DH, Haddad S, King VJ, Ott MJ, Straight RC, Jolles CJ (1989) Systemic immunosuppression induced by photodynamic therapy (PDT) is adoptively transferred by macrophages. Photochem Photobiol 49:453–458
108. Martin A, Tope WD, Grevelink JM, Starr JC, Fewkes JL, Flotte TJ, Deutsch TF, Anderson RR (1995) Lack of selectivity of protoporphyrin IX fluorescence for basal cell carcinoma after topical application of 5-aminolevulinic acid: implications for photodynamic treatment. Arch Dermatol Res 287:665–674
109. McCaughan JS Jr, Guy JT, Hicks W, Laufman L, Nims TA, Walker J (1989) Photodynamic therapy for cutaneous and subcutaneous malignant neoplasms. Arch Surg 124:211–216
110. McCullough JL, Weinstein GD (1998) Photodynamic therapy of psoriasis. In: Psoriasis (Roenigk HH Jr., Maibach HI, eds.), Marcel Dekker, 3rd ed., New York Basel Hong Kong, pp 757–760
111. Meffert H, Preš H, Diezel W, Sönnichsen N (1989) Antipsoriatische und phototoxische Wirksamkeit von Hämatoporphyrin-Derivat nach topischer Applikation und Bestrahlung mit sichtbarem Licht. Dermatol Monatsschr 175:28–34
112. Meijnders PJN, Star WM, De Bruijn RS, Treurniet-Donker AD, Van Mierlo MJM, Wijthoff SJM, Naafs B, Beerman H, Levendag PC (1996) Clinical results of photo-

dynamic therapy for superficial skin malignancies or actinic keratosis using topical 5-aminolevulinic acid. Las Med Sci 11:123–131

113. Milanesi C, Zhou C, Biolo R, Jori G (1990) Zn(II)-phthalocyanine as a photodynamic agent for tumours. II. Studies on the mechanism of photosensitised tumour necrosis. Br J Cancer 61:846–850

114. Moan J (1986) Porphyrin photosensitization and phototherapy. Photochem Photobiol 43:681–690

115. Monfrecola G, Dánna F, Delfino M (1987) Topical hematoporphyrin plus UVA for treatment of alopecia areata. Photodermatol Photoimmunol Photomed 4:305–306

116. Morton CA, Whitehurst C, Moseley H, McColl JH, Moore JV, Mackie RM (1996) Comparison of photodynamic therapy with cryotherapy in the treatment of Bowen's disease. Br J Dermatol 135:766–771

117. Nelson JS (1993) Photodynamic therapy of port wine stain: preliminary clinical studies. In: Shapshay SM, Anderson RR, White JV, White RA, Bass LR (eds) Lasers in otolaryngology, dermatology, and tissue welding. Proc SPIE 1876:142–146

118. North J, Coombs R, Levy JG (1994) Photodynamic inactivation of free and cell-associated HIV-1 using the photosensitizer, benzoporphyrin derivative. J Acquir Immune Defic Syndr 7:891–898

119. Nseyo UO, Whalen RK, Duncan MR, Berman B, Lundahl SL (1990) Urinary cytokines following photodynamic therapy for bladder cancer. A preliminary report. Urology 36:167–171

120. Nugent LJ, Jain RK (1984) Extravascular diffusion in normal and neoplastic tissues. Cancer Res 44:238–244

121. Obochi MO, Canaan AJ, Jain AK, Richter AM, Levy JG (1995) Targeting activated lymphocytes with photodynamic therapy: susceptibility of mitogen-stimulated splenic lymphocytes to benzoporphyrin derivative (BPD) photosensitization. Photochem Photobiol 62:169–175

122. Ochsner M (1997) Photophysical and photobiological processes in the photodynamic therapy of tumours. J Photochem Photobiol B 39:1–18

123. Ortel B, Tanew A, Hönigsmann H (1993) Lethal photosensitization by endogenous porphyrins of PAM cells – modification by desferrioxamine. J Photochem Photobiol B Biol 17:273–278

124. Oseroff AR (1993) Photodynamic therapy. In: Lim HW, Soter NA (eds) Clinical photomedicine. Dekker, New York, pp 387–402

125. Pass HI (1993) Photodynamic therapy in oncology: mechanisms and clinical use. J Natl Cancer Inst 85:443–456

126. Peng Q, Warloe T, Moan J (1995) Topically-applied ALA-based PDT for nodulo-ulcerative basal cell carcinoma, IPA News 7:2

127. Peng Q, Warloe T, Berg K, Moan J, Kongshaug M, Giercksky KE, Nesland JM (1997) 5-Aminolevulinic acid-based photodynamic therapy. Clinical research and future challenges. Cancer 79:2282–2308

128. Pennington DG, Waner M, Knox A (1988) Photodynamic therapy for multiple skin cancers. Plast Reconstr Surg 82:1067–1071

129. Preš H, Meffert H, Sönnichsen N (1989) Photodynamische Therapie der Psoriasis palmaris et plantaris mit topisch appliziertem Hämatoporphyrin-Derivat und sichtbarem Licht. Dermatol Monatsschr 175:745–750

130. Qin B, Selman SH, Payne KM, Keck RW, Metzger DW (1993) Enhanced skin allograft survival after photodynamic therapy. Association with lymphocyte inactivation and macrophage stimulation. Transplantation 56:1481–1486

131. Raab O (1900) Über die Wirkung fluorescierender Stoffe auf Infusoria. Z Biol 39:524

132. Ratkay LG, Chowdhary RK, Iamaroon A, Richter AM, Neyndorff HC, Keystone EC, Waterfield JD, Levy JG (1998) Amelioration of antigen-induced arthritis in rabbits by induction of apoptosis of inflammatory cells with local application of transdermal photodynamic therapy. Arthritis Rheum 41:525–534

133. Rebeiz N, Arkins S, Rebeiz CA, Simon J, Zachary JF, Kelley KW (1996) Induction of tumor necrosis by δ-aminolevulinic acid and 1,10-phenantroline photodynamic therapy. Cancer Res 56:339–344

134. Rebeiz N, Rebeiz CC, Arkins S, Kelley KW, Rebeiz CA (1992) Photodestruction of tumor cells by induction of endogenous accumulation of protoporphyrin IX: enhancement by 1,10-phenanthroline. Photochem Photobiol 55:431–435

135. Reddan J, Anderson CY, Xu H, Hrabovsky S, Freye K, Fairchild R, Tubesing KA, Elmets CA (1999) Immunosuppressive effects of silicon phthalocyanine photodynamic therapy. Photochem Photobiol 70:72–77

136. Renschler MF, Yuen A, Panella TJ, Wieman TJ, Julius C, Panjehpour M, Taber S, Fingar V, Horning S, Miller RA, Lowe E, Engel J, Woodburn K, Young SW (1997) Photodynamic therapy trials with lutetium texaphyrin PCI-0123 (Lu-Tex). Photochem Photobiol 65:47S (Abstract)

137. Richert C, Wessels JM, Müller M, Kisters M, Benninghaus T, Goetz AE (1994) Photodynamic antitumor agents: beta-methoxyethyl groups give access to functionalized porphycenes and enhance cellular uptake and activity. J Med Chem 37:2797–2807

138. Richter AM, Jain AK, Canaan AJ, Waterfield E, Sternberg ED, Levy JG (1992) Photosensitizing efficiency of two regioisomers of the benzoporphyrin derivative monoacid ring A. Biochem Pharmacol 43:2349–2358

139. Rittenhouse-Diakun K, Van Leengoed H, Morgan J, Hryhorenko E, Paszkiewicz G, Whitaker JE, Oseroff AR (1995) The role of transferrin receptor (CD71) in photodynamic therapy of activated and malignant lymphocytes using the heme precursor delta-aminolevulinic acid (ALA). Photochem Photobiol 61:523–528

140. Robinson PJ, Carruth JAS, Fairris GM (1988) Photodynamic therapy: a better treatment for widespread Bowen's disease. Br J Dermatol 119:59–61

141. Rosenblum LA, Hoskwith B, Kramer SD (1937) Photodynamic action of methylene blue on poliomyelitis virus. Proc Soc Exp Biol Med 37:166–169

142. Rünger TM (1995) Genotoxizität, Mutagenität und Karzinogenität von UVA und UVB. Z Hautkr 70:877–881

143. Sacchini V, Melloni E, Marchesini R, Fabrizio T, Cascinelli N, Santoro O, Zunino F, Andreola S, Bandieramonte G (1987) Topical administration of tetrasodium-meso-tetraphenyl-porphinesulfonate (TPPS) and red light irradiation for the treatment of superficial neoplastic lesions. Tumori 73:19–23

144. Schaffner K, Vogel E, Jori G (1994) Porphycenes as photodynamic therapy agents. In: Jung EG, Holick MF (eds) Biologic effects of light 1993. De Gruyter, Berlin, pp 312–321

145. Schlag P, Hünerbein M, Stern J, Gahlen J, Graschew G (1992) Photodynamische Therapie – Alternative bei lokal rezidiviertem Mamma-Karzinom. Dt Ärztebl 89:680–687

146. Schmidt S, Wagner U, Oehr P, Krebs D (1992) Klinischer Einsatz der photodynamischen Therapie bei gynäkologischen Tumorpatienten – Antikörper-vermittelte photodynamische Lasertherapie als neues onkologisches Behandlungsverfahren. Zentralbl Gynäkol 114:307–311

147. Schuh M, Nseyo UO, Potter WR, Dao TL, Dougherty TJ (1987) Photodynamic therapy for palliation of locally recurrent breast carcinoma. J Clin Oncol 5:1766–1770

148. Schultz EW, Krueger AP (1930) Inactivation of staphylococcus bacteriophage by methylene blue. Proc Soc Exp Biol Med 26:100–101

149. Schwartz SK, Absolon K, Vermund H (1955) Some relationships of porphyrins, x-rays and tumours. Univ Minn Med Bull 27:7–8

150. Schweitzer VG, Visscher D (1990) Photodynamic therapy for treatment of AIDS-related oral Kaposi's sarcoma. Otolaryngol Head Neck Surg 102:639–649

151. Silver H (1937) Psoriasis vulgaris treated with hematoporphyrin. Arch Dermatol Syph 36:1118–1119

152. Sperduto PW, DeLaney TF, Thomas G, Smith P, Dachowski LJ, Russo A, Bonner R, Glatstein E (1991) Photodynamic therapy for chest wall recurrence in breast cancer. Int J Radiat Oncol Biol Phys 21:441–446
153. Star WM, Marijnissen HP, van den Berg Blok AE, Versteeg JA, Franken KA, Reinhold HS (1986) Destruction of rat mammary tumor and normal tissue microcirculation by hematoporphyrin derivative photoradiation observed in vivo in sandwich observation chambers. Cancer Res 46:2532–2540
154. Stender IM, Na R, Fogh H, Glaud C, Wulf HC (2000) Photodynamic therapy with 5-aminolaevulinic acid or placebo for recalcitrant foot and hand warts: randomized double-blind trial. Lancet 355:963–966
155. Stern R, Zierler S, Parrish JA (1982) Psoriasis and the risk of cancer. J Invest Dermatol 78:147–149
156. Svaasand LO, Tromberg BJ, Wyss P, Wyss-Desserich MT, Tadir Y, Berns MW (1996) Light and drug distribution with topically administered photosensitizers. Las Med Sci 11:261–265
157. Svanberg K, Andersson T, Killander D, Wang I, Stenram U, Andersson-Engels S, Berg R, Johansson J, Svanberg S (1994) Photodynamic therapy of non-melanoma malignant tumours of the skin using topical δ-amino levulinic acid sensitization and laser irradiation. Br J Dermatol 130:743–751
158. Szeimies RM, Abels C, Fritsch C, Karrer S, Steinbach P, Bäumler W, Goerz G, Goetz AE, Landthaler M (1995) Wavelength dependency of photodynamic effects after sensitization with 5-aminolevulinic acid in vitro and in vivo. J Invest Dermatol 105:672–677
159. Szeimies RM, Hein R, Bäumler W, Heine A, Landthaler M (1994) A possible new incoherent lamp for photodynamic treatment of superficial skin lesions. Acta Derm Venereol (Stockh) 74:117–119
160. Szeimies RM, Karrer S, Heine A, Hohenleutner U, Landthaler M (1995) Topical photodynamic therapy with 5-aminolevulinic acid in the treatment of arsenic-induced skin tumors. Eur J Dermatol 5:208–211
161. Szeimies RM, Karrer S, Sauerwald A, Landthaler M (1996b) Topical photodynamic therapy with 5-aminolevulinic acid in the treatment of actinic keratoses: a first clinical study. Dermatology 192:246–251
162. Szeimies RM, Landthaler M (1993) Treatment of Bowen's disease with topical photodynamic therapy. J Dermatol Treat 4:207–209
163. Szeimies RM, Landthaler M (1995) Topische photodynamische Therapie in der Behandlung oberflächlicher Hauttumoren. Hautarzt 46:315–318
164. Szeimies RM, Sassy T, Landthaler M (1994) Penetration potency of topical applied δ-aminolevulinic acid for photodynamic therapy of basal cell carcinoma. Photochem Photobiol 59:73–76
165. Taber SW, Fingar VH, Coots CT, Wieman TJ (1998) Photodynamic therapy using mono-L-aspartyl chlorin e$_6$ (Npe6) for the treatment of cutaneous disease: a phase I clinical study. Clin Cancer Res 4:2741–2746
166. Thiele B, Grotmann P, Hüttmann G, Diddens H, Hörauf H (1994) Topische photodynamische Therapie (TPDT) von Basaliomen: klinische, histologische und experimentelle Ergebnisse (erste Mitteilung). Z Hautkr 3:161–164
167. Tse DT, Kersten RD, Anderson RL (1984) Hematoporphyrin derivative photoradiation therapy in managing nevoid basal cell carcinoma syndrome. Arch Ophthalmol 102:990–994
168. Vogel E, Köcher M, Schmickler H, Lex J (1986) Porphycene – a novel porphin isomer. Angew Chem 98:262–264
169. von Tappeiner H, Jesionek A (1903) Therapeutische Versuche mit fluorescierenden Stoffen. Münch Med Wochenschr 47:2042–2044
170. Wainwright M (1998) Photodynamic antimicrobial chemotherapy (PACT). J Antimicrob Chemother 42:13–28

171. Waldow SM, Lobraico RV, Kohler IK, Wallk S, Fritts HT (1987) Photodynamic therapy for treatment of malignant cutaneous lesions. Lasers Surg Med 7:451–456

172. Walter AW, Pivnick EK, Bale AE, Kun LE (1997) Complications of the nevoid basal cell carcinoma syndrome : a case report. J Pediatr Hematol Oncol 19:258–262

173. Warloe T, Peng Q, Moan J, Qvist HL, Giercksky KE (1992) Photochemotherapy of multiple basal cell carcinoma with endogenous porphyrins induced by topical application of 5-aminolevulinic acid. In: Spinelli P, Dal Fante M, Marchesini R (eds) Photodynamic therapy and biomedical lasers. Elsevier Science, Amsterdam, pp 449–453

174. Weinstein GD, McCullough JL, Jeffes EW, Nelson JS, Fong NL, McCormick AJ (1994) Photodynamic therapy (PDT) of psoriasis with topical delta aminolevulinic acid (ALA): a pilot dose ranging study. Photodermatol Photoimmunol Photomed 10:92 (abstract)

175. Weinstein GD, McCullough JL, Nelson JS, Berns MW, McCormick AJ (1991) Low-dose photofrin II photodynamic therapy of psoriasis. Clin Res 39:509A (abstract)

176. Weishaupt KR, Gomer CJ, Dougherty TJ (1976) Identification of singlet oxygen as the cytotoxic agent in photo-inactivation of a murine tumor. Cancer Res 36:2326–2329

177. Wennberg AM, Lindholm LE, Alpsten M, Larkö O (1996) Treatment of superficial basal cell carcinomas using topically applied delta-aminolaevulinic acid and a filtered xenon lamp. Arch Dermatol Res 288:561–564

178. Wessels JM, Strauss W, Seidlitz HK, Rück A, Schneckenburger H (1992) Intracellular localization of meso-tetraphenylporphine tetrasulphonate probed by time-resolved and microscopic fluorescence spectroscopy. J Photochem Photobiol B Biol 12:275–284

179. Wilson BD, Mang TS, Cooper M, Stoll H (1989) Use of photodynamic therapy for the treatment of extensive basal cell carcinomas. Facial Plast Surg 6:185–189

180. Wilson BD, Mang TS, Stoll H, Jones C, Cooper M, Dougherty TJ (1992) Photodynamic therapy for the treatment of basal cell carcinoma. Arch Dermatol 128:1597–1601

181. Winkelman JW, Collins GH (1987) Neurotoxicity of tetraphenylporphinesulfonate $TPPS_4$ and its relation to photodynamic therapy. Photochem-Photobiol 46:801–807

182. Wolf P, Fink-Puches R, Cerroni L, Kerl H (1994) Photodynamic therapy for mycosis fungoides after topical photosensitization with 5-aminolevulinic acid. J Am Acad Dermatol 31:678–680

183. Wolf P, Fink-Puches R, Kerl H (1995) Photodynamic therapy for mycosis fungoides after topical photosensitization with 5-aminolevulinic acid. J Am Acad Dermatol 33:541

184. Wolf P, Kerl H (1995) Photodynamic therapy with 5-aminolevulinic acid: a promising concept for the treatment of cutaneous tumors. Dermatology 190:183–185

185. Wolf P, Rieger E, Kerl H (1993) Topical photodynamic therapy with endogenous porphyrins after application of 5-aminolevulinic acid. J Am Acad Dermatol 28:17–21

186. Wolford ST, Novicki DL, Kelly B (1995) Comparative skin phototoxicity in mice with two photosensitizing drugs: Benzoporphyrin derivative monoacid ring A and porfimer sodium (Photofrin). Fundam Appl Toxicol 24:52–56

187. Woodburn KW, Vardaxis NJ, Hill JS, Kaye AH, Phillips DR (1991) Subcellular localization of porphyrins using confocal laser scanning microscopy. Photochem Photobiol 54:725–732

188. Xiao-xi L, Wie W, Shuo-fan W, Chuan Y, Ti-Sheng C (1997) Treatment of capillary vascular malformation (port-wine stains) with photochemotherapy. Plast Reconstr Surg 99:1826–1830

189. Yamamoto N, Hoober JK, Yamamoto N, Yamamoto S (1992) Tumoricidal capacities of macrophages photodynamically activated with hematoporphyrin derivative. Photochem Photobiol 56:245–250

190. Yamamoto N; Sery TW; Hoober JK; Willett NP; Lindsay DD (1994) Effectiveness of photofrin II in activation of macrophages and in vitro killing of retinoblastoma cells. Photochem Photobiol 60:160–164
191. Zaidi SI; Oleinick NL; Zaim MT; Mukhtar H (1993) Apoptosis during photodynamic therapy-induced ablation of RIF-1 tumors in C3H mice: electron microscopic, histopathologic and biochemical evidence. Photochem Photobiol 58:771–776

12 Extracorporeal Photoimmunochemotherapy

Robert Knobler, Peter Heald

Contents

Extracorporeal photoimmunochemotherapy (ECP, photopheresis) was introduced in 1987 for the palliative management of cutaneous T-cell lymphoma (CTCL) [1]. ECP was shown to work in a multicenter trial that focused primarily on erythrodermic CTCL patients. As of 2000, this therapy has continued to be utilized in the management of CTCL along with multiple applications in T-cell-mediated diseases. As a result, this modality is available in over 100 centers in the United States, Europe, and Latin America. In this chapter, the procedure and its utilization will be reviewed, including the rapidly expanding role in the management of refractory acute and chronic graft-vs-host disease (GVHD) after bone marrow transplantation [2–30].

The procedure itself has been modified slightly since its first description [1]. Due to problems in obtaining consistent reproducible psoralen levels in the to-be treated plasma/Buffy coat fraction, the procedure is now utilizing drug delivery direct into the lymphocytes, rather than via oral administration. The other change is that the most recent lymphocyte harvest and irradiation device performs the therapy in successive cycles, equally dosing all lymphocytes with the same amount of ultraviolet (UV)A light in the presence of 8-methoxypsoralen (MOP). ECP is, on the average, repeated on 2 successive days at a frequency of every 2–4 weeks. It can, in selected non-responsive patients, be repeated for limited periods of time with much shorter intervals between treatment sets. During one treatment between 10% and 15% of the circulating T-cell pool is treated; the total UVA dose delivered per cell is 2 J/cm^2.

Since the multicenter study by Edelson and co-workers [1], a number of subsequent reports have basically confirmed the initial observations so that ECP can be considered as a first-line treatment for patients with the erythrodermic stage of CTCL [32–39]. Based on all the available literature, ECP appears to have a very low side-effect and toxicity profile in this as well as other indications so that evaluation of ECP for other indications in the last years has been explored at a number of centers extensively. The rationale for the expanded treatment spectrum was also supported by some experimental studies evaluating the effect of ECP on the immune system [40–54]. Under the assumption that ECP can suppress detrimental relevant T-cell clones and relevant associated peptides, a number of clinical investigations have been performed in order to evaluate the efficacy of ECP in inflammatory diseases other than CTCL where auto-reactive T-cells play a central role. Experience has been gained in a number of disease groups including systemic sclerosis, pemphigus vulgaris, rheumatoid arthritis, psoriasis arthritis, systemic lupus erythematosus, and atopic dermatitis. New studies suggest that ECP may also be of major clinical importance in the treatment of acute and chronic rejection in organ transplantation as well as GVHD after bone marrow transplantation [12, 23, 24, 27, 28] and possibly refractory steroid dependent inflammatory bowel disease (e.g., ulcerative colitis, Crohn's disease).

In addition to clinical studies evaluating possible other indications, improvements in the procedure should lead to decreased treatment costs, shorter treatment times and improved drug delivery associated with lower side effects [31].

Cutaneous T-Cell Lymphoma

CTCL was the first disease for which ECP was evaluated. Sufficient evidence in clinical studies as well as FDA approval for use of ECP for the palliative treatment of the Sézary Syndrome variant strongly support its value as the first line treatment in this disease.

In the first study by Edelson and co-workers published in 1987 [1], 27 of 37 patients responded either with a partial or a complete remission. In a follow-up study, the prolonged remissions induced by ECP suggested that ECP may also increase survival time from a median of 30 months to over 66 months [36]. Even in view of the existing controversy and statistical validity associated with comparing results to historical controls, the prolonged palliative effects appear to be of significance. Later studies appear to confirm the initial impressions of efficacy [17, 34, 39, 55, 56]. They show that ECP can be of significant value in the treatment of this disease and describe a response rate reaching up to 75 % with possible complete remissions of up to 25 % and no response in 25 %. Among the criteria that appear to help predict a better outcome in patients are a normal CD4/CD8 ratio, a normal absolute count of CD8$^+$ cells in the peripheral blood and short disease duration [38, 39]. Still, these factors in and of themselves are not always sufficient for predicting response and responders and non-responders can be found at both extremes.

As a monotherapy, the most common response of CTCL to ECP is a partial response. Immunosuppressive agents such as chemotherapy and systemic steroids may interfere with the therapeutic effects of ECP. Thus, debulking the disease with radiation therapy may be of significance: in one report, there was an increase in the complete response rate when a total-skin electron beam was combined with ECP therapy [57]. Another modality used in combination with

ECP is further immunostimulation with interferon injections. One report suggested that the synergy between the two immunomodulating therapies was strong enough to consider initiating both modalities simultaneously [58]. One case of CTCL with pronounced blood and lymph node involvement remitted with the combination modality [59]. The practical approach to incorporating these observations into everyday practice has been to consider multimodality therapy at the initiation of treatment. If there is marked leukemic involvement or tumors present, the patient will not achieve a complete remission from ECP monotherapy. Those patients should be considered for adjunctive therapy at the start. In patients with erythroderma, monotherapy should be considered for 3–6 months before adding adjunctive modalities to maximize the clinical response. Clearly prospective randomized studies in the future should help define the value of this type of combination therapy in overall survival time and response.

Photopheresis for Other T-Cell-Mediated Diseases

Limited data on current and past small clinical trials suggest a possible place for photopheresis in the management of other T-cell-mediated diseases such as systemic sclerosis, pemphigus vulgaris, rheumatoid arthritis, and to a lesser degree, systemic lupus erythematosus, dermatomyositis, psoriasis arthritis, and atopic dermatitis. From the available published literature, treatment of organ transplant recipients, who have been sensitized to donor antigens, appears effective and, if confirmed in large designed trials, will be of considerable potential benefit to organ transplant recipients of heart, kidney, lung, and liver. Recent data also suggest an important role for photopheresis in the treatment of GVHD after bone marrow transplantation. Improvement in drug delivery systems and the elucidation of the mechanisms that contribute to the observed effects should help in the design of better treatment protocols and pinpoint its long- and short-term role in the area of therapeutics.

Pemphigus Vulgaris

Pemphigus vulgaris was among the first autoimmune diseases that were evaluated after the initial success with cutaneous T-cell lymphoma. The first positive results were summarized in a paper by Rook et al. [5] who reported their observations in a preliminary trial with response in 3 out of 4 patients suffering from drug-resistant pemphigus vulgaris. Initially, all 4 patients in this pilot study showed dramatic improvement of their disease with significant reduction in specific antibody titers and clinical symptoms. The major benefit of ECP therapy in pemphigus was the lack of toxicity and the lack of adverse interactions with other medications. Remissions of significant duration (up to 6 months) with concomitant substantial reduction in glucocorticoid and immunosuppressive reduction was obtained in 3 of the 4 patients treated. Two subsequently published reports as well as experiences in our own centers confirm this effect.

Liang et al. reported on a 31-year-old patient who, under treatment with photopheresis, underwent a near complete remission with significant reduction in concomitant immunosuppressive therapy [21]. Gollnick et al. reported on a 37-year-old female patient with a 5-year history of severe therapy-resistant disease [8]. Lack of response and associated severe side effects under treatment with corticosteroids (40–300 mg/day), azathioprine (100–150 mg/day), and intermittent methotrexate (25 mg/week) required treatment with additional ECP. Within 4 ECP cycles, serum antibodies against IgG fell from a titer of 1:800 to 1:100, and by the sixth cycle 95 % of the cutaneous and mucosal lesions cleared to a large extent.

Based on these reported six cases and the observed responses under ECP therapy there appears to be sufficient evidence to justify a multicenter randomized phase III trial for use in selected therapy refractory patients. The relative rarity of this condition and even less of the refractory type will make larger studies very difficult to carry out since it may not be possible to enroll an adequate number of patients to satisfy requirements for statistical significance. In practice, a refractory pemphigus patient should be considered for a 3- to 4-month trial of ECP therapy. The results should continue to be reported along with any effect of ECP on pemphigus antibody titers and the ability to taper immunosuppressive medications. The latter two parameters represent the improvements ECP may bring to a patient with refractory pemphigus.

Progressive Systemic Sclerosis

Progressive systemic sclerosis (PSS) or scleroderma, is an autoimmune disease characterized by excess collagen deposition within the skin and visceral organs (e.g., heart, lungs, kidneys, gastrointestinal tract). The similarities of PSS to sclerotic GVHD suggest that it may be a T-cell-mediated problem. Early T-lymphocyte infiltration of affected organs as well as presence of autoreactive antibodies support the argument for its autoimmune nature. The pilot study of ECP involved two PSS patients with therapy refractive rapidly progressive disease [60]. The pilot study of ECP involved two PSS patients with therapy refractive rapidly progressive disease [60], both of which showed some improvement.

Encouraged by these observations, a single-blinded, randomized eight-center trial was conducted, comparing photopheresis to D-penicillamine. Seventy-nine patients with systemic sclerosis of recent onset (mean symptom duration, 1.83 years) and documented progressive cutaneous involvement 6 months prior to the study were entered into this parallel group, single-blinded, clinical trial. ECP was delivered on two consecutive days at intervals of 4 weeks and compared to D-pencillamine at a maximum dose of 750 mg/day. The extent and severity of skin involvement was evaluated by blinded clinical examiners using accepted modalities for skin evaluation [61], surface area involvement, oral aperture, and hand closure. Skin changes were evaluated by repeat biopsies. For evaluation of pulmonary involvement and course, lung function tests were performed at regular intervals. Serology markers were also followed at baseline and after 6 and 12 months of treatment. Exclusion criteria for patients participating in the study included, prior to randomization: past D-penicillamine failure and extensive life-compromising internal organ involvement.

In the 10-month study period, ECP was demonstrated to be superior to increasing doses of D-penicillamine. It showed a reversal of pathological cutaneous changes and arrested progression. Fifty-six patients were able to undergo at least 6 months of therapy, 31 with ECP and 25 with D-penicillamine. Forty-seven completed 10 months of therapy of which 29 were with ECP. At the first evaluation point, namely 6 months, 21 of 31 (68 %) of the patients on ECP showed significant skin softening as opposed to 8 of 25 (32 %) who received D-penicillamine only. At 6 months, 3 out of 31 (10 %) of the patients on ECP reported significant worsening of their skin score while 8 of 25 (32 %) on D-penicillamine had significant progression. All patients on ECP were able to complete the study while 25 % of the patients on D-penicillamine had to be dropped from the study due to side effects and progression of disease.

These observations have recently been questioned by controlled studies which showed that ECP did not result in any advantage over placebo treatment. Therefore, ECP is no longer recommended for the treatment of PSS.

Similarly a small study on eight patients by Zachariae et al. [4] made an observation that clearly encourages extreme caution in treating patients with severe PSS with ECP monotherapy after initial immunosuppressive therapy.

Rheumatoid Arthritis

In the search for more effective therapies associated with a low side-effect profile, Malawista et al. [19] proceeded with a pilot study on seven patients suffering from therapeutically resistant rheumatoid arthritis. As in similar diseases of an "autoimmune" nature, the investigators were motivated by the potential implications of ECP where one may be able to elicit an immune response to non-monoclonal, presumably pathogenic, circulating T-cells. In this short 6-month study, the patients were also treated using monthly intervals between two successive treatments followed by biweekly intervals in non-responders. In 4 of the 7 patients improvement was first noted after 4 months of treatment which, most likely, rules out the well-known placebo effect seen in many patients with this type of disease. In this sense, the observation that those patients that did respond all had recurrence of disease activity several months after being off ECP further supports its possible influence on the disease course. The authors report that in 4 of the 7 studied patients, improvement of joint counts and joint scores was initially noted after 12 and 16 weeks therapy. In 3 of the 4 patients where improvement could be documented, the above measures improved by a mean of 71 % and 80 % of baseline values respectively. Other less-direct measures of clinical response were variable in their improvement, e.g., grip strength in 2 of the 7 patients, 50-foot walking time one patient, morning stiffness for 2 patients. This small, preliminary study suggests that ECP may be beneficial in the short term for selected patients with rheumatoid arthritis, and it involves less toxicity than the drugs currently used for this disease. Double-blind placebo controlled trials, perhaps with a different treatment schedule, with and without the aid of other drugs, are certainly mandatory before a final recommendation can be given for ECP in rheumatoid arthritis and related disorders including psoriasis arthritis [10, 11, 25] and lyme arthritis [18], where positive reports also suggest benefit from ECP.

Transplantation and Graft-Vs-Host Disease

One of the most exciting developing areas where photoimmunotherapy may prove to be of importance is in the area of organ transplantation. A number of groups have been able to demonstrate in small clinical trials that ECP can be a valuable adjunct in the control and prevention of organ transplant rejection without the classical side effects commonly associated with currently used immunosuppressive therapy. Constanzo-Nordin and co-workers at Loyola University evaluated the effect of photopheresis on seven heart transplant (HT) patients on triple immunosuppression (cyclosporine, corticosteroids, and aza-thioprine) who had nine episodes of non-hemodynamically compromising moderate rejection [23]. Eight of these nine episodes of rejection were successfully reversed by photopheresis as assessed by endomyocardial biopsy (EMB) performed 1 week after treatment. In addition, immunohistochemical analysis of these biopsies revealed that post-treatment cell counts for T-cells, B-cells, and macrophages were reduced when compared to values before ECP, and they corresponded to the picture of histopathological resolution of rejection. In the follow-up study, ECP was evaluated for its potential to reverse International Society for Heart and Lung Transplantation (ISHLT) rejection grades 2, 3A, and 3B without hemodynamic compromise. Sixteen patients were randomized to be treated either by photopheresis or corticosteroid therapy. In this study, ECP reversed eight of nine rejection episodes and corticosteroids of seven. The median time from initiation of treatment to rejection reversal was 25 days in the ECP group and 17 days in the corticosteroid group. The authors conclude from these preliminary short-term results in prospectively randomized patients that ECP may be as effective as corticosteroids for treating ISHLT rejection grades 2, 3A, and 3B with a lower side-effects profile [24].

Rose and co-workers at Columbia University evaluated the effect of ECP on four patients: two multiple transplant patients with pre-existent high levels of panel reactive antibodies, and two multiparous women who were considered at risk of sensitization. ECP was added to conventional immunosuppressive therapy [26]. A reduction in the high levels of panel reactive antibodies, a reduction of the number of rejection episodes, and no infection complications in this small group were observed. Specifically, a fall in the panel of reactive lymphocytotoxic antibody levels was observed in two of the patients in whom they were detected before transplantation, and reversal lymphocytotoxic antibody expression was observed in the other two patients. These authors noted that a potential area of investigation for ECP should include its impact on the progression of the reversal of acute rejection episodes. Following these observations, two additional European groups have confirmed the results of these initial preliminary studies. In the first group, Dall Ámico and co-workers treated four patients who, due to multiple acute rejections after heart transplantation, needed additional corticosteroids. Photopheresis, when combined with conventional immunosuppressive therapy, helped to control repeat rejection episodes and thus contributed to the reduction of steroid use [62]. A second group from the University of Munich, Germany, used photopheresis for adjunct immunosuppression in the first 6 months after heart transplantation [63]. Fifteen patients after orthotopic heart transplantation were included in this study; these 15 patients were divided into 3 groups: the first group received standard triple drug immunosuppression (cyclosporine, azathioprine, glucocorticoids); the second group received adjunct treatment with ten single-day ECP treatments; and the third group received 20 ECP treatment courses, whereby each treatment consisted of two back-to-back treatments. Photopheresis was performed in the two latter groups within 24 h after transplantation with a higher frequency in the early postoperative period and later on at 4-week intervals for a total of 6 months. In this study the authors were able to show that the total number of acute rejection episodes within the first 4 weeks after transplantation was more impressive in the third group with standard back-to-back treatments than with the single treatments. Both photopheresis groups were more effective than the control group by reducing the rejection episodes by more than 50 % [64]. In this last study, the photoreactive drug 8-MOP was administered extracorporeally in the manner described by Knobler et al. [31], even though the number of patients per group was small and the concentration of the drug was below what present studies suggest as optimal levels for ECP efficacy (~100 ng/ml). These observations, when taken together with the other reported studies, certainly suggest an important role of this treatment modality in the field of organ transplantation. Recently, a multicenter-, prospective-, parallel-designed study was performed to assess the safety and efficacy of 6 months of maintenance ECP. Included were 60 primary cardiac recipients at 12 clinical sites. Patients were randomized (stratified and balanced intra-center by age and gender) to receive either triple drug therapy alone (standard) or in conjunction with ECP. Even though survival in both groups was similar, 94 % [3, 31] in the EPC group vs 96 % [26, 27] in the standard group, the study stood out by the result that the ECP group had a 2.13 times greater likelihood of being rejection free vs the standard group. ECP thus was shown to be able to significantly decrease cardiac rejection episodes without increasing the incidence of infections [64]. This study certainly supports immunomodulatory effects ascribed to ECP and its possible future use in the areas of pulmonary, kidney, small bowel, and bone marrow (GVHD) transplantation where standard immunosuppressive therapy is less successful [12, 13, 27–30], or is associated with significant life-threatening side effects. On-going trials in these areas should help set the stage for the appropriate indication for ECP in this area.

Systemic Lupus Erythematosus

As in other autoimmune diseases, systemic lupus erythematosus (SLE) is a T-cell-mediated disease for which no specific side-effect-free therapy is available;

nonspecific immunosuppressive therapy that includes long-term use of cortico-steroids and cytotoxic drugs is required to control the disease. As previously pointed out, these drugs on long-term use can lead to limiting and often debili-tating side effects and complications. In order to evaluate the safety, feasibility, and efficacy of ECP in the management and treatment of SLE, an open 2-year clinical trial on 10 patients was performed [6, 7]. Ten patients who met the crite-ria of the American Rheumatism Association (ARA) for lupus erythematosus were entered into this trial. For the purposes of this pilot study, patients were included if their systemic involvement was not life-threatening and if they had

1. mild-to-moderate disease adequately controlled with conventional treatment, including non-steroidal anti-inflammatory drugs (NSAIDs), low-dose ste-roids, chloroquine, oral azathioprine, or oral cyclophosphamide and
2. repeated, consecutive flares of disease activity upon attempted reduction or elimination of these medications within 3 months prior to inclusion. Eight of the ten patients were able to complete the trial. In seven of eight patients, response to treatment was significant.

The clinical activity score decreased from a median of 7 (range 1–9) to a median of 1 (range 0–5) ($p<$ 0.05). The utilized score (SIS) was a validated score, which had been compared to other known SLE scoring systems; the laboratory abnor-malities did not change significantly but, as noted by the authors, were mild at the outset. As with other small studies, the reported study demonstrates the potential safe use of ECP in SLE. The results with respect to clinical improve-ment were encouraging, particularly with regard to the arthritic and cutaneous manifestations. Perhaps the most interesting observation in this study is that ECP can be used in patients with known photosensitivity without inducing an exacerbation. Again, one can recommend that this therapeutic approach be fur-ther evaluated, not only in the treatment of selected cases [20] but also in con-trolled clinical trials, before recommendations can be made.

Oral Lichen Planus

The similarities between lichen planus and GVHD may reflect a common patho-genic feature. Another common feature shared between these two similar clini-cal pictures is that they are both ECP-responsive. Becherel reported a series of patients with severe refractory erosive oral lichen planus. Responses occurred within the 6-month trial of therapy [65]. Minimal toxicity was observed. Since that report, there have been no follow-up studies published, although at our treatment center we have treated one severe oral lichen planus patient who had a prompt remission after two cycles of ECP. The mechanism underlying this response is unclear; our patient had an additional diagnosis of hepatitis C. There is an association between lichen planus and hepatitis C infection. Addi-tionally, it has been shown that ECP can elicit beneficial responses in hepatitis C patients who are resistant to interferon injections [66]. It is possible that by enhancing the immune response against this chronic viral infection that the parainfectious phenomenon of oral lichen planus also improved.

Multiple Sclerosis

With therapeutic impacts beyond that achievable with interferons in many clinical situations, it was hoped that ECP might also be able to impact the apparently T-cell-mediated crippling disease multiple sclerosis. In a well-controlled, double-blind study, 16 patients were treated with ECP or sham ECP. No changes in the neurological or MRI assessments were noted in the 1-year follow-up study [67].

Summary

The control of mature T cells in the disease CTCL should allow clinicians an avenue for controlling T cells in other T-cell-mediated diseases. With minimal acute and chronic toxicity, this treatment modality can have significant positive effects on a number of conditions, including the cutaneous manifestations of progressive systemic sclerosis, therapy-resistant pemphigus vulgaris, acute rejection in heart transplantation, both acute and chronic GVHD, rheumatoid arthritis, systemic lupus erythematosus, psoriasis arthritis, and lichen planus. This innovative approach to the treatment of T-cell-mediated diseases has certainly opened new avenues of therapy in photoimmunology not restricted to the diseases discussed in this paper. The very low side-effect profile of this therapy certainly makes it more attractive than the chemotherapeutic and immunosuppressive substances that are currently used. Once the mechanisms of action are understood, a more rational approach to the utilization of this modality will benefit patients. That responsibility is not on the basic scientists alone. Appropriate studies investigating combination therapies and varying treatment schedules can lead to meaningful advances in maximizing the impact of ECP.

References

1. Edelson RL, Berger C, Gasparro F, Jegasothy B, Heald P, Wintroub B, Vonderheid E, Knobler R, Wolff K, Plewig G, McKiernan G, Christensen I, Oster M, Hoenigsmann H, Wilford H, Kokoschka E, Rehle T, Perez M, Stingl G, Laroche L (1987) Treatment of cutaneous T-cell lymphoma by extracorporeal photochemotherapy. N Engl J Med 316:297–303
2. Rook AH, Freundlich B, Jegasothy BV, Perez ML, Barr WG, Jiminez SA, Rietschel RL, Wintroub B, Kahaleh B, Varga J, Heald PW, Steen V, Massa MC, Murphy GF, Perniciaro C, Istfan M, Ballas SK, Edelson RL (1992) Treatment of systemic sclerosis with extracorporeal photochemotherapy – results of a multicenter trial. Arch Dermatol 128:337–346
3. DiSpaltro F, Cotrill C, Cahill C, Degnan E, Mulford J, Scarborough D, Franks A, Klainer A, Bisaccia E (1993) Extracorporeal photochemotherapy in progressive systemic sclerosis. Int J Dermatol 32:1–5
4. Zachariae H, Bjerring P, Heickendorff L, Moller B, Wallevik K (1992) Photopheresis and systemic sclerosis. Arch Dermatol 128:1651–1653
5. Rook AH, Jegasothy BV, Heald P, Nahass GT, Ditre C, Witmer WK, Lazarus GS, Edelson RL (1990) Extracorporeal photochemotherapy for drug-resistant pemphigus vulgaris. Ann Intern Med 112:303–305

6. Knobler RM, Graninger W, Graninger W, Lindmaier A, Trautinger F, Smolen J (1992) Extracorporeal photochemotherapy for the treatment of systemic lupus erythematosus. A Pilot Study. Arthritis Rheum 35:319–324
7. Knobler RM, Graninger M, Lindmaier A, Trautinger F (1991) Photophereses for the treatment of lupus erythematosus. Ann NY Acad Sci 636:340
8. Gollnick H, Owsianowski M, Taube K, Orfanos C (1993) Unresponsive severe generalized pemphigus vulgaris successfully controlled by extracorporeal photopheresis. J Am Acad Dermatol 28:122–124
9. Prinz B, Nachbar F, Plewig G (1994) Treatment of severe atopic dermatitis with extracorporeal photopheresis. Arch Dermatol Res 287:48–52
10. Wilfert H, Hönigsmann H, Steiner G, Smolen J, Wolff K (1990) Treatment of psoriatic arthritis by extracorporeal photochemotherapy. Br J Dermatol 122:225–232
11. Vahlquist C, Larsson M, Ernerudh J, Berlin G, Skogh T, Vahlquist A (1996) Treatment of psoriatic arthritis with extracorporeal photochemotherapy and conventional psoralen-ultraviolet A irradiation. Arthritis Rheum 39(9):1519–1523
12. Owsianowski, M, Gollnick H, Siegert W, Schwerdtfeger R, Orfanos EE (1994) Successful treatment of chronic graft-versus-host diseaese with extracorporeal photopheresis. Bone Marrow Transpl 14:845–848
13. Gerber M, Gmeinhart B, Volc-Platzer B, Kahls P, Greinix R, Knobler R (1997) Complete remission of lichen-planus-like graft-versus-host disease (GVHD) with extracorporeal photochemotherapy (CP). Bone Marrow Transplant 19:517–519
14. DeWilde A, DiSpaltro F, Geller A, Szer L, Klainer A, Bisaccia E (1992) Extracorporeal photochemotherapy as adjunctive treatment in juvenile dermatomyositis. A case report. Arch Dermatol 128:1656–1657
15. Rosetti F, Zulian F, Dall'Amico R, Messina C, Montini G, Zacchello F (1995) Extracorporeal photochemotherapy as single therapy for extensive cutaneous, chronic graft-versus-host disease. Transplantation 59:149–151
16. Vonderheid EC, Kang C, Kadin M, Bigler RD, Griffin TD, Rogers TJ (1990) Extracorporeal photopheresis in psoriasis vulgaris: clinical and immunologic observations. J Am Acad Dermatol 23:703–712
17. Zachariae H, Bjerring P, Brodthagen U, Sogaard H (1995) Photopheresis in the red man or pre-sezary syndrome. Dermatology 190:132–135
18. Randazzo J, DiSpaltro F, Cottrill C, Klainer A, Steere A, Bisaccia E (1994) Successful treatment of a patient with chronic lyme arthritis with extracorporeal photochemotherapy. J Am Acad Dermatol 30:908–910
19. Malawista S, Trock D, Edelson R (1991) Treatment of rheumatoid arthritis by extracorporeal photochemotherapy: a pilot study. Arthritis Rheum 34:646–654
20. Licht-Mbalyohere A, Heller A, Stadler R (1996) Extracorporeal photochemotherapy of therapy-refractory cases of systemic lupus erythematosus with urticarial vasculitis and pemphigus foliaceus. Eur J Dermatol 6:106–109
21. Liang G, Nahas G, Kerdel FA (1992) Pemphigus vulgaris treated with photopheresis. J Am Acad Dermatol 26:779–780
22. Berkson M, Lazarus GS, Uberti-Benz M, Rook AH (1991) Extracorporeal photochemotherapy: a potentially useful treatment for scleromyxedema. J Am Acad Dermatol 25:724
23. Costanzo-Nordin MR, Hubbell EA, O'Sullivan EJ, Johnson MR, Mullen GM, Heroux AL, Kao WG, McManus BM, Pifarre R, Robinson JA (1992) Successful treatment of heart transplant rejection with photopheresis. Transplantation 53:808–815
24. Costanzo-Nordin MR, Hubbell EA, O'Sullivan EJ, Johnson MR, Mullen GM, Heroux AL, Kao WG, McManus BM, Pifarre R, Robinson JA (1992) Photopheresis versus corticosteroids in the therapy of heart transplant rejection. Circulation 86:242–250
25. Hilliquin P, Andreu G, Heshmati F, Menkes CJ (1993) Treatment of refractory rheumatoid arthritis by extracorporeal photochemotherapy. Rheumatol Rev 60:125–130

26. Rose EA, Barr ML, Xu H, Peoino P, Murphy MP, McGovern MA, Ratner AJ, Watkins JF, Marboe CC, Berger CL (1992) Photochemotherapy in human heart transplant recipients at high risk for fatal rejection. J Heart Lung Transpl 11:746–750
27. Sunder-Plassman G, Druml W, Steininger R, Hönigsmann H, Knobler R (1995) Renal allograft rejection controlled by photopheresis. Lancet 346:506
28. Wolfe J, Tomaszewski J, Grosman R, Gottlieb S, Naji A, Brayman K, Kobrin S, Rook A (1996) Reversal of acute renal allograft rejection by extracorporeal photopheresis: a case presentation and review of the literature. J Clin Apheresis 11:36–41
29. Slovis BS, Loyd JE, King LE (1995) Photopheresis for chronic rejection of lung allografts. N Engl J Med 332:962
30. Andreu G, Achkar A, Couteil JP, Guillemain R, Heshmati F, Amrein C, Chevalier P, Guinvarch A, Dore MF, Capron F et al (1995) Extracorporeal photochemotherapy treatment for acute lung rejection episode. J Heart Lung Transplant 14(4):793–796
31. Knobler RM, Trautinger F, Graninger W, Macheiner W, Gruenwald C, Neumann R, Ramer W (1993) Parenteral administration of 8-methoxypsoralen in photopheresis. J Am Acad Dermatol 28:580–584
32. Knobler RM, Edelson RL (1986) Cutaneous T-cell lymphoma. Med Clin North Am 70:109–138
33. Knobler RM (1987) Photopheresis – extracorporeal irradiation of 8-MOP containing blood – a new therapeutic modality. Blut 54:247–250
34. Armus S, Keyes B, Cahill C, Berger C, Crater D, Scarborough D, Klainer A, Bisaccia E (1990) Photopheresis for the treatment of cutaneous T-cell lymphoma. J Am Acad Dermatol 23:898–902
35. Heald PW, Perez MI, Christensen I, Dobbs N, McKiernan G, Edelson RL (1989) Photopheresis therapy of cutaneous T-cell lymphoma: the Yale-New Haven Hospital Experience. Yale J Biol Med 62:629–638
36. Heald P, Rook A, Perez M, Wintroub B, Knobler R, Jegasothy B, Gasparro F, Berger C, Edelson R (1992) Treatment of erythrodermic cutaneous T-cell lymphoma with extracorporeal photochemotherapy. J Am Acad Dermatol 27:427–433
37. Heald P, Knobler R, LaRoche L (1994) Photoinactivated lymphocyte therapy of cutaneous T-cell lymphoma. Dermatol Clin 12:443–449
38. Knobler R (1995) Photopheresis and the red man syndrome. Dermatology 190:97–98
39. Zic J, Arzubiaga C, Salhany KE, Parker RA, Wilson D, Stricklin GP, Greer J, King LE Jr (1992) Extracorporeal photopheresis for the treatment of cutaneous T-cell lymphoma. J Am Acad Dermatol 27:729–736
40. Berger CL, Perez MM, Laroche L, Edelson R (1990) Inhibition of autoimmune disease in a murine model of systemic lupus erythematosus induced by exposure to syngeneic photoinactivated lymphocytes. J Invest Dermatol 94:52–57
41. Berger CL Wang N, Christensen I, Longley J, Heald P, Edelson RL (1996) The immune response to class I-associated tumor-specific cutaneous T-cell lymphoma antigens. J Invest Dermatol 107:392–397
42. Edelson R (1988) Light activated drugs. Sci Am 259:68–75
43. Gasparro FP, Song J, Knobler RM, Edelson RL (1986) Quantitation of psoralen photoadducts in DNA isolated from lymphocytes treated with 8-methoxypsoralen and ultraviolet a radiation (extracorporeal photopheresis). Curr Probl Dermatol 15:67–84
44. Gasparro F, Dall'Amico R, O'Malley M, Heald PW, Edelson RL (1990) Cell mem-brane DNA: a new target for psoralen photoadduct formation. Phochem Photobiol 52:315–321
45. Perez M, Edelson R, Laroche L, Berger C (1989) Inhibition of antiskin allograft immunity by infusions with syngeneic photoinactivated effector lymphocytes. J Invest Dermatol 92:669–676
46. Vowels BR, Cassin M, Boufal MH, Walsh LJ, Rook AJ (1992) Extracorporeal photochemotherapy induces the production of tumor necrosis factor-α by monocytes:

implications for the treatment of cutaneous T-cell lymphoma and systemic sclerosis. J Invest Dermatol 96:686–692

47. Gasparro FP, Berger CL, Edelson RL (1984) Effect of monochromatic UVA light and 8-methoxypsoralen on human lymphocyte response to mitogen. Photodermatol 1:10–17

48. Santella RM, Dharmaraja N, Gasparro FP, Edelson RL (1985) Monoclonal antibodies to DNA modified by 8-methoxypsoralen and ultraviolet a light. Nucleic Acids Res 13:2533–2544

49. Schmitt I, Moor A, Patrignelli R, Chimenti S, Beijersbergen van Henegouwen G, Edelson R, Gasparro F (1995) Increased surface expression of class I MHC molecules on immunogenic cells derived from the xenogenization of P815 mastocytoma cells with 8-methoxypsoralen and long-wavelenght ultraviolet radiation. Tissue Antigens 46:45–49

50. Sumpio BE, Phan SM, Gasparro FP, Deckelbaum LI (1993) Control of smooth muscle cell proliferation by psoralen photochemotherapy. J Vasc Surg 17:1010–1016

51. Trautinger F, Knobler RM, Macheiner W, Grünwald C, Miksche M (1991) Release of oxygen-free radicals by neutrophils is reduced by photopheresis. Ann NY Acad Sci 636:383–385

52. Van Iperen HP, Beijersbergen van Henegouwen GMJ (1992) Animal model for extracorporeal photochemotherapy based on contact hypersensitivity. J Photochem Photobiol B Biol 15:361–366

53. Yamane Y, Lobo FM, John LA, Edelson RL, Perez MI (1992) Suppression of anti-skin-allograft response by photodamaged effector cells – the modulating effects of prednisone and cyclophosphamide. Transplantation 54:119–124

54. Rook A, Prystowsky M (1991) Combined therapy for sezary syndrome with extracorporeal photochemotherapy and low-dose interferon alfa therapy. Arch Dermatol 127:1535–1540

55. Duvic M, Hester P, Lemak A (1996) Photopheresis therapy for cutaneous T-cell lymphoma. J Am Acad Dermatol 35:573–579

56. Zic J, Stricklin G, Greer J, Kinney M, Shyr Y, Wilson D, Kind Jr. L (1996) Long term follow-up with cutaneous T-cell lymphoma treated with extracorporeal photochemotherapy. J Am Acad Dermatol 356:935–945

57. Gottlieb S, Wolfe T, Fox F, DeNardo B, Macey W, Bromley P, Lessin S, Rook A (1996) Treatment of cutaneous T-cell lymphoma with extracorporeal photopheresis monotherapy and in combination with recombinant interferon alpha: a 10 year experience at a single institution. J Am Acad Dermatol 35:946–957

58. Haley H, Davis D, Sams W (1999) Durable loss of a malignant T-cell clone in a stage IV cutaneous T-cell lymphoma patient treated with high dose interferon and photopheresis. J Am Acad Dermatol 41:880–883

59. Wilson LD, Licata AL, Braverman IM, Edelson RL, Heald PW, Feldman AM, Kacinski BM (1995) Systemic chemotherapy and extracorporeal photochemotherapy for T3 and T4 cutaneous T-cell lymphoma patients who have achieved a complete response to total skin electron beam therapy. Int J Radiat Oncol Biol Phys 32:987–995

60. Rook AH, Freundlich B, Nahass G, Washko R, Macelis B, Skolnicki M, Bromley P, Winter W, Jegasothy B (1989) Treatment of autoimmune disease with extracorporeal photochemotherapy: progressive systemic sclerosis. Yale J Biol Med 16:639–645

61. Kahale MB, Suttany GL, Smith EA et al (1986) A modified scleroderma skin scoring method. Clin Exp Rheumatol 4:367–369

62. Dall'Amico R, Livi U, Montini G. et al (1994) Successful treatment of heart transplant (HT) patients with multiple rejection. J Heart Lung Transplant 2:S81

63. Meiser BM, Kur F, Reichenspurner H et al (1994) Reduction of the incidence of rejection by adjunct immunosuppression with photochemotherapy after heart transplantation. Transplant 57:563–568

64. Barr ML (1996) Immunomodulation in transplantation with photopheresis. Artif Org 20/8:971–973
65. Becherel P, Bussel A, Chosidow O, Rabian C, Piette J, Frances C (1998) Extracorporeal photochemotherapy for chronic erosive lichen planus (letter). Lancet 351(9105):805
66. O'Brien C, Henzel B, Moonka D, Inverso J, Rook A. (1999) Extracorporeal photopheresis alone and with interferon alpha 2a in chronic hepatitis C patients who failed previous interferon therapy. Dig Dis Sci 44:1020–1026
67. Rostami A, Sater R, Bird S, GalettaS, Farber R, Kamon M, Silberberg D, Grossman R, Pfohl D (1999) A double blind, placebo controlled trial of extracorporeal photopheresis in chronic progressive multiple sclerosis. Multiple Sclerosis 5:198–203

13 Ultraviolet-A1 Phototherapy: Indications and Mode of Action

Jean Krutmann, Helger Stege, Akimichi Morita

Contents

Introduction

In 1981, Mutzhas et al. reported the development of an irradiation device which almost exclusively emitted in the long-wave ultraviolet (UV)A range, i.e., UVA-1 (340–400 nm) [35]. The combination of a metal halide lamp with a novel filtering system offered, for the first time, the unique possibility to expose human skin to high doses of UVA-1 radiation without causing a sunburn reaction. Soon thereafter, UVA-1 irradiation devices proved to be useful in photoprovocation testing for patients with UVA-sensitive photodermatoses, in particular polymorphic light eruption. It took, however, more than a decade before the therapeutic potential of these novel irradiation devices was recognized and systematically exploited. In 1992, Krutmann and Schöpf reported that exposure to high doses of UVA-1 radiation was beneficial for patients with severe acute atopic dermatitis [21]. These observations prompted a continually growing interest in the therapeutic use of UVA-1 radiation. As a consequence, there is now a substantial body of literature to suggest that for selected indications UVA-1 phototherapy is superior to conventional phototherapeutic modalities [26]. A major difference between UVA-1 and UVB or UVA/UVB radiation is given by the fact that with UVA-1 phototherapy it has been possible to achieve therapeutic responses by penetrating deep into the dermis without the usual side effects caused by less penetrating UVB and UVB-like wavelengths in the UVA-2 region [15]. In addition, UVA-1 radiation has some unique immunomodulatory features indicating that, under appropriate circumstances, it might prove superior even when compared with psoralen plus UVA (PUVA) therapy [23]. UVA-1 phototherapy was used first to treat patients with atopic dermatitis, but it has since been

Table 1. Indications for UVA-1 therapy

Indication	Type of study	Comment
Atopic dermatitis	Several open studies, 1 multicenter trial	Established indication
Urticaria pigmentosa	2 open studies	Promising results, "long-lasting effects" Controlled study lacking
Localized scleroderma	2 open studies	Very promising, "breakthrough" Controlled comparative studies needed
Systemic sclerosis	1 open study	Very promising, "breakthrough", controlled comparative studies needed
CTCL	2 open studies, 1 comparative study	Promising multicenter trial ongoing
Psoriasis/HIV+	1 open study	Very promising, "therapy of choice" Larger studies required
Psoriasis/HIV –	Case report	Disappointing
Alopecia areata	Unpublished study	Not effective
Solar urticaria	Several cases	Not effective
Lichen planus	Several cases	Not effective

found to be efficacious in several other skin diseases, such as localized and systemic scleroderma, in which other therapeutic options are limited. This development has been fostered by studies in which the photobiological and molecular basis of UVA-1 phototherapy was analyzed. Currently, the indications for UVA-1 phototherapy fall into four major categories: T-cell-mediated skin diseases, mast cell-mediated skin diseases, connective tissue diseases, and phototherapy in HIV+ patients (Table 1).

UVA-1 Phototherapy for T-Cell-Mediated Skin Diseases

In vitro studies have demonstrated that UVA-1 radiation is a potent inducer of apoptosis in human T lymphocytes [8]. At a molecular level, UVA-1 radiation-induced apoptosis differs from apoptosis observed in UVB-irradiated or PUVA-treated cells because it is mediated through a pathway that does not require protein synthesis. This so-called preprogrammed cell death or early apoptosis appears to be highly specific for UVA-1 radiation and is mediated through the generation of singlet oxygen. The in vivo relevance of these in vitro findings is suggested by the observation that UVA-1 phototherapy of patients with atopic dermatitis resulted in apoptosis of skin-infiltrating T-helper cells [32]. The appearance of apoptotic T cells was then followed by their depletion from lesional skin, a reduction in the in situ expression of the proinflammatory T-cell-derived cytokine interferon-γ, and clearing of atopic eczema [11, 12]. Therefore, it is now generally believed that UVA-1 radiation-induced T-helper cell apoptosis constitutes the basis of UVA-1 phototherapy in patients with atopic dermatitis. As a clinical consequence, UVA-1 phototherapy has been extended to the treatment of other T-cell-mediated skin diseases including cutaneous T-cell lymphoma [37].

UVA-1 Phototherapy for Atopic Dermatitis

The therapeutic efficacy of UVA-1 radiation in the management of patients with atopic dermatitis was first evaluated in an open study in patients with acute, severe exacerbations [22]. They were exposed daily to 130 J/cm^2 at an irradiation intensity of 70 mW/s for 15 consecutive days (Fig. 1). Therapeutic effectiveness was assessed by a clinical scoring system as well as by monitoring serum levels of eosinophil cationic protein [3, 6]. The latter represents a laboratory parameter that can be measured objectively and which has been shown to correlate well with disease activity. In that study, UVA-1 phototherapy was found to be highly efficient in promptly inducing clinical improvement. This was associated with a concomitant reduction in elevated serum levels of eosinophil cationic protein.

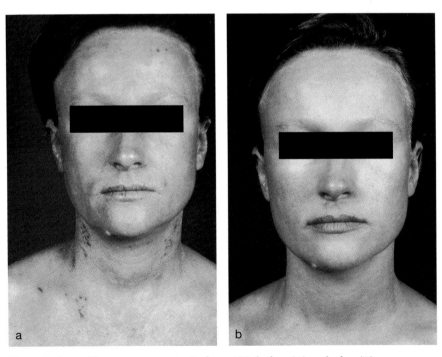

Fig. 1. Patient with acute, severe atopic dermatitis before (**A**) and after (**B**) 15 exposures to 130 J/cm^2 UVA-1

Patients treated with UVA-1 were compared to subjects who had been treated with UVA/UVB phototherapy, which at that time was considered the best phototherapy for atopic dermatitis available. Significant differences were observed in favor of UVA-1 phototherapy, indicating that UVA-1 phototherapy was the phototherapy of choice for patients with severe atopic dermatitis.

During the subsequent years there have been numerous reports confirming these original observations [18, 20, 30]. It should be noted that in their pilot study, Krutmann et al. employed UVA-1 phototherapy as a monotherapy, thereby suggesting that it might represent a therapeutic alternative to the gold standard in the treatment of severe atopic dermatitis, glucocorticosteroids [22]. Indeed, a direct comparison of UVA-1 phototherapy with a standardized topical glucocorticosteroid treatment revealed that for the treatment of patients with severe, exacerbated atopic dermatitis UVA-1 phototherapy was at least equivalent to topical glucocorticosteroids [25]. To date, this study is also the only one to provide a multicenter evaluation of the therapeutic efficacy of UVA-1 phototherapy by studying a larger number of patients with severe atopic dermatitis ($n = 53$) in a controlled randomized fashion. Patients were treated with UVA-1 (10×130 J/cm^2), UVA/UVB (minimal erythema dose-dependent), or topical flucortolone. After ten treatments, patients in all three groups had improved, but improvement was significantly greater in UVA-1-irradiated or fluocortolone-treated patients compared to UVA/UVB phototherapy. Significant reductions in serum levels of eosinophil cationic protein were only observed after glucocorticosteroid or UVA-1 therapy. The multicenter trial thus confirmed the original observation that UVA-1 phototherapy was of great benefit for patients with severe atopic dermatitis.

There is currently a debate whether the therapeutic efficacy of UVA-1 for this indication is dose-dependent. Recent studies indicate that similar to a high-dose regimen with 130 J/cm^2, a medium UVA-1 dosage schedule is superior to UVA/UVB [18]. Also, therapeutic efficacy within the UVA-1 range seems to be dose-dependent, because irradiations with 50 J/cm^2 were superior to a low-dose regimen (20 J/cm^2) [20]. Very recently, a high-dose protocol (130 J/cm^2 was found to be superior to a medium-dose regimen (50 J/cm^2), which again was more efficient than a low-dose schedule (20 J/cm^2) (J.C. Simon et al., submitted for publication). Thus, the use of low doses of UVA-1 does not offer any advantage over conventional phototherapeutic modalities such as UVA/UVB or 311 nm UVB and should therefore be discouraged. In contrast, medium- and high-dose UVA-1 are clearly superior to conventional phototherapy, but for achieving an optimal therapeutic response, a high-dose regimen with 130 J/cm^2 seems to be necessary.

UVA-1 Phototherapy of Cutaneous T-Cell Lymphoma

Cutaneous T-cell lymphoma (CTCL) is a neoplasm of helper T cells that initially manifests in the skin. The most common form is mycosis fungoides. Helper T cells in mycosis fungoides are located intraepidermally and below the epidermis as band-like dermal infiltrates. Topical treatment of patch and plaque CTCL thus requires modalities capable of penetrating into the dermis. For stage IA and IB CTCL, the treatment of choice is PUVA therapy, which, similar to UVA-1 radiation, induces T-cell apoptosis [26]. From a theoretical point of view, UVA-1 phototherapy is an alternative to PUVA for this indication because UVA-1 radiation reaches deeper layers of the dermis at higher intensities compared with PUVA and because UVA-1 phototherapy avoids the unwanted side effects resulting from the photosensitizer methoxypsoralen.

Plettenberg et al. used UVA-1 phototherapy as a monotherapy in three patients with histologically proven CTCL, stages IA and IB [37]. For daily, whole-body UVA-1 irradiations, patients were exposed to 130 J/cm^2 ($n = 2$) or 60 J/cm^2 ($n = 1$) UVA-1 radiation (Fig. 2). In each of the three patients, skin lesions began to resolve after only a few UVA-1 radiation exposures. Complete clearance was observed between 16 and 20 exposures, regardless of whether the high- or medium-dose regimen was used. These clinical data were corroborated by histological evaluation. In all three patients, histological features of mycosis fungoides were present prior to therapy, whereas after UVA-1 phototherapy, the epidermis looked almost normal and only a few lymphocytic infiltrates were left in the dermis. In a second study, ten patients with early stages of CTCL were treated with daily doses of 100 J/cm^2 UVA-1. In 10/10 patients, complete remissions were observed after a total of 20–25 exposures [2]. In a recent comparative study, CTCL patients were randomly assigned to either UVA-1 ($n = 10$) or PUVA

Fig. 2a, b. Patient with CTCL stage 1A before (**a**) and after (**b**) UVA-1 photo-therapy (20×130 J/cm^2)

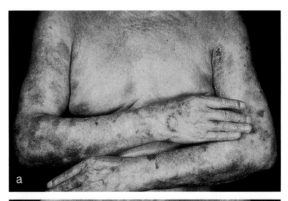

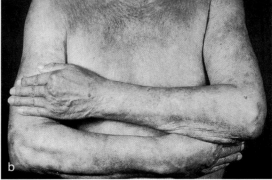

($n = 10$) therapy [38]. Again, UVA-1 phototherapy was found to be efficient in the treatment of early stages of CTCL, and no significant differences in favor of PUVA therapy were observed.

The current mainstay for the treatment of stage IA to IB CTCL is PUVA therapy. From a practical point of view, UVA-1 phototherapy has significant advantages over PUVA because unwanted side effects resulting from the systemic application of the photosensitizer are completely avoided. Therefore, an international (Duesseldorf, Vienna, Brescia, Muenster, Nagoya, and Heidelberg) multicenter trial has been initiated to compare the efficacy of UVA-1 and PUVA therapy for early stages of CTCL in a controlled study. This trial will also provide information about the duration of remission-free intervals that can be achieved with UVA-1 phototherapy. The UVA-1 dose being used in this study is in the medium- rather than the high-dose range and has been extrapolated from in vitro studies [34]. In these experiments, neoplastic T cells were shown to be significantly more sensitive to UVA-1 radiation-induced apoptosis when compared with normal T cells. This is in line with the previous notion that exposure to 60 J/cm^2 UVA-1 was equally effective to a 130 J/cm^2 UVA-1 regimen for patients with CTCL. The optimal dose for treating CTCL patients might thus differ from the one to be used for atopic dermatitis patients.

UVA-1 Phototherapy for Urticaria Pigmentosa

Induction of apoptosis in skin-infiltrating cells and their subsequent depletion from skin is thought to represent the major mechanisms of action of UVA-1 phototherapy for yet another indication, urticaria pigmentosa. In initial studies, skin sections from patients before and after UVA-1 therapy were assessed for effects on mast cells by histochemical and immunohistochemical techniques [9]. It was found that UVA-1 phototherapy reduced the density of dermal mast cells, and that this decrease was closely linked to significant clinical improvement. These studies indicated that changes in the number, and possibly function, of dermal mast cells may contribute to the clinical effects of this treatment. It was therefore not surprising to learn that UVA-1 therapy proved to be of benefit for patients suffering from cutaneous mastocytosis. In a pilot study, four adult patients with severe generalized urticaria pigmentosa were treated with a high-dose UVA-1 regimen, which was used as a monotherapy [46]. UVA-1 phototherapy was given once daily five times per week for two consecutive weeks. The initial dose was 60 J/cm^2 UVA-1; subsequently the daily dose was 130 J/cm^2 UVA-1 per body half. In all patients, UVA-1 therapy induced a prompt improvement of cutaneous symptoms, which was reflected by a reduction of increased histamine in 24-hour urine to normal levels. In addition to skin symptoms, two patients presented with systemic manifestations of urticaria pigmentosa such as diarrhea and migraine. After ten treatments, relief from systemic symptoms was noted and elevated serum serotonin was reduced to normal in both patients. No relapse occurred in any of the patients for more than 2 years after cessation of UVA-1 therapy. This is in contrast to PUVA therapy for urticaria pigmentosa, which is characterized by recurrence after 5–8 months. The long-lasting effectiveness of UVA-1 for urticaria pigmentosa has recently been confirmed in a second study [48]. In total, 15 patients with urticaria pigmentosa were treated using a high-dose UVA-1 regimen. Of the patents, 14 of 15 showed a prompt response to UVA-1 phototherapy and were free of cutaneous and/or systemic symptoms after cessation of phototherapy. A 2-year follow-up of these patients revealed that 8 months after phototherapy, 100 % of UVA-1-treated patients were still in full remission. Remission free intervals of 1 year were observed for 70 % and of 18 months for 40 % of these patients.

Differences in the recurrence rate between UVA-1- and PUVA-treated urticaria pigmentosa patients might be explained by the fact that UVA-1 therapy is associated with a reduction in numbers of dermal mast cells, which has not been observed after PUVA therapy [4, 10, 19]. This hypothesis is supported by recent in vivo studies that demonstrate a significant decrease in the number of dermal mast cells in UVA-1-, but not in PUVA-treated, patients. By employing a double-staining technique, it could also be demonstrated that lesional skin of patients with urticaria pigmentosa constitutively contained a low percentage of apoptotic mast cells, and that this percentage was significantly increased by UVA-1 phototherapy [48]. In contrast, PUVA therapy did not cause mast cell apoptosis. Taken together these studies indicate that UVA-1 phototherapy, by virtue of its capacity to induce apoptosis in skin-infiltrating mast cells, is capable of depleting these cells from the skin of urticaria pigmentosa patients. As a consequence, therapeutic responses to UVA-1 phototherapy are longer lasting and therefore, UVA-1 phototherapy has the potential to replace PUVA as the therapy of choice for urticaria pigmentosa patients.

UVA-1 Phototherapy for Connective Tissue Disease

Patients with localized scleroderma develop one or multiple, circumscribed, ivory-white, indurated plaques, which may be up to 20 cm in diameter and are frequently surrounded by an inflammatory halo known as the lilac ring [40]. Although the disease has a self-limited course, sclerosis of skin lesions may cause significant morbidity and discomfort. It is possible that sclerotic skin lesions lead to muscle atrophy and thereby disfiguration of the trunk or face. They may also extend over joints and cause flexion contractures with functional impairment. Numerous modalities including penicillin, penicillamine, antimalarial drugs, cyclosporin A, interferon-γ, and topical or systemic glucocorticosteroids have been employed, but in general, there is no effective curative or symptomatic therapy for localized scleroderma.

In this regard, it is of particular interest that sclerosis of skin lesions appears to result from an increased synthesis of type I and type III collagen [7, 27, 39]. Evidence has been provided that a major cause for this excessive collagen deposition is a malfunction of dermal fibroblasts, in particular a decreased collagenase I expression [50]. It is possible to increase synthesis of collagenase I in cultured human dermal fibroblasts by in vitro exposure to UVA-1 radiation [36, 41]. In these studies, UVA-1 radiation-induced collagenase production was associated with a dose-dependent upregulation of collagenase I mRNA expression,

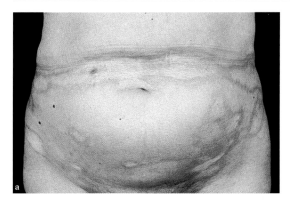

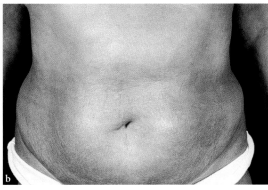

Fig. 3a, b. Sclerotic plaques
in the abdominal region of a
patient with localized scleroderma before (a) and after
(b) UVA-1 phototherapy
(30 × 130 J/cm² UVA-1)

and maximal induction was achieved in vitro by UVA-1 radiation doses, which
are equivalent to those used in high-dose UVA-1 phototherapy of atopic dermatitis or urticaria pigmentosa patients. It has therefore been hypothesized that
UVA-1 radiation, by virtue of its capacity to increase collagenase I expression,
may have beneficial effects for patients with localized scleroderma [16, 47]. This
hypothesis has been tested in an open study, in which 10 patients with histologically proven localized scleroderma were exposed 30 times to 130 J/cm² of UVA-1
radiation [47] (Fig. 3). In all patients, UVA-1 therapy softened sclerotic plaques,
and complete clearance was observed in 4 out of 10 patients. In addition, 20-
MHz sonography revealed that UVA-1 therapy significantly reduced thickness
and increased elasticity of plaques (Fig. 4). These changes were not due to spontaneous remission of skin lesions in these patients because they could only be
observed in UVA-1-irradiated, but not in unirradiated, control plaques of the
same patients. It has also been suggested that similar therapeutic effects can be
achieved by exposing patients with localized scleroderma to low doses (20 J/
cm²) of UVA-1 radiation [13, 17]. Direct comparison of low- versus high-dose
UVA-1 phototherapy, however, revealed that high-dose UVA-1 therapy was superior to low-dose UVA-1 therapy for all parameters assessed (clinical evaluation,
thickness of plaques, and cutaneous elastometry) [47]. Patients were followed
up for a total of 3 months after cessation of therapy. Termination of UVA-1 ther-

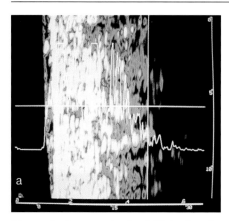
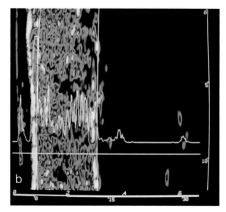

Fig. 4a, b. Sonography (20-MHz) of a sclerotic plaque of a patient with localized scleroderma before (a) and after (b) UVA-1 phototherapy (30 × 130 J/cm² UVA-1)

apy was not associated with a loss of the beneficial effects achieved in any of these patients. Accordingly, in 6/7 patients, skin thickness values obtained at the end of the follow-up period were identical to those measured immediately after the last high-dose UVA-1 irradiation. In one patient, a partial relapse of skin symptoms was observed, but skin thickness after the 3-month follow-up period was still significantly below values obtained before phototherapy was started. In none of the patients, further improvement of skin symptoms was observed after UVA-1 therapy was stopped.

The precise mechanism(s) by which UVA-1 therapy may act in localized scleroderma are currently unknown. The rationale for employing a high-dose UVA-1 radiation regimen for this indication was based on previous in vitro observations that UVA-1 irradiation induced collagenase I expression in cultured human dermal fibroblasts in a dose-dependent manner [36, 41]. This concept is strongly supported by recent studies in which sequential biopsies before and after high-dose UVA-1 therapy were obtained from sclerotic skin lesions of patients with localized scleroderma. UVA-1 radiation-induced clinical improvement and reduction of skin thickness were found to be associated with about a 20-fold upregulation of collagenase I mRNA expression in irradiated sclerotic plaques [47]. Taken together these studies strongly indicate that UVA-1 phototherapy is effective for localized scleroderma. Effectiveness is UVA-1 dose-dependent and associated with induction of collagenase I expression.

In addition to localized scleroderma, UVA-1 phototherapy has also been reported to be of benefit for patients with systemic sclerosis. Morita et al. exposed lesional skin on the forearms of 5 patients with systemic sclerosis to single doses of 60 J/cm² UVA-1 [33]. In all patients, UVA-1 phototherapy treated skin lesions were markedly softened after 10–30 exposures. Clinical improvement was associated with an increase in joint passive range of motion values, skin temperature, and cutaneous elasticity.

Histological evaluation of skin specimens obtained before and after therapy revealed loosening of collagen bundles and the appearance of small collagen fibers. A half-side comparison in one patient revealed that improvement of these parameters was only observed in UVA-1-treated, but not in unirradiated control skin [33]. This study further supports the concept that UVA-1 phototherapy is a valuable treatment option for patients suffering from scleroderma. The fact that currently no other treatment options with proven efficacy for the management of diseases associated with skin sclerosis are available should further stimulate the interest in UVA-1 phototherapy.

It should be noted that in addition to UVA-1 therapy, systemic as well as topical PUVA therapy have been reported to be of benefit for patients with localized scleroderma and systemic sclerosis [31, 42]. Future studies will therefore have to compare UVA-1 versus PUVA therapy for both therapeutic efficacy and unwanted side effects. At least in the in vitro situation, PUVA treatment, but not UVA-1 irradiation, induced terminal differentiation of cultured human fibroblasts, indicating that PUVA therapy may be associated with a greater risk for photoaging. In addition, clinical improvement in patients with systemic sclerosis required an average of 50 PUVA treatments given over a period of 4–5 months [31]. In contrast, UVA-1 phototherapy required a total of 30 irradiations to achieve maximal therapeutic effects [34]. Since UVA-1, in contrast to PUVA therapy, was given on a daily basis, the total treatment time was reduced to 1–1.5 months, and UVA-1 phototherapy thus yielded beneficial effects much faster than PUVA.

UVA-1 Phototherapy for HIV-Positive Patients

The safety of UVB or PUVA in the treatment of patients with skin disorders remains controversial. On the one hand, clinical studies have not shown dramatic adverse effects on immune status or plasma viral load. On the other hand, laboratory studies have clearly demonstrated that UVB or PUVA can activate HIV in cultured cells and in vivo in transgenic animals. The debate has been further stimulated by recent studies in which HIV-1 (gag) expression was analyzed in a semiquantitative manner in human skin using a PCR-based assay. It was observed that UVB administered in vivo in suberythemogenic doses can activate the virus in lesional skin and non-lesional skin of seropositive patients with psoriasis or eosinophilic folliculitis. Previous in vitro studies have demonstrated that the only wavelength range within the UV that does not activate the HIV promoter is UVA-1 [51]. Since psoriasis is currently being regarded as a T-cell-mediated skin disease and since UVA-1 phototherapy has proven to be highly effective for the treatment of T-cell-mediated inflammatory responses in human skin, it was obvious to assess whether UVA-1 phototherapy can be used for the treatment of psoriasis in HIV+ individuals. In an open, uncontrolled trial, HIV+ patients ($n = 3$) showed a beneficial response to UVA-1 phototherapy, which was given on a daily base as a high-dose regimen [5] (Fig. 5). Prior to initiation of whole-body UVA-1 phototherapy, the safety of UVA-1 phototherapy in HIV+ patients was assessed. For this purpose, paired lesional and non-lesional skin specimens were obtained from all patients after a single exposure to UVB (150 mJ/cm^2), UVA-1 (130 J/cm^2) or sham irradiation. By employing the

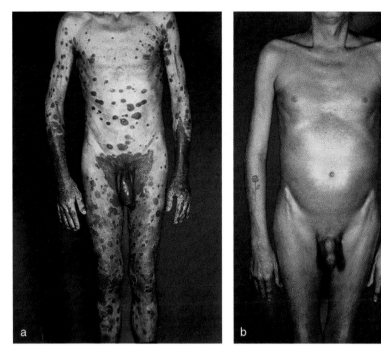

Fig. 5a, b. HIV+ patient with psoriasis before (a) and after (b) UVA-1 phototherapy $(20 \times 130 \text{ J/cm}^2)$

quantitative PCR-based HIV assay it was observed that UVB-treated skin showed a 6- to 15-fold increase in HIV count compared to unirradiated skin. By contrast, there were no differences in the HIV count of UVA-1 treated versus unirradiated skin. Moreover, complete clearance of psoriasis was observed in these patients after 20–30 UVA-1 irradiations. Importantly, there were also no increments in the skin viral counts of HIV+ patients with psoriasis after UVA-1 phototherapy (up to 41 total-body UVA-1 radiation exposures). These studies indicate, that (1) UVA-1 is an effective treatment for psoriasis in HIV+ patients and (2) that UVA-1, unlike UVB, does not activate HIV in human skin. At least from the perspective of safety, UVA-1 phototherapy therefore seems to represent the phototherapy of choice in HIV+ patients.

Miscellaneous Indications for UVA-1 Phototherapy

In an open pilot study, 12 patients with an acute exacerbation of their chronic vesicular dyshidrotic hand eczema were subjected to a local UVA-1 phototherapy [43]. Palms and backs of hands were exposed to 15 UVA-1 irradiations with a dose of 40 J/cm^2 per day over a period of 3 weeks. After 1 week of treatment, all but one patient reported a marked relief of itch. After the 3-week treatment period, significant clinical improvement was noted in 10/12 patients. This report is consistent with the observed therapeutic efficacy of UVA-1 phototherapy for atopic dermatitis and other T-cell-mediated skin diseases [24, 32]. Local UVA-1 phototherapy may thus prove to be an effective therapeutic option in the management of patients with chronic vesicular hand eczema.

A recent case report indicates that UVA-1 phototherapy is of benefit for patients with keloids and hypertrophic scars [1]. A 37-year-old man (skin type IV) with a 17-year history of a stable chest keloid secondary to severe acne was treated 22 times with single exposures of 130 J/cm^2 UVA-1. Only two thirds of the keloid were treated, whereas the remaining third served as the unirradiated control. Already after 3 weeks, and even more so after 6 weeks, of UVA-1 phototherapy, marked softening and flattening of the irradiated, but not the unirradiated parts of the keloid were noted. Histological evaluation revealed the reappearance of normal looking collagen and elastic fibers in this keloid after phototherapy. These very preliminary but exciting results indicate that UVA-1 phototherapy could be of great help to patients with large scars such as burn scars for whom surgical remodeling or intralesional corticosteroid injection can be difficult.

Combined UVA-1 radiation and acitretin therapy has been reported as a treatment option in one patient with pityriasis rubra pilaris [14]. From this case report, the relative contribution of UVA-1 and acitretin to the therapeutic response remains unclear.

It has been suggested that daily low-dose UVA-1 irradiation is beneficial to patients with lupus erythematosus. In support of this concept has been the publication of an open study with 10 patients with systemic lupus erythematosus who were treated with single doses of 6 J/cm^2 UVA-1 for various durations (15 days to 8 months) [28]. There was a decrease in clinical indices of disease activity as well as in titers of anti-SSA or antinuclear antibodies. This study has recently been confirmed in an 18-week, 2-phase study [29]. During the initial 6-week prospective, double-blind, placebo-controlled phase, 26 female patients were divided into two groups. Group A patients were exposed to 6 J/cm^2 UVA-1 and group B patients for an equal amount of time to visible light. Each group was subsequently crossed over for 3 weeks. This was followed by a second phase of 12 weeks, in which patients and physicians were unblinded and patients were treated with progressively decreasing levels of UVA-1 radiation. In patients from group A, disease activity was significantly decreased after 3 weeks of UVA-1 therapy but relapsed to baseline levels after 3 weeks of visible light treatment. In contrast, group B patients showed no significant response to the initial three weeks of visible light treatment nor to the following 3 weeks of UVA-1 therapy. In both groups, however, significant improvement of clinical symptoms was detected after 6 weeks of UVA-1 phototherapy, which was given under uncontrolled conditions in phase 2. These single center studies, however, have not yet been confirmed by other groups. Also, treatment of a UV-sensitive autoimmune disease such as lupus erythematosus with UVA-1 phototherapy may not be without risk, in particular when UVA-1 is used at higher doses for SCLE patients who might develop a systemic form due to phototherapy [45].

Side Effects of UVA-1 Phototherapy

UVA-1 phototherapy may not be performed in patients with UVA-sensitive photo-dermatoses or photosensitive atopic dermatitis. It is necessary to exclude these diseases prior to initiation of phototherapy. This can easily be accomplished by photo-provocation testing. Except for eczema herpeticum, no acute side effects have been observed in any patient treated with UVA-1. No other side effects have been observed, although its potential carcinogenic risk is a concern. Exposure of hairless albino Skh-hr1 mice to high doses of UVA-1 radiation has been shown to induce squamous cell carcinoma [49]. The actual contribution of UVA-1 radiation to the development of malignant melanoma in humans is under debate and at this point cannot be excluded [44]. These theoretical concerns are mainly relevant for atopic dermatitis patients who usually are at a younger age. Until more is known about UVA-1 phototherapy, its use in patients with atopic dermatitis should be limited to periods of acute exacerbation and one treatment cycle should not exceed 10–15 exposures once or twice a year. As a general rule, children should not be treated with UVA-1 phototherapy except for severe cases of scleroderma where other treatment options do not exist [13]. For other indications such as CTCL, urticaria pigmentosa, and connective tissue diseases, the benefits achieved by UVA-1 phototherapy probably outweigh its potential long-term risks. In order to approach this problem in a more systematic fashion, the European Follow-Up Study for UVA-1 Phototherapy (EFUP-Study) patients has been launched. This longitudinal, prospective study aims toward monitoring each UVA-1-treated patient, after his central registration, for any signs of an increased skin cancer risk over the years.

Perspectives

UVA-1 phototherapy has almost always been used as a monotherapy in order to unambiguously prove its efficacy. Combination regimens integrating UVA-1 phototherapy are, however, of obvious clinical interest and practical benefit because they should allow for the maximization of therapeutic efficacy and safety at the same time. Combinations of interest include the use of UVA-1 together with topical steroids or novel immunosuppressants for atopic dermatitis, or UVA-1 with systemic retinoids or interferon-α for CTCL.

Analysis of the mechanism of action of UVA-1 phototherapy has led to a rapid expansion of its indication spectrum. It is anticipated that this development will continue within the near future. In this regard, it has been of particular interest to learn that the generation of singlet oxygen by UVA-1 radiation represents a central photobiological mechanism required for the achievement of therapeutic effects [32]. It is thus conceivable to assume that strategies directed at the amplification of singlet-oxygen-mediated effects as well as the development of alternative modes for singlet oxygen generation in human skin, e.g., through the use of radiation spectra, which are even more selective than UVA-1, will prove to be superior to UVA-1 phototherapy as it is currently being employed. All these efforts will eventually contribute to the further development of UVA-1 phototherapy as one of the driving forces of modern photomedicine.

References

1. Asawonando P, Khoo LSW, Fitzpatrick TB, Taylor CR (1999) UVA-1 for keloid. Arch Dermatol 135:348–349
2. Calzavara Pinton P (2000) High-dose UVA1 therapy of large plaques and nodular lesions of cutaneous T-cell lymphoma. J Am Acad Dermatol (in press)
3. Costa C, Rillet A, Nicolet M, Saurat JH (1989) Scoring atopic dermatitis: the simpler the better. Acta Derm Venereol (Stockh) 69:41–47
4. Christophers E, Hönigsmann H, Wolff K, Langner A (1978) PUVA treatment of urticaria pigmentosa. Br J Dermatol 98:701–702
5. Cruz P Jr, Dougherty I, Dawson B, Krutmann J (2000) Unlike UVB, UVA-1 radiation does not activate HIV in human skin. J Invest Dermatol (in press)
6. Czech W, Krutmann J, Schöpf E, Kapp A (1992) Serum eosinophil cationic protein is a sensitive measure for disease activity in atopic dermatitis. Br J Dermatol 126:351–355
7. Fleischmajer R (1993) Localized and systemic scleroderma. In: Lapiere CM, Krieg T (eds) Connective tissue diseases of the skin. Dekker, New York, pp 295–313
8. Godar DE (1999) UVA 1 radiation mediates singlet-oxygen and superoxide-anion production which trigger two different final apoptotic pathways: the S and P site of mitochondria. J Invest Dermatol 112:3–12
9. Grabbe J, Welker P, Humke S, Grewe M, Schöpf E, Henz BM, Krutmann J (1996) High-dose UVA1 therapy, but not UVA/UVB therapy, decreases IgE binding cells in lesional skin of patients with atopic eczema. J Invest Dermatol 107:419–423
10. Granerus G, Roupa G, Swanbeck G (1981) Decreased urinary histamine levels after successful PUVA treatment of urticaria pigmentosa. J Invest Dermatol 76:1–3
11. Grewe M, Gyufko K, Schöpf E, Krutmann J (1994) Lesional expression of interferon-γ in atopic eczema. Lancet 343:25–26
12. Grewe M, Bruijnzeel-Koomen CAFM, Schöpf E, Thepen T, Langeveld-Wildschut AG, Ruzicka T, Krutmann J (1998) A role for Th1 and Th2 cells in the immunopathogenesis of atopic dermatitis. Immunol Today 19:359–361
13. Gruss C, Strucker M, Kobyletzki G, Kerscher M, Altmeyer P (1997) Low dose UVA1 phototherapy in disabling pansclerotic morphea. Br J Dermatol 136:293–294
14. Herbst RA, Vogelbruich M, Ehnis A, Kiehl P, Kapp A, Weiss J (2000) Combined ultraviolet A1 radiation and acitretin therapy as a treatment option for pityriasis rubra pilaris. Br J Dermatol 142:574–575
15. Jekler J, Larkö O (1990) Combined UV-A-UV-B versus UVB phototherapy for atopic dermatitis. J Am Acad Dermatol 22:49–53
16. Kerscher M, Dirschka T, Volkenandt M (1995) Treatment of localized scleroderma by UVA1 phototherapy. Lancet 346:1166
17. Kerscher M, Volkenandt M, Gruss C, Reuther T, Kobyletzki G, Freitag M, Dirschka T, Altmeyer P (1998) Low-dose UVA₁ phototherapy for treatment of localized scleroderma. J Am Aacd Dermatol 38:21–26
18. Kobyletzki G, Pieck C, Hoffmann K, Freitag M, Altmeyer P (1999) Medium-dose UVA1 cold-light phototherapy in the treatment of severe atopic dermatitis. J Am Acad Dermatol 41:931–937
19. Kolde G, Frosch PJ, Czarnetzki BM (1984) Response of cutaneous mast cells to PUVA in patients with urticaria pigmentosa: histophotometric, ultrastructural, and biochemical investigations. J Invest Dermatol 83:175–178
20. Kowalzick L, Kleinhenz A, Weichenthal M, Ring J (1995) Low dose versus medium dose UVA-1 treatment in severe atopic dermatitis. Acta Derm Venereol (Stockh) 75:43–45
21. Krutmann J, Schöpf E (1992) High-dose UVA1 therapy: a novel and highly effective approach for the treatment of patients with acute exacerbation of atopic dermatitis. Acta Derm Venereol (Stockh) 176:120–122

22. Krutmann J, Czech W, Diepgen T, Niedner R, Kapp A, Schöpf E (1992) High-dose UVA1 therapy in the treatment of patients with atopic dermatitis. J Am Acad Dermatol 26:225–230
23. Krutmann J (1995) UVA1-induced immunomodulation. In: Krutmann J, Elmets CA (eds) Photoimmunology. Blackwell Science, Oxford, pp 246–256
24. Krutmann J (1996) Phototherapy for atopic dermatitis. Dermatol Ther 1:24–31
25. Krutmann J, Diepgen T, Luger TA, Grabbe S, Meffert H, Sönnichsen N, Czech W, Kapp A, Stege H, Grewe M, Schöpf E (1998) High-dose UVA1 therapy for atopic dermatitis: results of a multicenter trial. J Am Acad Dermatol 38:589–593
26. Krutmann J (1999) Therapeutic photomedicine: phototherapy. In: Freedberg IM, Eisen AZ, Wolff K, Austen KF, Goldsmith LA, Katz SI, Fitzpatrick TB (eds) Fitzpatrick's dermatology in general medicine, 5th edn. McGraw-Hill, New York, pp 2870–2879
27. LeRoy EC (1979) Increased collagen synthesis by scleroderma skin fibroblasts in vitro. J Clin Invest 54:880–889
28. McGrath H Jr (1994) Ultraviolet-A1 irradiation decreases clinical disease activity and autoantibodies in patients with systemic lupus erythematosus. Clin Exp Rheumatol 12:129–135
29. McGrath Jr H, Martinez-Osuna P, Lee FA (1996) Ultraviolet A-1 (340–400 nm) irradiation in systemic lupus erythematosus. Lupus 5:269–274
30. Meffert H, Soennichsen N, Herzog M, Hutschenreuther A (1992) UVA-1 cold light therapy of severe atopic dermatitis. Dermatol Monatsschr 78:291–296
31. Morita A, Sakakibara S, Sakakibara N, Yamauchi R, Tsuji T (1995) Successful treatment of systemic sclerosis with topical PUVA. J Rheumatol 22:2361–2365
32. Morita A, Werfel T, Stege H, Ahrens C, Karmann K, Grewe M, Grether-Beck S, Ruzicka T, Kapp A, Klotz LO, Sies H, Krutmann J (1997) Evidence that singlet oxygen-induced human T helper cell apoptosis is the basic mechanism of ultraviolet-A radiation phototherapy. J Exp Med 186:1763–1768
33. Morita A, Kobayashi K, Isomura I, Tsuji T, Krutmann J (2000) Ultraviolet A-1 (340–400 nm) phototherpy for systemic sclerosis. J Am Acad Dermatol 43:670–674
34. Morita A, Yamauchi Y, Yasuda Y, Tsuji T, Krutmann J (2000) Malignant T-cells are exquisitely sensitive to ultraviolet A-1 (UVA-1) radiation-induced apoptosis. J Invest Dermatol 114:751
35. Mutzhas MF, Hölzle E, Hofmann C, Plewig G (1981) A new apparatus with high radiation energy between 320–460 nm: physical description and dermatological applications. J Invest Dermatol 76:42–47
36. Petersen MJ, Nasen C, Craig S (1992) Ultraviolet A irradiation stimulates collagenase production in cultured human fibroblasts. J Invest Dermatol 99:440–442
37. Plettenberg H, Stege H, Megahed M, Ruzicka T, Hosokawa Y, Tsuji T, Morita A, Krutmann J (1999) Ultraviolet A1 (340–400 nm) phototherapy for cutaneous T-cell lymphoma. J Am Acad Dermatol 41:47–50
38. Plettenberg H, Stege H, Mang R, Ruzicka T, Krutmann J (2001) A comparison of Ultraviolet A-1 and PUVA therapy for early stages of cutaneous T-cell lymphoma. Photodermatol Photoimmunol Photomed (in press)
39. Rodnan GP, Lipinski I, Luksick J (1979) Skin collagen content in progressive systemic sclerosis (scleroderma) and localized scleroderma. Arthritis Rheum 22:130–140
40. Rosenwasser TA, Eisen AZ (1993) Scleroderma. In: Fitzpatrick TB, Eisen AZ, Wolff K, Freedberg IM, Austen KF (eds) Dermatology in general medicine, 4th edn. McGraw-Hil, New York, pp 2156–2167
41. Scharffetter K, Wlaschek M, Hogg A, Bolsen K, Schothorst A, Goerz G, Krieg T, Plewig G (1991) UVA irradiation induces collagenase in human dermal fibroblasts in vitro and in vivo. Arch Dermatol Res 283:506–511
42. Scharfetter-Kochanek K, Goldermann R, Lehmann P, Hölzle E, Goerz G (1995) PUVA therapy in disabling pansclerotic morphea of children. Br J Dermatol 132:830–831

43. Schmidt T, Abeck D, Boeck K, Mempel M, Ring J (1998) UVA1 irradiation is effective in treatment of chronic vesicular dyshidrotic hand eczema. Acta Derm Venereol (Stockh) 78:318–319
44. Setlow RB, Grist E, Thompson K, Woodhead AD (1993) Wavelengths effective in induction of malignant melanoma. Proc Natl Acad Sci USA 90:6666–6670
45. Soennichsen N, Meffert H, Kunzelmann V (1993) UV-A-1 Therapie bei subakut-kutanem Lupus erythematodes. Hautarzt 44:723–725
46. Stege H, Schöpf E, Ruzicka T, Krutmann J (1996) High-dose-UVA1 for urticaria pigmentosa. Lancet 347:64
47. Stege H, Humke S, Berneburg M, Klammer M, Grewe M, Grether-Beck S, Dierks K, Goerz G, Ruzicka T, Krutmann J (1996) High-dose ultraviolet A1 radiation therapy of localized scleroderma. J Am Aacd Dermatol 36:938–943
48. Stege H, Budde M, Kürten V, Ruzicka T, Krutmann J (1999) Induction of apoptosis in skin-infiltrating mast cells by high-dose ultraviolet A-1 radiation phototherapy in patients with urticaria pigmentosa. J Invest Dermatol 112:561
49. Sterenbroigh HCJM, van der Leun JC (1990) Tumorigenesis by a long wavelength UV-A source. Photochem Photobiol 51:325–330
50. Takeda K, Hahamochi A, Ueki H, Nakata M, Oishi Y (1994) Decreased collagenase expression in cultured systemic sclerosis fibroblasts. J Invest Dermatol 103:359–363
51. Zmudzka BZ, Olvey KM, Lee W, Beer JZ (1994) Reassessment of the differential effects of ultraviolet and ionizing radiation on HIV promoter: the use of cell survival as the basis for comparisons. Photochem Photobiol 59:643–649

IV Photoprotection in daily practice

14 Acute and Chronic Photodamage from Solar Radiation, Phototherapy, and Photochemotherapy

Henry W. Lim, Kristi J. Robson

Contents

Photodamage

Exposure of human skin to ultraviolet radiation (UVR) results in several distinct and well-characterized pathophysiological processes that may be divided into acute and chronic categories. Photodamage refers to the destructive effects that ultraviolet radiation produces on the structure of exposed human skin. The acute cutaneous effect of UVR exposure is the sunburn reaction, which is an inflammatory response. Chronic effects result in photoaging. In addition, exposure to UVR has been implicated in the development of some forms of skin cancers. All effects known to occur as a consequence of exposure to natural sunlight also are seen in individuals exposed to phototherapy and photochemotherapy. This chapter focuses on photodamage induced by UVR in general, followed by that induced by UVB and UVA-1 phototherapy and PUVA photochemotherapy. Effects of UVR on the immune system is described in detail in Chap. 2 (this volume).

Clinical and Histological Changes of Acute Photodamage

The most prominent cutaneous effect of acute UVR is the erythema of sunburn. The other signs of inflammation are also typically present, which include increased pain, warmth, and swelling. In addition to inflammation, the acute responses of the skin to UVR include increases in pigmentation and thickness of the epidermis, altered immunity, and vitamin D synthesis [1]. When ultraviolet light reaches the skin, portions are scattered and reflected in the stratum corneum, parts are absorbed in the epidermis, and part is transmitted [2]. The depth of penetration of UVR is dependent upon the wavelength: longer wavelengths penetrate deeper than shorter wavelengths. Most of the shorter UVB radiation is absorbed in the epidermis. However, about 50 % of incident UVA radiation reaches a depth of 0.1–0.2 mm in the papillary dermis [2, 3].

The relative effectiveness of different wavelengths to induce erythema is known as the erythema action spectrum [4]. The most erythemogenic wavelengths are UVC and shorter wavelength UVB, with a decrease in effectiveness as wavelength increases [1]. For example, approximately 1,000 times more energy is required to produce erythema at 320 nm compared to 290 nm [4]. The degree of erythema produced is also influenced by skin pigmentation, skin thickness, and environmental conditions such as season, latitude, altitude, and time of day [1, 4]. The mechanism of UV-induced erythema is not fully known, but it is postulated that DNA is the chromophore responsible for initiating the erythema after UVB exposure [1]. This is based in part on the similarities between the action spectrum for the frequency of pyrimidine dimer formation induced in the DNA of human skin and the erythema action spectrum. The chromophore for erythema caused by UVA is not known [1].

The epidermis is most affected by UVB exposure. Studies performed in persons under the age of 30 revealed damaged keratinocytes as early as 30 min after irradiation, and became most numerous at 24 h [1]. The damaged keratinocytes were primarily located in the lower half of the epidermis, and by 72 h were confined to the superficial layers [1, 5]. The damaged keratinocytes are believed to represent apoptotic cells, and histologically they have a pale, eosinophilic appearance, often with a pyknotic nucleus [2]. Other epidermal changes included infrequent intercellular edema and a mild exocytosis of lymphocytes. The most prominent dermal changes involved the superficial vascular plexus with endothelial cell enlargement, which was noted at 30 min and progressively increased over 24 h, and perivenular edema, which was present 1 h after exposure and was prominent after 4 h. Endothelial cell activation and perivenular edema were also noted in the vessels of the reticular dermis and subcutaneous fat. A reduction in the number of dermal mast cells was also seen, with return to normal levels by 24 h. The skin of persons older than 60 contained fewer sunburn cells, and dyskeratotic cells were still seen at 72 h. The alterations in mast cells were not as extensive, minor vascular changes were present up to 24 h, and endothelial cell alterations were prominent only at 72 h [1]. In younger subjects, the number of epidermal Langerhans cells was reduced 3–4 h after irradiation, and the number remained near zero from 24 to 72 h [1, 6]. In older subjects, the Langerhans cell number fell less rapidly initially, but also reached low levels by

24 h. In all ages, the number of mononuclear cells exceeded the number of neutrophils in the dermal infiltrate at all times examined [1]. Mononuclear cells reached a plateau 11–21 h after exposure, with increased levels up to 48 h. Neutrophils were seen immediately after exposure, peaked at 4 h after exposure, and then decreased in number. Macrophages increased with a peak level at 24 h [1].

Histopathological changes after 2.5 minimal erythema doses (MEDs) of UVA have shown variation in the size and staining properties of keratinocytes, often with perinuclear vacuoles and mild intercellular edema [7]. In contrast to the sunburn cells seen after UVB exposure, dyskeratotic cells were absent. Langerhans cells declined to approximately one-fifth of their number prior to exposure, and no thickening of the stratum corneum was seen [7]. A slight-to-moderate lymphocytic infiltrate in both the papillary and reticular dermis was seen; it was far greater than the neutrophilic infiltrate. Endothelial cell enlargement was observed immediately after exposure and became more extensive over the subsequent 24 h [1]. Slight hypogranulation of mast cells, along with slight perivenular edema, were frequently noted [7]. In addition, small foci of interstitial fibrin deposition were seen at 24 and 48 h [1]. In a study using an exposure of 4 MEDs of UVA, there was necrosis and loss of endothelial cells in some of the superficial capillary venules and vessels in the superficial venular plexus. This was accompanied by a prominent neutrophilic infiltrate along with mononuclear cells in the upper and mid dermis [1, 8].

Several different mediators appear to play a role in the erythema response induced by UVR. UVB- and UVA-induced erythema is associated with elevated histamine levels in aspirates of suction blister fluids from irradiated skin. Histamine causes increased vascular permeability and vasodilation, which may play an early role in the erythema response. However, H1 and H2 antihistamines do not block UV-light induced erythema, so other mediators must also be important in the inflammatory response to UVR [2]. These other mediators may include eicosanoids (arachidonic acid, PGD2, PGE2, and 6-keto-PGF1α), kinins, cytokines, as well as other chemotactic factors [1].

Cytokines may play an important role in the erythema response from UVR. Exposure of cultured human keratinocytes to UVB resulted in increased levels of interleukin (IL)-1α and IL-1β mRNA at 6 h [1, 9]. Studies measuring IL-1 in vitro after UVB exposure have shown varying results with either a decrease, increase, or no change in IL-1 level [1, 10]. Exposure of human skin to 2 MEDs of UVB has resulted in an elevation of serum IL-6 levels which peaked at 12 h and persisted over 72 h [1, 11]. Studies have also shown an elevation of IL-8, IL-10, tumor necrosis factor (TNF)-α, and granulocyte-macrophage colony stimulating factor (GM-CSF) after UVB exposure [10, 12]. Exposure to 3 MEDs was associated with increased levels of transforming growth factor (TGF)-α at 30 min, normal levels at 4 h, and increased levels at 24 h. UVR has also been shown to affect adhesion molecules. UVR increases expression of intercellular adhesion molecule (ICAM)-1 on keratinocytes 48–96 h after exposure [13]. After 2 MEDs of UVB, endothelial leukocyte adhesion molecule (ELAM)-1, but not vascular cell adhesion molecule (VCAM)-1 was expressed on endothelial cells of the superficial venular plexus at 24 h, with decreases by 72 h [1, 14].

Clinical and Histological Changes of Chronic Photodamage

Over the course of the lifetime of an individual, photodamage accumulates contributing significantly to the discolored and wrinkled appearance of aged skin. This accumulation of photodamage, referred to as photoaging, historically has been differentiated from the intrinsic and predetermined degenerative aging process. However, recent evidence suggests that at least some of the underlying changes and pathophysiology characteristic of these two processes may be more similar than once was thought. Similarly, recent studies suggest that treatments once thought specific for photoaged skin may be effective for the treatment of chronologically aged skin as well.

The accumulation of photodamage has been referred to as photoaging or dermatoheliosis. In photoaged skin, many changes are superimposed on the normal aging process which include deep wrinkling and furrowing, roughness or dryness, laxity and sagging, sallowness, mottled hyperpigmentation and hypopigmentation, and a tendency to form malignant and premalignant lesions [2]. Individuals may develop comedones and infundibular follicular cysts in the periorbital region, which is known as Favre-Racouchot syndrome. Sun-induced deep furrowing on the back of the neck, referred to as cutis rhomboidalis nuchae is also commonly seen. Pigmentary changes include solar lentigines and ephelides and in severely sun-damaged skin, atypical intraepidermal proliferations of melanocytes or even lentigo maligna melanoma can occur [2].

Most of the histopathological changes associated with chronic UVR exposure are found in the middle to upper portions of the dermis. Histologically these sections appear "swollen" and contain many extra components not found in normal or chronologically aged skin. This material stains strongly with elastic tissue-specific stains; thus, its accumulation is known as solar elastosis. Indeed this accumulation of elastotic material is considered one of the histological hallmarks of photoaged skin [15]. In addition to elastin, elastotic material contains many other extracellular matrix components including fibrillin, proteoglycans, and hyaluronic acid. UVR also induces profound changes in collagen structure and regulation in the dermis, where the collagen network appears sparse and degraded in areas of solar damage. Interestingly, both the rate of new collagen synthesis and the degradation of existing collagen appear to be affected by UVR exposure [16–18]. Thus, UVR somehow induces dysregulation and disorganization of the normal ultrastructural components of the dermal extracellular matrix, contributing in large part to the histological changes and visual appearance of photoaged skin.

Other histological changes in photoaged skin include acanthosis of the epidermis, which is in contrast with the normal epidermal thinning and dermal-epidermal flattening that occur with intrinsic aging. Epidermal atrophy is associated with end-stage photoaging. Along with acanthosis, cellular atypia and loss of polarity also occur [19]. Staining with silver nitrate demonstrates irregular distribution of melanin in the basal cell layer with areas of hyperpigmentation alternating with areas of hypopigmentation. Melanocytes increase in size and number, and Langerhans cells decrease in number and become less functional [19]. The cutaneous vasculature is also affected, with many vessels becoming completely obliterated along with destruction of the horizontal plexuses. Ultrastructurally, vascular basement membranes are greatly duplicated. Mast cells are increased and are partially degranulated, and histiocytes and other mononuclear cells are increased [19].

Pathophysiology and Biochemical Mechanisms of Photodamage

Based on the observation that elastotic material accumulates in photoaged skin, recent studies have investigated the regulation of elastin gene expression in the dermis. Northern analysis demonstrates that elastin mRNA levels are elevated in fibroblast cultures derived from chronically sun-exposed sites on human skin as compared with control fibroblast cultures obtained from sun-protected sites [20]. These increased elastin mRNA levels correlated with increased elastin protein as demonstrated by immunohistochemical staining of paired biopsies taken from sun-exposed and sun-protected areas of the same individual [20]. Further studies utilizing the human elastin gene promoter linked to a chloramphenicol acetyl transferase (CAT) reporter gene demonstrated that UVR directly stimulates transcriptional activation of the elastin gene in a transient transfection system [20]. These same investigators have developed a transgenic mouse model that expresses the CAT reporter gene under control of the human elastin promoter [15, 21]. Exposure of these mice to UVR results in a dose-dependent increase in dermal CAT activity, reflecting UVR induction of human elastin promoter activity [15, 21]. In addition to its importance as an in vivo model of cutaneous photoaging, this transgenic system will likely be useful for the rapid screening of compounds that protect against photodamage [22].

In addition to the role of UVR in regulating elastin gene expression, other investigations have focused on its role in regulating collagen metabolism. As was discussed above, UVR induces profound changes in dermal collagen structure, affecting both the rate of new collagen synthesis and degradation of existing collagen [16–18]. The changes in collagen degradation have been demonstrated to be due in large part to the induction of matrix metalloproteinase (MMP) activity by UVR and the subsequent degradation of extracellular matrix proteins including denatured collagen and native collagen fibers [23, 24]. In addition to collagen, it is likely that MMPs degrade other extracellular matrix components including fibronectin, elastic fibers, and proteoglycans [25]. This activation of MMPs occurs within hours of UVR exposure and at levels well below the MED [24, 26]. On the biochemical level, UVR has been shown to activate cell surface growth factor receptors, which results in the subsequent activation of intracellular signal transduction pathways and induction of AP-1 transcription factor activity [24, 26]. Among the many transcriptional targets of AP-1 are several members of the MMP family, including collagenase, gelatinase, metalloelastase, and stromelysin [26–30].

These observations have led to the following hypothesis proposed by Voorhees and colleagues regarding the pathophysiology of photodamage induced by UVR. Exposure of skin to UVR induces dermal MMP activity resulting in subtle degradation of collagen and other extracellular matrix components. This breakdown is likely followed by synthesis of new collagen and "wound" repair, which like all types of adult wound healing is imperfect and results in scarring. This sequence of events is repeated countless times throughout the lifetime of an individual. The resulting subtle dermal scars remain clinically undetectable for many years, but with repeated UVR exposure eventually become apparent histologically, and ultimately result in visually evident photoaging [23, 24, 26].

Effects of Retinoids on Collagen and the Extracellular Matrix

It is now both well-established and accepted that use of topical retinoids is an effective therapy for the treatment of photoaging, however only recently have the underlying biochemical mechanisms begun to be elucidated. As was discussed previously, UVR affects both the rate of synthesis and degradation of collagen [16–18]. Interestingly, retinoid therapy appears to alter both of these effects of UVR. Retinoids stimulate the growth of fibroblasts and keratinocytes in skin and monolayer culture, and stimulate synthesis of the ECM proteins collagen and fibronectin in epithelial cell culture, fibroblast culture, and human skin [17, 31, 32]. Retinoids also inhibit the UVR-induced induction of MMP activity, possibly in part by repressing AP-1 [23, 24, 26, 31, 33, 34]. Thus by both promoting the synthesis of collagen and other ECM proteins, and by inhibiting their breakdown, retinoid therapy reverses some of the dermal photodamage induced by UVR. Additionally, it has recently been shown that human skin from sun-protected areas responds to retinoid treatment equally well compared with skin from sun-exposed areas [31]. These interesting results suggest that retinoid therapy, recently thought specific for photoaged skin, may also be effective for the treatment of chronologically aged skin; and furthermore that the underlying changes and pathophysiology characteristic of two aging processes may be more similar than once was thought.

Ultraviolet Radiation and DNA Damage

The sun emits radiation in wavelengths ranging from the X-ray to the infrared. By convention the ultraviolet portion of the solar spectrum is divided into four main parts: UVA-1 (340–400 nm), UVA-2 (320–340 nm), UVB (290–320 nm), and UVC (200–290 nm). The shorter wavelengths of UVR are absorbed by nucleic acids and proteins. The most frequent DNA photoproducts produced by UVR are cyclobutane pyrimidine dimers, and pyrimidine (6–4) pyrimidone photoproducts which are formed by the covalent association of adjacent pyrimidines (cytosine and thymine) (Fig. 1) [35–37]. Cyclobutane dimers are formed when the double bonds between the C5 and C6 carbon atoms of adjacent pyrimidines become saturated, which produces a four-member ring structure. Alternatively, in the (6–4) photoproduct, the C6 position of the 5' pyrimidine is covalently linked to the C4 position of its adjacent 3' pyrimidine. Cyclobutane dimers are more common than pyrimidine (6–4) pyrimidone photoproducts, but the ratio between the two can vary depending on the nucleotides flanking

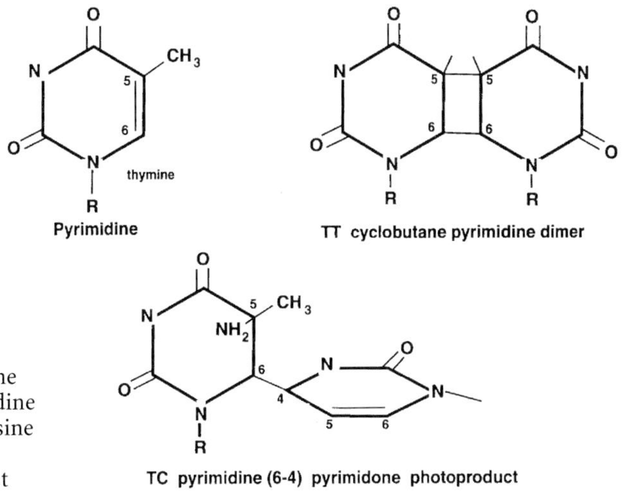

Fig. 1. Structures of thymine, thymine-thymine (TT) cyclobutane pyrimidine dimer, and thymine-cytosine (TC) pyrimidine (6–4) pyrimidone photoproduct

the lesion site [35]. Both photoproducts distort the DNA helix such that it appears to contain an abasic site, and an adenine is inserted opposite the damaged pyrimidine (usually cytosine) during subsequent DNA replication [36]. Thus, the most common mutation induced by UVR is C→T (cytosine to thymine), occurring in about 70 % of instances [36]. Replacement of both cytosines results in the CC→TT change, which occurs in about 10 % of instances, and is considered to be specific for UVR-induced mutations [36]. The frequency of pyrimidine dimer formation is greatest at wavelengths near 300 nm and decreases at both longer and shorter wavelengths [38]. UVR also causes other types of DNA damage such as single-strand breaks, other mutations, DNA-protein crosslinks, unstable pyrimidine photohydrates, and chromosomal translocations mediated by reactive oxygen species. Photoproducts involving purine bases in double-stranded DNA occur at very low frequencies [35, 36].

In general, it has been assumed that most of the harmful effects from solar radiation are from UVB, however, the UVA spectrum can produce the same negative effects when given in equivalent biological doses. Accumulated doses of UVA are also capable of inducing DNA damage such as pyrimidine dimer formation [39]. In a recent study, equivalent biological doses of UVA1, UVA-1+2, and solar simulating radiation were found to induce pyrimidine dimer formation equally [40]. UVC is a potent mutagen in vitro, but is of no clinical significance as it is attenuated by the ozone layer before reaching Earth's surface. The transmission of solar radiation through the skin also sharply decreases below wavelengths of 300 nm [35, 38].

Molecular Evidence Implicating Ultraviolet Radiation in the Development of Skin Cancer

Mutations involving the p53 tumor suppressor gene have been linked strongly to UV exposure. The p53 gene encodes a 53 kDa DNA binding protein involved in many cellular functions including transcription, cell cycle inhibition, and apoptosis [41]. Inactivation of p53 plays an important role in induction of many types of human cancer, and p53 mutations are among the most frequently observed genetic lesions in human cancers [37, 41, 42]. From a dermatological standpoint, p53 mutations have been found in over 90 % of cutaneous squamous cell carcinomas (SCCs), in about 50 % of basal cell carcinomas (BCCs), and in sun-damaged skin, actinic keratoses, and Bowen's disease (squamous cell carcinoma in situ) [37, 43–46].

Interestingly the specific p53 mutations found in skin cancers differ from those found in other types of cancers. As discussed above, the most common UV-induced mutations are C→T and CC→TT, of which the latter is considered diagnostic of UV-induced DNA damage [36, 46–50]. Mutations to p53 in SCC are not random and occur most often where one cytosine or thymine is adjacent to another. About two-thirds of the base changes are C→T, and many are CC→TT [36]. Additionally the mutations tend to cluster at nine mutation "hotspots," many of which are sites of slow photoproduct excision repair [36, 49]. The proportion of p53 CC→TT mutations is negligible in non-cutaneous types of cancer [46].

After these UV-associated p53 mutations were described, the question arose whether these mutations are important in tumor induction or are they merely passive indicators of UV exposure. It appears that sun exposure of normal skin causes many p53 mutations that serve as an initiation process that starts cells on the pathway to cancer [37]. Studies have shown that non-cancerous skin adjacent to skin cancers contains p53 mutations that are distinct from those present in skin cancers [46]. DNA sequence analysis of nine p53 mutations found in normal skin demonstrated that all resulted in an amino acid change in the p53 protein [51, 52]. The fact that no silent mutations were detected strongly suggests that the resultant alterations were not due to chance alone; and that these mutations might offer some selective growth advantage to the initiated cells [37].

The p53 protein is normally unstable and is either absent or barely detectable in normal cells [37, 48]. Many mutations in p53 gene produce a functionally inactive protein that has a significantly prolonged half-life that can be detected by immunohistochemical staining. One study investigating p53 protein staining in sun-exposed and sun-protected skin from normal human donors found clonal patches of p53-mutated keratinocytes that were larger and more numerous in sun-exposed skin, and were estimated to involve up to 4 % of the epidermis [46, 52]. The actual mutation frequency in the skin can be estimated based on the p53 staining and averages 30 clones/cm² in sun-exposed skin [36]. The clonal arrangement of these mutated cells is indicative of proliferation; however most clones apparently never progress which may be due to clonal regression or failure of additional required mutations to occur. These observations suggest that p53 mutations arise early in the sequence of UV-induced skin carcinogenesis.

The exact role that p53 mutations play in UV-induced skin cancers is a subject of considerable current investigation. Wild-type p53 protein is thought to suppress tumor formation through regulation of both the cell cycle and apoptosis, thus limiting DNA damage either by promoting DNA repair or helping to eliminate damaged cells [43, 46]. In the skin, the protective role of p53 protein is underscored by the observation that UVR increases its expression, resulting in the arrest of cells at the G1/S step of the cell cycle and allowing DNA repair to occur prior to replication and cell division [43, 44, 53]. Another interesting and important observation is that p53 is necessary for formation of "sunburn cells," which are keratinocytes that die by apoptosis following UV exposure [53]. In mice engineered to be deficient for the p53 gene, very few sunburn cells were induced by UVR, demonstrating that p53 is required for these presumably damaged cells to die by apoptosis [53]. This observation led to the following hypothesis proposed by Brash and colleagues regarding the role of p53 in the development of actinic keratoses and SCC [53]. Exposure of skin to UVR occasionally results in the production of DNA photoproducts that either usually become repaired, or else induce apoptosis of the affected cells through a p53-dependent pathway. However, when a mutation arises in the p53 gene itself, the affected cell becomes less likely to die from apoptosis, despite accumulating photodamage. Repeated UV exposure results in apoptosis of surrounding cells; in a sense selecting for the slow clonal expansion of the p53 mutant cell that may eventually become an actinic keratosis. Thus in this hypothesis, UVR functions as both a tumor initiator (through the p53 mutation) and as a tumor promoter (through clonal selection of the mutated cell) [53].

In addition to p53 that is mutated in about one half of BCCs, recent work has identified another gene that plays an important role in the development of BCC. A genetic defect was identified in persons with basal cell nevus syndrome, an autosomal dominant disorder characterized by a high frequency of developmental anomalies as well as the development of multiple cutaneous BCCs, especially on sun-exposed skin [54]. The gene involved, PTCH, is the human homologue of the Drosophila patched (PTC) gene and is found on chromosome 9q22.3 [37]. PTCH encodes a transmembrane protein that represses transcription of genes encoding members of the TGF-β and Wnt families of signaling proteins [36, 37, 54, 55]. Another recent study demonstrated PTCH gene mutations in 16 of 37 sporadic BCCs [56]. Seven of these PTCH mutations were C→T or CC→TT substitutions indicating that the PTCH gene may play an important role in sunlight induction of BCC.

There has also been molecular evidence implicating UVR with melanoma. Mutations of the CDKN2 tumor suppressor gene, which encodes the cyclin dependent kinase inhibitor p16, have been implicated in a wide range of human malignancies, including melanoma [57]. Mutations of this gene have been demonstrated in the germ line of familial melanoma cases, somatically in melanoma cell lines, and in sporadic melanoma [58]. In one study, a high proportion of both C→T transitions and CC→TT tandem mutations was found in the CDKN2 gene in 30 melanoma cell lines, suggesting one possible target of UVR in melanoma [58]. Interestingly p53 mutations are found very infrequently in melanoma in contrast to nonmelanocytic skin cancers.

The association of extreme sun sensitivity and skin cancer susceptibility in patients with the genetic disorder xeroderma pigmentosum (XP) also provides evidence linking UVR to the development of skin cancer. XP patients have a risk of developing skin cancer about 1,000 times that of the general population [37, 59]. XP patients are highly susceptible to UV-induced mutations, which results from a generalized defect in the repair of both cyclobutane dimers and 6–4 photoproducts [59]. Seven different repair genes (XP-A to XP-G) involved in XP have been cloned, and it is estimated that as many as eleven different enzymes may be important [37, 59]. Cockayne's syndrome and trichothiodystrophy both show UVR hypersensitivity and hypermutability similar to XP. However, neither disorder exhibits an increase in skin cancer [59]. These findings suggest that defective DNA repair of UV-induced DNA damage is not analogous with increased skin cancer risk, and that other factors may be important. It has been demonstrated that cells from patients with Cockayne's syndrome, unlike cells from XP patients, are not globally deficient in DNA repair; 6–4 pyrimidine-pyrimidone photoproduct repair remains intact, which may be responsible for cancer resistance [59].

In addition to UV-induced DNA damage, UV-induced immunosuppression may also play a role in skin cancer development. Murine studies have shown exposure to low-dose UVR prevents rejection of UV-induced tumors whereas these tumors were promptly rejected when transplanted into mice that were not pre-exposed with UVR. In addition to inducing skin cancers, UVR appears to hinder the ability to mount an immune response against UV-induced tumor antigens [59].

Epidemiology of Ultraviolet Radiation and Melanoma

The most important risk factor for the development of melanoma appears to be sun exposure. However, the relationship between UVR and melanoma is complex. There are several inconsistencies with a simple linear relationship between the two [60, 61]. For example, the sites most frequently affected are generally not the areas that receive the highest cumulative sun exposure. Melanoma has a relative peak incidence in mid life, which is an unexpected pattern from a life-long exposure to an environmental agent, and melanoma occurs more frequently in indoor versus outdoor workers [60]. In fact, some studies have even proposed that long-term occupational exposure may be protective against melanoma. Despite these findings, however, there is significant epidemiological evidence linking ultraviolet light exposure and melanoma.

The first epidemiological data that supported a possible association between sun exposure and melanoma was published in Australia in 1956 in which the observation was made that the lower the latitude, the higher the mortality from melanoma [61, 62]. There have been several studies that have documented an increased rate of melanoma with closer proximity to the equator where the amount of solar radiation is greater [63]. This effect has been demonstrated in populations from Australia and New Zealand, Scandinavia, and the Caucasian population of the United States [61, 64, 65]. It is important that the population examined be homogeneous with respect to pigmentation, as studies when this was not controlled for have not demonstrated this latitude gradient.

Studies that compare the increase in melanoma in immigrants to regions with higher levels of solar radiation have also provided strong evidence for a relationship between ultraviolet light exposure and melanoma. Several studies have documented an increase in melanoma in the immigrants in comparison to individuals in their native land [66]. For example, in an Australian study, when the incidence of melanoma in migrants from Great Britain and in native Australians was compared, it was found that immigrants who migrated to Australia before age 10 had a similar risk to native individuals [67]. Early immigrants also had a fourfold increase in the risk of developing melanoma compared to those arriving after the age of 15. Therefore, migration in childhood appears to be important in terms of increasing the risk of melanoma [66].

Other studies have found that sun exposure in childhood and adolescence is an important risk factor for melanoma [61]. In a study in Denmark, an increased relative risk was demonstrated for people with five or more sunburns before the age of 15 compared to those with no sunburns. No significant association was seen for individuals who experienced sunburns occurring in early adulthood or in the 10 years prior to diagnosis [68].

Lack of pigmentation has been shown to be a risk factor for melanoma. The majority of melanomas occur in the Caucasian population [69]. The incidence of melanoma in Blacks living within a similar geographical region is between 1/10th and 1/20th of that of Caucasians [66, 70]. The incidence of melanoma in Asians is also less than that of Caucasians. The sites involved for melanoma in Blacks and Asians in general are in sun-protected areas. It is postulated that the low incidence of melanoma in these populations is due to a protective effect of melanin against solar radiation [66]. Results regarding skin cancers from the National Cancer Institute's Surveillance, Epidemiology, and End Results (SEER) population based database from 1973 and 1987 revealed a 13- and 23-fold higher rate of invasive and in situ melanoma in Caucasians than Blacks [71]. Most melanomas in Blacks occurred on the lower limb, and the age-adjusted population-based incidence of melanoma in this location during the study period decreased slightly in Blacks, whereas it increased by 38 % in Caucasians [71].

Within the Caucasian population, those with fair skin are at a greater risk for melanoma. Case control studies have established blue eyes, blond or red hair, and pale skin as risk factors [60, 66, 72, 73]. The relative risk for blond hair ranges from 1.4 to 7.1 and from 2.9 to 4.7 for red hair [61]. Some authors, however, have not found an association between hair color and melanoma [74]. Others have found that sun sensitivity may be more closely associated with an increased risk than individual pigmentary characteristics [75].

A history of sunburns, especially in childhood, has been associated with an increased risk of melanoma in many case-control studies [76–79]. However, the number of sunburns that an individual sustains has not been shown to be consistently associated with melanoma [61]. For example, some authors have found the tendency to sunburn to be more strongly associated with melanoma than the frequency of sunburn [80]. Others have not been able to demonstrate a relationship between frequency of sunburn and melanoma after confounders, such as hair color and skin reaction to sunlight, were controlled for [81]. These studies suggest that skin pigmentation characteristics are more important risk factors than the number of sunburns.

It has been hypothesized that the risk of melanoma is related to episodes of intermittent, intense sun exposure of normally unexposed skin [61]. This hypothesis is used as a basis to explain why melanomas occur most frequently on the trunk in men and the lower extremities in women, instead of areas that receive maximum sun exposure such as the head and neck [61]. This theory has also been used to explain the increased incidence of melanoma in individuals from higher socioeconomic class, and in indoor workers [63]. This assumes that intermittent and intense sun exposure leads to greater stimulation of the normal function of melanocytes, resulting in proliferation and an increase in melanin production. Repeated stimulation is postulated to encourage tumor production. Long-term constant dose exposure may involve less melanocyte stimulation than repeated, intermittent exposures, and may lead to a constant degree of suntan and epidermal thickening which may provide protection against episodes of increased sun exposure.

This hypothesis has been supported by studies which have shown the risk of melanoma is apparently not increased by total or occupational exposure but is increased with increasing recreational exposure of untanned skin to intense sunlight. In the Western Canada Melanoma Study, significant increases in risk were noted with increasing amount of sun exposure received through recreation or vacation [82]. A moderate amount of occupational exposure was associated with increased risk, but greater occupational exposure resulted in no further increase, and in men, a decrease was seen. No obvious relationship was seen between melanoma and total sunlight exposure [82]. These findings were independent of hair and skin color, freckles, ethnic origin, and socioeconomic status. In this study, lentigo maligna melanoma, which has been reported to be more closely associated with cumulative sun exposure, was excluded [61].

The histological subtypes of melanoma appear to differ with respect to location and pattern of sun exposure. Superficial spreading melanomas (SSM) have been associated with recreational patterns of sun exposure and are predominantly found on the trunk and extremities, sites that are intermittently exposed [61, 71]. In contrast, lentigo maligna melanoma (LMM) occurs most commonly on the head and neck, which is skin that is chronically exposed to the sun, and in some studies has been shown to be associated with occupational patterns of sun exposure [61, 71]. In addition, LMM has been shown to progressively increase with age, which supports an association with cumulative sun exposure, while SSM peaks in middle age and then declines [83]. Acral lentiginous melanoma occurs on sites generally protected from sunburn by thick keratin (palms and soles), and is the most common subtype in races with darker pigmentation. This suggests that the acral lentiginous subtype may be associated with etiologic factors other than UV exposure [71].

Epidemiology of Ultraviolet Radiation and Nonmelanotic Skin Cancer

The epidemiological evidence linking nonmelanocytic skin cancers, especially SCC, with UVR is very strong. There is an increased incidence of skin cancer in sunny climates, it occurs more frequently in fair-skinned individuals, and these skin cancers typically arise on sun-exposed areas [84, 85]. The roles of ethnic origin, pigmentary traits, and sun sensitivity as risk factors for both BCC and SCC were examined in a case-control study in western Australia [86]. The risk of both cancers was higher in native-born Australians than in migrants, and the risk of BCC decreased with increasing age at arrival in Australia. The inability to tan was the strongest pigmentary risk factor for both BCC and SCC. Indicators of sun damage such as actinic keratoses, facial telangiectasia, and solar elastosis of the neck were associated with both BCC and SCC. Another case control study of 145 cases of cutaneous SCC showed people who migrated to Australia early in life had a higher risk than immigrants who arrived later in life [87]. Among Australian-born subjects of British or northern European ancestry, the skin's sensitivity to sunlight was strongly associated with SCC. This sensitivity to sunlight was more strongly associated with risk than individual pigmentary traits. The risk of SCC also increased strongly with increasing evidence of cutaneous solar damage and was most strongly associated with the number of actinic keratoses.

Some authors have postulated that intermittent sun exposure rather than cumulative sun exposure, may play a greater role in the induction of BCC. A review of 7,685 cases of BCC and 3,049 cases of SCC showed that the risk for SCC increased more steeply with age than for BCC, suggesting that continuous exposure may be more important in SCC formation [88]. A case control study in western Australia in 1988 examined the relationship of pattern and timing of sun exposure to BCC [89]. A statistically significant association was noted between the risk of BCC and intermittent sun exposure, which was based on the amount of exposure on non-working days relative to that over the whole week. However, after a certain amount of UV exposure, there was no further increase in the risk of BCC with continuing increases in sun exposure This risk increased considerably with increasing intermittency in poor tanners, but not at all in good tanners. It was postulated that good tanners may have protective effects such as increased melanization, which may provide an element of protection from the sun, even on an intermittent basis in comparison to those with poor tanning ability [89]. No association was observed between mean annual cumulative summer sunlight exposure and the risk of BCC in the examination of 226 BCC cases from Canada [90]. However, a significant increased risk was seen in patients with increased recreational sun exposure in adolescence and childhood.

It has been recently proposed that BCC subtypes may differ with regard to the role of sun exposure [91]. A review was performed with 1,711 patients who had a total of 2,990 BCCs that were histologically differentiated [92]. Superficial BCCs were found more commonly in younger subjects and were most commonly seen on the trunk in males and lower extremities in females. Nodular BCC occurred mainly in the head and neck region in older subjects. It is hypothesized that because the superficial BCCs were more commonly seen on the trunk or legs, which are areas not constantly exposed to UVR, that intermittent sun exposure may be more important than cumulative exposure with this histological subtype of BCC. In contrast, as nodular BCCs are seen most frequently on the head and neck, this suggests that chronic sun exposure may be more important to the development of nodular BCCs [92].

Photodamage Related to UVB (Broadband and Narrowband) and UVA-1 Phototherapy

Acute Photodamage. This is cutaneous erythema or sunburn response secondary to exposure to UVB. Broadband UVB-induced erythema appears in 3–5 h, peaks at 12–24 h, and resolves in 72 h [93]. Narrowband UVB erythema has a steep dose-response curve, namely, a small increase in dose could result in a significant increase in the erythema [94]. Narrowband UVB induces a more intense and rapid delayed tanning response compared to broadband UVB. UVB-induced erythema can be minimized by performing MED determination, and increasing the treatment dose gradually. Patients should always wear protective eye goggles during therapy to prevent conjunctivitis and keratitis.

Chronic Side Effects. Photoimmunological effects of UVB and UVA-1 are discussed elsewhere in this volume. Potential chronic effects of UVB phototherapy include photoaging and photocarcinogenesis. Currently, it is increasingly common to employ rotational therapy, where different therapeutic modalities are used for varying periods of time in the same patient to minimize the long-term side effects of each modality. Therefore, photoaging is usually not a prominent clinical feature of broadband UVB therapy. To minimize photoaging, UVB exposure to the face is usually limited.

No conclusive epidemiological data exist on the risk of skin cancer development in patients treated with broadband UVB. Two 25-year retrospective reviews of 305 patients, and 260 patients treated with Goeckerman therapy did not show an increase in skin cancer [95, 96]. Similar result was obtained in another study involving 85 patients [97]. However, in study of 983 patients drawn from the U.S. PUVA Cooperative Study database, high exposure to sunlamp treatments was associated with increase risk of nonmelanoma skin cancers [98]. In another study involving 892 patients from the same database, patients exposed to high levels UVB radiation had an increased risk of genital tumors [99]. Therefore, the genital should be shielded during treatment, and efforts should be made to minimize the total cumulative UVB dose.

Because narrowband UVB has been in use only since the late 1980s, the long-term side effects of this treatment modality are not known. Compared to broadband UVB, up to tenfold higher doses of narrowband UVB are needed to produce erythema, edema, and sunburn cell formation. Using the single-cell gel electrophoresis (the comet assay), when therapeutically equivalent doses were compared, there were only minimal differences in the amount of DNA damage produced by these two light sources [100]. As narrowband UVB is clinically more effective than broadband UVB in that the MED equivalents needed to achieve therapeutic response using narrowband are less than broadband, it suggests that narrowband UVB phototherapy is not more carcinogenic than broadband UVB.

As discussed elsewhere in this volume, since the early 1990s, UVA-1 phototherapy has been employed successfully for the treatment of localized scleroderma, atopic dermatitis, urticaria pigmentosa, generalized granuloma annulare, and mycosis fungoides [101–103]. Because of the relatively short follow-up period and the small number of patients who had been exposed to this treatment, at present, the long-term effects of this therapeutic modality is not known.

Photodamage Related to Photochemotherapy (PUVA)

Photochemistry of Psoralens. In vitro, the absorption maximum of psoralens is in the UVC and UVB range. In vivo, the erythema action spectrum was initially determined to be from 320 nm to 370 nm, with a peak at 360 nm [104]; this has lead to the development of UVA fluorescent lamps with peak emission at 350–355 nm that are currently used for PUVA therapy [105]. Later studies showed that shorter wavelengths (320–340 nm) were more effective in inducing erythema and in clearing psoriasis [106, 107]. With the availability of narrowband UVB (311 nm) fluorescent tubes, studies have been performed that show psoralen 311-nm UVB (PUVB) is as effective as conventional PUVA in the treatment of psoriasis, although the long-term safety of this treatment modality is not yet known [108, 109].

Psoralens readily intercalate with DNA base pairs, primarily because of their hydrophobicity and planar structure (Fig. 2) [110]. Formation of pyrimidine-psoralen adducts is initiated by the absorption of a UVA photon by the psoralen

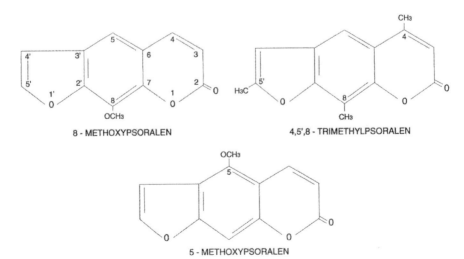

Fig. 2. Commonly used psoralens

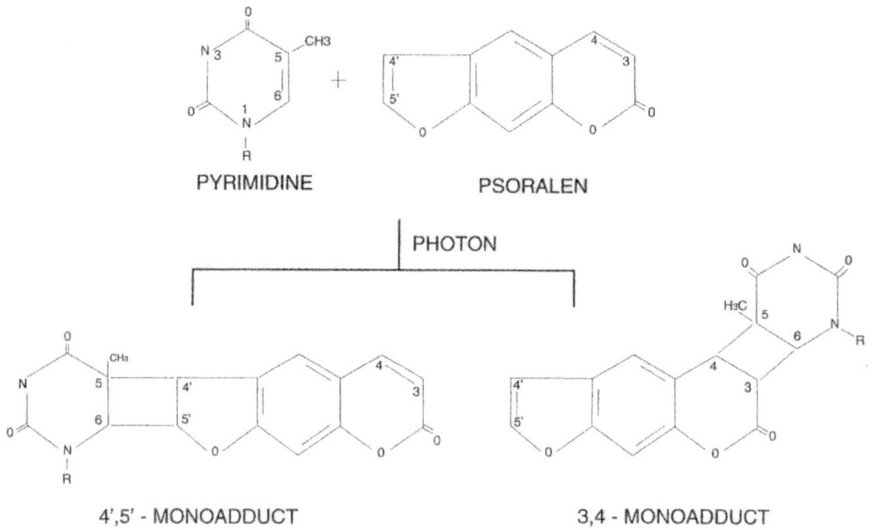

Fig. 3. Formation of monofunctional adduct between psoralen and pyrimidine base of DNA

molecule, resulting in the formation of covalent linkage with a pyrimidine base in DNA to form a cyclobutane addition product (monoadduct) (Fig. 3). Adduct formation occurs 10–20 times more efficiently with thymine moiety, compared to cytosine [110]. Following the formation of a monofunctional adduct, absorption of a second UVA photon results in a second cycloadduct formation with a pyrimidine base in the opposite strand of DNA (Fig. 4) [111]. This bifunctional adduct therefore crosslinks the two strands of DNA, resulting in suppression of cell proliferation; this is thought to be the mechanism of action of PUVA in psoriasis. Consequences of bifunctional adduct formation are either cell death or mutagenic transformation due to the error-prone DNA repair process that needs to occur [112]. Examination of mutations in the p53 tumor suppressor gene in squamous cell carcinomas obtained from PUVA patients showed that many of mutations were not the PUVA type (T→A), rather, they were characteristic of UVB mutations (C→T, and CC→TT); this finding suggests that PUVA may enhance progression of UVB-induced tumors [110, 113, 114].

Acute Photodamage. Psoralen and UVA-induced erythema appears at 24–36 h, and peaks at 36–48 h; it may be delayed to 72–96 h, and takes 7 days to resolve. In some patients, pruritus, which may be intense, develops within a few hours after PUVA. Photo-onycholysis and friction blisters have been also reported. Phototoxicity necessitating the temporary cessation of therapy has been reported in 10 % of patients [115]. Exposure of unprotected eyes will result in conjunctivitis and keratitis; these are totally avoidable with proper eye protection.

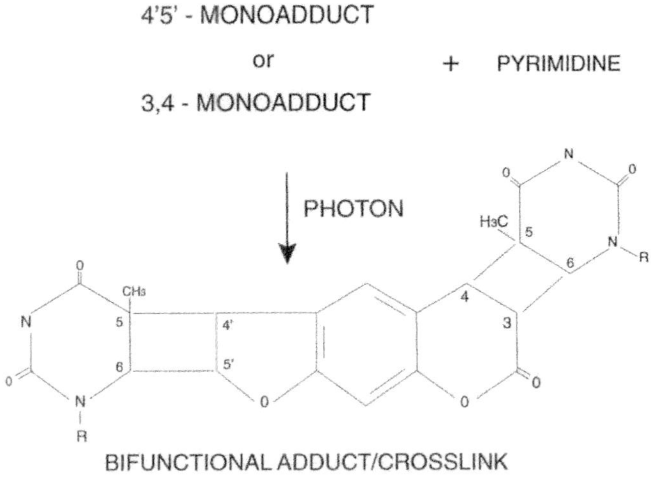

4'5' - MONOADDUCT

or   +   PYRIMIDINE

3,4 - MONOADDUCT

PHOTON

BIFUNCTIONAL ADDUCT/CROSSLINK

Fig. 4. Formation of bifunctional adduct between psoralen and pyrimidine bases from complementary strands of DNA, resulting in cross-linking

Subacute Phototoxicity. This rather uncommon side effect presents as tingling or burning sensation, followed by the appearance of psoriasiform dermatitis on areas exposed to PUVA. It occurs more commonly in patients with skin types I and II who have had prolonged PUVA therapy [116].

Chronic Photodamage. Clinically significant changes induced by long-term PUVA therapy includes photoaging and photocarcinogenesis. PUVA-induced photoaging manifests as wrinkling, telangiectasia, and lentigines [117]. There is no evidence that these lentigines would undergo malignant transformation. The risk of development of basal cell carcinoma, squamous cell carcinoma, and melanoma has been reviewed [118]. In some but not in all studies, there is a small increased risk of basal cell carcinoma on the trunk [119]. Meta-analysis of 8 studies (all with more than 150 patients, and a greater than 5-year follow-up) showed that the incidence of squamous cell carcinoma in patients exposed to high-dose PUVA (with more than 200 treatments or 2,000 J/cm^2) was 14-fold higher than those with low-dose (less than 100 treatments or 1,000 J/cm^2) [120]. Additional risk factors include prior exposure to arsenic, ionizing radiation, and methotrexate [118, 119, 121, 122]. Increased incidence of genital tumors was observed in patients of the United States PUVA Cooperative Study group; specifically, PUVA-treated male patients with a history of exposure to high doses of UVB had a risk of genital tumors 4.6 times higher than in other patients [99]. However, medical record review of 32,599 PUVA patients treated in 11 centers in Europe failed to find any increase in these tumors [123].

Similar discrepancy has been reported with PUVA-associated melanoma. A 21-year follow-up evaluation of 1,380 patients of the U.S. PUVA Cooperative Study showed an increased risk of melanoma in patients with skin types II and

III; in all patients, melanoma developed more than 5 years after cessation of PUVA [118, 124]. However, a review of 4,799 Swedish patients who had received PUVA between 1974 and 1985, with an average follow-up period of 15.9 years for the 2,343 men, and 16.2 years for the 2,456 women, failed to show any increased risk of melanoma [125]. Analysis of a subcohort of 1,867 patients followed for 15–21 years also did not show an increase in melanoma. It should be noted that 20% of the Swedish patients received bath PUVA. This factor, together with the differences in the selection criteria for initiation of PUVA therapy, difference in the treatment protocol, and the use of other therapeutic agents (methotrexate, tar, cytotoxic agents, etc.) may account for these different observations across the Atlantic.

Summary

Exposure of skin to UVR, including to phototherapy and photochemotherapy, has many consequences ranging from sunburn to photoaging to the induction of skin cancer. Recent work has begun to elucidate the underlying biochemical pathophysiology of these processes, and genetic and epidemiological data link UVR strongly with the development of skin cancer. Specific DNA mutations serve as markers for further characterizing the role of UVR in carcinogenesis, and UVR-induced immunosuppression has been shown likely to play a role in skin cancer induction. Besides leading to a greater understanding of basic photobiology and the consequences of UVR exposure, these and further investigations will serve to guide the prevention and treatment of diseases of ultraviolet exposure.

References

1. Soter NA (1993) Acute effects of ultraviolet radiation on the skin. In: Lim H, Soter N (eds) Clinical photomedicine. Dekker, New York, pp 75–93
2. Coopman SA, Garmyn M, Gonzalez-Serva A, Glogau RG (1996) Photodamage and photoaging. In: Arndt KA, Leboit PE, Robinson JK, Wintroub BU (eds) Cutaneous medicine and surgery: an integrated program in dermatology. Saunders, Philadelphia, pp 732–750
3. Gilchrest BA (1990) Actinic injury. Annu Rev Med 41:199–210
4. McGregor JM, Hawk JLM (1999) Acute effects of ultraviolet radiation on the skin. In: Freedberg IM, Eisen AZ, Wolff K, Austen KF, Goldsmith LA, Katz SJ, Fitzpatrick TB (eds) Fitzpatrick's dermatology in general medicine. McGraw-Hill, New York, pp 1555–1561
5. Rosario R, Mark GJ, Parrish JA, Mihm MC Jr (1979) Histological changes produced in skin by equally erythemogenic doses of UV-A, UV-B, UV-C and UV-A with psoralens. Br J Dermatol 101:299–308
6. Gilchrest BA, Murphy GF, Soter NA (1982) Effect of chronologic aging and ultraviolet irradiation on Langerhans cells in human epidermis. J Invest Dermatol 79:85–88
7. Gilchrest BA, Soter NA, Hawk JL, Barr RM, Black AK, Hensby CN, Mallet AI, Greaves MW, Parrish JA (1983) Histologic changes associated with ultraviolet A– induced erythema in normal human skin. J Am Acad Dermatol 9:213–219

8. Margolis RJ, Sherwood M, Maytum DJ, Granstein RD, Weinstock MA, Parrish JA, Gange RW (1989) Longwave ultraviolet radiation (UVA, 320–400 nm)-induced tan protects human skin against further UVA injury. J Invest Dermatol 93:713–718

9. Kupper TS, Chua AO, Flood P, McGuire J, Gubler U (1987) Interleukin 1 gene expression in cultured human keratinocytes is augmented by ultraviolet irradiation. J Clin Invest 80:430–436

10. Granstein RD (1999) Photoimmunology. In: Freedberg IM, Eisen AZ, Wolff K, Austen KF, Goldsmith LA, Katz SJ, Fitzpatrick TB (eds) Fitzpatrick's dermatology in general medicine. McGraw-Hill, New York, pp 1562–1573

11. Urbanski A, Schwarz T, Neuner P, Krutmann J, Kirnbauer R, Kock A, Luger TA (1990) Ultraviolet light induces increased circulating interleukin-6 in humans. J Invest Dermatol 94:808–811

12. Schwarz A, Bhardwaj R, Aragane Y, Mahnke K, Riemann H, Metze D, Luger TA, Schwarz T (1995) Ultraviolet-B-induced apoptosis of keratinocytes: evidence for partial involvement of tumor necrosis factor-alpha in the formation of sunburn cells. J Invest Dermatol 104:922–927

13. Krutmann J, Kock A, Schauer E, Parlow F, Moller A, Kapp A, Forster E, Schöpf E, Luger TA (1990) Tumor necrosis factor beta and ultraviolet radiation are potent regulators of human keratinocyte ICAM-1 expression. J Invest Dermatol 95:127–131

14. Norris P, Poston RN, Thomas DS, Thornhill M, Hawk J, Haskard DO (1991) The expression of endothelial leukocyte adhesion molecule-1 (ELAM-1), intercellular adhesion molecule-1 (ICAM-1), and vascular cell adhesion molecule-1 (VCAM-1) in experimental cutaneous inflammation: a comparison of ultraviolet B erythema and delayed hypersensitivity. J Invest Dermatol 96:763–770

15. Uitto J, Bernstein EF (1998) Molecular mechanisms of cutaneous aging: connective tissue alterations in the dermis. J Invest Dermatol Symp Proc 3:41–44

16. Bernstein EF, Chen YQ, Kopp JB, Fisher L, Brown DB, Hahn PJ, Robey FA, Lakkakorpi J, Uitto J (1996) Long-term sun exposure alters the collagen of the papillary dermis. Comparison of sun-protected and photoaged skin by northern analysis, immunohistochemical staining, and confocal laser scanning microscopy. J Am Acad Dermatol 34:209–218

17. Griffiths CE, Russman AN, Majmudar G, Singer RS, Hamilton TA, Voorhees JJ (1993) Restoration of collagen formation in photodamaged human skin by tretinoin (retinoic acid). N Engl J Med 329:530–535

18. Talwar HS, Griffiths CE, Fisher GJ, Hamilton TA, Voorhees JJ (1995) Reduced type I and type III procollagens in photodamaged adult human skin. J Invest Dermatol 105:285–290

19. Havlik NL, Fitzpatrick TB, Kligman AM, Kligman LH (1999) Geriatric Dermatology. In: Freedberg IM, Eisen AZ, Wolff K, Austen KF, Goldsmith LA, Katz SI, Fitzpatrick TB (eds) Fitzpatrick's dermatology in general medicine. McGraw-Hill, New York, pp 1707–1723

20. Bernstein EF, Chen YQ, Tamai K, Shepley KJ, Resnik KS, Zhang H, Tuan R, Mauviel A, Uitto J (1994) Enhanced elastin and fibrillin gene expression in chronically photodamaged skin. J Invest Dermatol 103:182–186

21. Bernstein EF, Brown DB, Urbach F, Forbes D, Del Monaco M, Wu M, Katchman SD, Uitto J (1995) Ultraviolet radiation activates the human elastin promoter in transgenic mice: a novel in vivo and in vitro model of cutaneous photoaging. J Invest Dermatol 105:269–273

22. Bernstein EF, Brown DB, Takeuchi T, Kong SK, Uitto J (1997) Evaluation of sunscreens with various sun protection factors in a new transgenic mouse model of cutaneous photoaging that measures elastin promoter activation. J Am Acad Dermatol 37:725–729

23. Fisher GJ, Datta SC, Talwar HS, Wang ZQ, Varani J, Kang S, Voorhees JJ (1996) Molecular basis of sun-induced premature skin ageing and retinoid antagonism. Nature 379:335–339

24. Fisher GJ, Wang ZQ, Datta SC, Varani J, Kang S, Voorhees JJ (1997) Pathophysiology of premature skin aging induced by ultraviolet light. N Engl J Med 337:1419–1428
25. Matrisian LM (1992) The matrix-degrading metalloproteinases. Bioessays 14:455–463
26. Fisher GJ, Voorhees JJ (1998) Molecular mechanisms of photoaging and its prevention by retinoic acid: ultraviolet irradiation induces MAP kinase signal transduction cascades that induce Ap-1-regulated matrix metalloproteinases that degrade human skin in vivo. J Invest Dermatol Symp Proc 3:61–68
27. Angel P, Imagawa M, Chiu R, Stein B, Imbra RJ, Rahmsdorf HJ, Jonat C, Herrlich P, Karin M (1987) Phorbol ester-inducible genes contain a common cis element recognized by a TPA-modulated trans-acting factor. Cell 49:729–739
28. Angel P, Karin M (1992) Specific members of the Jun protein family regulate collagenase expression in response to various extracellular stimuli. Matrix Suppl 1:156–164
29. Sato H, Seiki M (1993) Regulatory mechanism of 92 kDa type IV collagenase gene expression which is associated with invasiveness of tumor cells. Oncogene 8:395–405
30. Quinones S, Buttice G, Kurkinen M (1994) Promoter elements in the transcriptional activation of the human stromelysin-1 gene by the inflammatory cytokine, interleukin 1. Biochem J 302:471–477
31. Varani J, Fisher GJ, Kang S, Voorhees JJ (1998) Molecular mechanisms of intrinsic skin aging and retinoid-induced repair and reversal. J Invest Dermatol Symp Proc 3:57–60
32. Federspiel SJ, DiMari SJ, Howe AM, Guerry-Force ML, Haralson MA (1991) Extracellular matrix biosynthesis by cultured fetal rat lung epithelial cells. IV. Effects of chronic exposure to retinoic acid on growth, differentiation, and collagen biosynthesis. Lab Invest 65:441–450
33. Chen JY, Penco S, Ostrowski J, Balaguer P, Pons M, Starrett JE, Reczek P, Chambon P, Gronemeyer H (1995) RAR-specific agonist/antagonists which dissociate transactivation and AP1 transrepression inhibit anchorage-independent cell proliferation. EMBO J 14:1187–1197
34. Schule R, Rangarajan P, Yang N, Kliewer S, Ransone LJ, Bolado J, Verma IM, Evans RM (1991) Retinoic acid is a negative regulator of AP-1-responsive genes. Proc Natl Acad Sci USA 88:6092–6096
35. Kanjilal SAH (1996) Molecular mechanisms of photocarcinogenesis: the role of ras and p53 alterations. In: Arndt KA, Leboit PE, Robinson JK, Wintroub BU (eds) Cutaneous medicine and surgery: an integrated program in dermatology. Saunders, Philadelphia, pp 1363–1377
36. Brash DE (1997) Sunlight and the onset of skin cancer. Trends Genet 13:410–414
37. Kraemer KH (1997) Sunlight and skin cancer: another link revealed. Proc Natl Acad Sci USA 94:11–14
38. Freeman SE, Hacham H, Gange RW, Maytum DJ, Sutherland JC, Sutherland BM (1989) Wavelength dependence of pyrimidine dimer formation in DNA of human skin irradiated in situ with ultraviolet light. Proc Natl Acad Sci USA 86:5605–5609
39. Young AR, Potten CS, Nikaido O, Parsons PG, Boenders J, Ramsden JM, Chadwick CA (1998) Human melanocytes and keratinocytes exposed to UVB or UVA in vivo show comparable levels of thymine dimers. J Invest Dermatol 111:936–940
40. Burren R, Scaletta C, Frenk E, Panizzon RG, Applegate LA (1998) Sunlight and carcinogenesis: expression of p53 and pyrimidine dimers in human skin following UVA I, UVA I + II and solar simulating radiations. Int J Cancer 76:201–216
41. Levine AJ (1997) p53, the cellular gatekeeper for growth and division. Cell 88:323–331
42. Gasparro FP (1998) p53 in dermatology. Arch Dermatol 134:1029–1032
43. Li G, Ho VC, Berean K, Tron VA (1995) Ultraviolet radiation induction of squamous cell carcinomas in p53 transgenic mice. Cancer Res 55:2070–2074

44. Campbell C, Quinn AG, Ro YS, Angus B, Rees JL (1993) p53 mutations are common and early events that precede tumor invasion in squamous cell neoplasia of the skin. J Invest Dermatol 100:746–748

45. Rehman I, Takata M, Wu YY, Rees JL (1996) Genetic change in actinic keratoses. Oncogene 12:2483–2490

46. Ananthaswamy HN, Loughlin SM, Ullrich SE, Kripke ML (1998) Inhibition of UV-induced p53 mutations by sunscreens: implications for skin cancer prevention. J Invest Dermatol Symp Proc 3:52–56

47. Nakazawa H, English D, Randell PL, Nakazawa K, Martel N, Armstrong BK, Yamasaki H (1994) UV and skin cancer: specific p53 gene mutation in normal skin as a biologically relevant exposure measurement. Proc Natl Acad Sci USA 91:360–364

48. Berg RJ, van Kranen HJ, Rebel HG, de Vries A, van Vloten WA, van Kreijl CF, van der Leun JC, de Gruijl FR (1996) Early p53 alterations in mouse skin carcinogenesis by UVB radiation: immunohistochemical detection of mutant p53 protein in clusters of preneoplastic epidermal cells. Proc Natl Acad Sci USA 93:274–278

49. Tornaletti S, Pfeifer GP (1994) Slow repair of pyrimidine dimers at p53 mutation hotspots in skin cancer. Science 263:1436–1438

50. Ullrich SE (1995) Cutaneous biologic responses to ultraviolet radiation. Curr Opin Dermatol 2:225–230

51. Ren ZP, Hedrum A, Ponten F, Nister M, Ahmadian A, Lundeberg J, Uhlen M, Ponten J (1996) Human epidermal cancer and accompanying precursors have identical p53 mutations different from p53 mutations in adjacent areas of clonally expanded non-neoplastic keratinocytes. Oncogene 12:765–773

52. Jonason AS, Kunala S, Price GJ, Restifo RJ, Spinelli HM, Persing JA, Leffell DJ, Tarone RE, Brash DE (1996) Frequent clones of p53-mutated keratinocytes in normal human skin (see comments). Proc Natl Acad Sci USA 93:14025–14029

53. Ziegler A, Jonason AS, Leffell DJ, Simon JA, Sharma HW, Kimmelman J, Remington L, Jacks T, Brash DE (1994) Sunburn and p53 in the onset of skin cancer. Nature 372:773–776

54. Johnson RL, Rothman AL, Xie J, Goodrich LV, Bare JW, Bonifas JM, Quinn AG, Myers RM, Cox DR, Epstein EH Jr, Scott MP (1996) Human homolog of patched, a candidate gene for the basal cell nevus syndrome. Science 272:1668–1671

55. Oro AE, Higgins KM, Hu Z, Bonifas JM, Epstein EH Jr, Scott MP (1997) Basal cell carcinomas in mice overexpressing sonic hedgehog. Science 276:817–821

56. Gailani MR, Stahle-Backdahl M, Leffell DJ, Glynn M, Zaphiropoulos PG, Pressman C, Unden AB, Dean M, Brash DE, Bale AE, Toftgard R (1996) The role of the human homologue of Drosophila patched in sporadic basal cell carcinomas. Nat Genet 14:78–81

57. Liu Q, Neuhausen S, McClure M, Frye C, Weaver-Feldhaus J, Gruis NA, Eddington K, Allalunis-Turner MJ, Skolnick MH, Fujimura FK et al (1995) CDKN2 (MTS1) tumor suppressor gene mutations in human tumor cell lines. Oncogene 11:2455

58. Pollock PM, Yu F, Qiu L, Parsons PG, Hayward NK (1995) Evidence for u.v. induction of CDKN2 mutations in melanoma cell lines. Oncogene 11:663–668

59. Grossman D, Leffell DJ (1997) The molecular basis of nonmelanoma skin cancer: new understanding. Arch Dermatol 133:1263–1270

60. Armstrong BK, Kricker A (1995) Skin cancer. Dermatol Clin 13:583–594

61. Katsambas A, Nicolaidou E (1996) Cutaneous malignant melanoma and sun exposure. Recent developments in epidemiology. Arch Dermatol 132:444–450

62. Lancaster HO (1956) Some geographical aspects of mortality from melanoma in Europeans. Med J Aust 1:1082–1087

63. Gallagher RP, Elwood JM, Yang CP (1989) Is chronic sunlight exposure important in accounting for increases in melanoma incidence? Int J Cancer 44:813–815

64. Magnus K (1977) Incidence of malignant melanoma of the skin in the five Nordic countries: significance of solar radiation. Int J Cancer 20:477–485

65. Moan J, Dahlback A (1992) The relationship between skin cancers, solar radiation and ozone depletion. Br J Cancer 65:916–921
66. Langley RG, Sober AJ (1997) A clinical review of the evidence for the role of ultraviolet radiation in the etiology of cutaneous melanoma. Cancer Invest 15:561–567
67. Holman CD, Armstrong BK (1984) Cutaneous malignant melanoma and indicators of total accumulated exposure to the sun: an analysis separating histogenetic types. J Natl Cancer Inst 73:75–82
68. Osterlind A, Hou-Jensen K, Moller Jensen O (1988) Incidence of cutaneous malignant melanoma in Denmark 1978–1982. Anatomic site distribution, histologic types, and comparison with non-melanoma skin cancer. Br J Cancer 58:385–391
69. Rhodes AR, Weinstock MA, Fitzpatrick TB, Mihm MC Jr, Sober AJ (1987) Risk factors for cutaneous melanoma. A practical method of recognizing predisposed individuals. JAMA 258:3146–3154
70. Reintgen DS, McCarty KM Jr, Cox E, Seigler HF (1982) Malignant melanoma in black American and white American populations. A comparative review. JAMA 248:1856–1859
71. Elder DE (1995) Skin cancer. Melanoma and other specific nonmelanoma skin cancers. Cancer 75:245–256
72. Beral V, Evans S, Shaw H, Milton G (1983) Cutaneous factors related to the risk of malignant melanoma. Br J Dermatol 109:165–172
73. Dubin N, Pasternack BS, Moseson M (1990) Simultaneous assessment of risk factors for malignant melanoma and non-melanoma skin lesions, with emphasis on sun exposure and related variables. Int J Epidemiol 19:811–819
74. Garbe C, Kruger S, Stadler R, Guggenmoos-Holzmann I, Orfanos CE (1989) Markers and relative risk in a German population for developing malignant melanoma. Int J Dermatol 28:517–238
75. Weinstock MA, Colditz GA, Willett WC, Stampfer MJ, Bronstein BR, Mihm MC Jr, Speizer FE (1991) Melanoma and the sun: the effect of swimsuits and a "healthy" tan on the risk of nonfamilial malignant melanoma in women. Am J Epidemiol 134:462–470
76. Elder DE (1989) Human melanocytic neoplasms and their etiologic relationship with sunlight. J Invest Dermatol 92:297S–303S
77. Elwood JM, Whitehead SM, Davison J, Stewart M, Galt M (1990) Malignant melanoma in England: risks associated with naevi, freckles, social class, hair colour, and sunburn. Int J Epidemiol 19:801–810
78. Green A, Siskind V, Bain C, Alexander J (1985) Sunburn and malignant melanoma. Br J Cancer 51:393–397
79. Weinstock MA, Colditz GA, Willett WC, Stampfer MJ, Bronstein BR, Mihm MC Jr, Speizer FE (1989) Nonfamilial cutaneous melanoma incidence in women associated with sun exposure before 20 years of age. Pediatrics 84:199–204
80. Elwood JM, Gallagher RP, Davison J, Hill GB (1985) Sunburn, suntan and the risk of cutaneous malignant melanoma – the Western Canada Melanoma Study. Br J Cancer 51:543–549
81. Holman CD, Armstrong BK, Heenan PJ (1986) Relationship of cutaneous malignant melanoma to individual sunlight- exposure habits. J Natl Cancer Inst 76:403–414
82. Elwood JM, Gallagher RP, Hill GB, Pearson JC (1985) Cutaneous melanoma in relation to intermittent and constant sun exposure – the Western Canada Melanoma Study. Int J Cancer 35:427–433
83. Holman CD, Mulroney CD, Armstrong BK (1980) Epidemiology of pre-invasive and invasive malignant melanoma in Western Australia. Int J Cancer 25:317–323
84. Quinn AG (1997) Ultraviolet radiation and skin carcinogenesis. Br J Hosp Med 58:261–264
85. Gallagher RP, Hill GB, Bajdik CD, Coldman AJ, Fincham S, McLean DI, Threlfall WJ (1995) Sunlight exposure, pigmentation factors, and risk of nonmelanocytic skin cancer. II. Squamous cell carcinoma. Arch Dermatol 131:164–169

86. Kricker A, Armstrong BK, English DR, Heenan PJ (1991) Pigmentary and cutaneous risk factors for non-melanocytic skin cancer – a case-control study. Int J Cancer 48:650–662
87. English DR, Armstrong BK, Kricker A, Winter MG, Heenan PJ, Randell PL (1998) Case-control study of sun exposure and squamous cell carcinoma of the skin. Int J Cancer 77:347–353
88. Franceschi S, Levi F, Randimbison L, La Vecchia C (1996) Site distribution of different types of skin cancer: new aetiological clues. Int J Cancer 67:24–28
89. Kricker A, Armstrong BK, English DR, Heenan PJ (1995) Does intermittent sun exposure cause basal cell carcinoma? a case-control study in Western Australia. Int J Cancer 60:489–494
90. Gallagher RP, Hill GB, Bajdik CD, Fincham S, Coldman AJ, McLean DI, Threlfall WJ (1995) Sunlight exposure, pigmentary factors, and risk of nonmelanocytic skin cancer. I. Basal cell carcinoma. Arch Dermatol 131:157–163
91. McCormack CJ, Kelly JW, Dorevitch AP (1997) Differences in age and body site distribution of the histological subtypes of basal cell carcinoma. A possible indicator of differing causes. Arch Dermatol 133:593–596
92. Bastiaens MT, Hoefnagel JJ, Bruijn JA, Westendorp RG, Vermeer BJ, Bouwes Bavinck JN (1998) Differences in age, site distribution, and sex between nodular and superficial basal cell carcinoma indicate different types of tumors. J Invest Dermatol 110:880–884
93. Gilchrest BA, Soter NA, Stoff JS, Mihm MC Jr (1981) The human sunburn reaction: histologic and biochemical studies. J Am Acad Dermatol 5:411–422
94. Coven TR, Burack LH, Gilleaudeau R, Keogh M, Ozawa M, Kreuger JG (1997) Narrowband UV-B produces superior clinical and histopathological resolution of moderate-to-severe psoriasis in patients compared with broadband UV-B. Arch Dermatol 133:1514–1522
95. Maughan WZ, Muller SA, Perry HO, Pittelkow MR, O'Brien PC (1980) Incidence of skin cancers in patients with atopic dermatitis treated with coal tar: a 25-year follow-up study. J Am Acad Dermatol 3:612–615
96. Pittelkow MR, Perry HO, Muller SA, Maughan WZ, O'Brien PC (1981) Incidence of skin cancers in psoriatic patients treated with coal tar: a 25-year follow-up study. Arch Dermatol 117:465–468
97. Larkö O, Swanbeck G (1982) Is UVB treatment safe? A study of extensively UVB treated psoriasis patients compared with a matched control group. Acta Derm Venereol (Stockh) 62:507–512
98. Stern RS, Zierler S, Parrish JA (1980) Skin carcinoma in patients with psoriasis treated with topical tar and artificial ultraviolet radiation. Lancet 1:732–735
99. Stern RS (1990) Genital tumors among men with psoriasis exposed to psoralens and ultraviolet A radiation (PUVA) and ultraviolet B radiation. N Engl J Med 322:1093–1097
100. Tzung TY, Runger TM (1998) Assessment of DNA damage induced by broadband and narrowband UVB in cultured lymphoblasts and keratinocytes using the comet assay. Photochem Photobiol 67:647–650
101. Krutmann J (1997) High-dose ultraviolet A1 (UVA-1) phototherapy: does it work? Photodermatol Photoimmunol Photomed 13:78–81
102. Plettenberg H, Stege H, Megahed M, Ruzicka T, Hosokawa Y, Tsuji T, Morita A, Krutmann J (1999) Ultraviolet A1 (340–400 nm) phototherapy for cutaneous T-cell lymphoma. J Am Acad Dermatol 41:47–50
103. Abeck D, Schmidt T, Fesq H, Strom K, Mempel M, Brockow K, Ring J (2000) Long-term efficacy of medium-dose UVA1 phototherapy in atopic dermatitis. J Am Acad Dermatol 42:254–257
104. Buck HW, Magnus IA, Porter AD (1960) The action spectrum of 8-methoxypsoralen for erythema in human skin. Br J Dermatol 72:249–255

105. Morison WL (1993) Photochemotherapy. In: Lim HW, Soter NA (eds) Clinical photo-medicine. Dekker, New York, pp 327–346
106. Cripps DJ, Lowe NJ, Lerner AB (1982) Action spectra of topical psoralens: a reevalua-tion. Br J Dermatol 107:77–82
107. Brücke J, Tanew A, Ortel B, Hönigsmann H (1991) Relative efficacy of 335 and 365 nm radiation in photochemotherapy of psoriasis. Br J Dermatol 124:372–374
108. Ortel B, Perl S, Kinaciyan T, Calzavara-Pinton PG, Hönigsmann H (1993) Compari-son of narrow-band (311 nm) UVB and broad-band UVA after oral or bath-water 8-methoxypsoralen in the treatment of psoriasis. J Am Acad Dermatol 29:736–740
109. De Berker DAR, Sakuntabhai A, Diffey BL, Matthews, JNS, Farr PM (1997) Compari-son of psoralen-UVB and psoralen-UVA photochemotherapy in the treatment of psoriasis. J Am Acad Dermatol 36:577–581
110. Gasparro FP (1998) p53 in dermatology. Arch Dermatol 134:1029–1032
111. Gonzalez E (1995) PUVA for psoriasis. Dermatol Clin 13:851–866
112. Kochevar IE (1993) Basic principles in photomedicine and photochemistry. In: Lim H, Soter N (eds) Clinical Photomedicine. Marcel Dekker, Inc., New York, pp 1–18
113. Wang XM, McNiff JM, Klump V, Asgari M, Gasparro FP (1997) An unexpected spec-trum of p53 mutations from squamous cell carcinomas in psoriasis patients treated with PUVA. Photochem Photobiol 66:294–299
114. Nataraj AJ, Wolf P, Cerroni L, Ananthaswamy HN (1997) p53 mutations in squamous cell carcinomas from psoriatic patients treated with psoralen + UVA (PUVA): rela-tive frequency of PUVA-versus-UV-signature mutations. J Invest Dermatol 109:238–243
115. Morison WL, Marwaha S, Beck L (1997) PUVA-induced phototoxicity: incidence and causes. J Am Acad Dermatol 36:183–185
116. Morison WL (1997) Subacute phototoxicity caused by treatment with oral psoralen plus UV-A. Arch Dermatol 133:1609
117. Stern RS, Parrish JA, Fitzpatrick TB, Bleich HL (1985) Actinic degeneration in asso-ciation with long-term use of PUVA. J Invest Dermatol 84:135–138
118. Morison WL, Baughman RD, Day RM, Forbes PD, Hoenigsmann H, Krueger GG, Lebwohl M, Lew R, Naldi L, Parrish JA, Piepkorn M, Stern RS, Weinstein GD, Whit-more SE (1998) Consensus workshop on the toxic effects of long-term PUVA therapy. Arch Dermatol 134:595–601
119. Stern RS, Laird N (1994) The carcinogenic risk of treatments for severe psoriasis. Cancer 73:2759–2764
120. Stern RS, Lunder EJ (1998) Risk of squamous cell carcinoma and methoxsalen (pso-ralen) and UV-A radiation (PUVA): a meta-analysis. Arch Dermatol 134:1582–1585
121. Stern RS, Lange R (1988) Non-melanoma skin cancer occurring in patients treated with PUVA five to ten years after first treatment. J Invest Dermatol 91:120–124
122. Henseler T, Christopher E, H(nigsmann H, Wolff K (1987) Skin tumors in the Euro-pean PUVA study. J Am Acad Dermatol 16:108–116
123. Wolff K, Hönigsmann H (1991) Genital carcinomas in psoriasis patients treated with photochemotherapy. Lancet 337:439
124. Stern RS, Nichols KT, Vakeva LH (1997) Malignant melanoma in patients treated for psoriasis with methoxsalen (psoralen) and ultraviolet A radiation (PUVA). N Engl J Med 336:1041–1045
125. Lindelöf, B., Sigurgeirsson B, Tegner E, Larko O, Johannesson A, Berne B, Ljunggren B, Andersson T, Molin L, Nylander-Lundqvist E, Emtestam L (1999) PUVA and can-cer risk: the Swedish follow-up study. Br J Dermatol 141:108–112

15 Photoprotection

Peter Wolf, Antony Young

Contents

Principles of Topical Sunscreens

The efficacy of a classic topical sunscreen is due to its incorporated active ingredients, i.e., chemical ultraviolet radiation (UV)-absorbing filters and physical UV-blocking agents [1]. The molecules of chemical substances (Fig. 1) such as aminobenzoates, cinnamates, salicylates, benzophenones, and camphor derivatives can absorb (Fig. 2a) quanta of UV radiation energy (i.e., photons) due to their molecular structure and, therefore, are promoted from their energy ground state to an excited state. The absorbed energy is then transferred to surrounding molecules, cells, and tissues by heat primarily and emission of fluorescence or phosphorescence. The photoprotective capacity of a sunscreen product relates to the absorption peaks and absorption waveband ranges of each UV-absorbing chemical or the composite absorption spectrum of all chemicals used

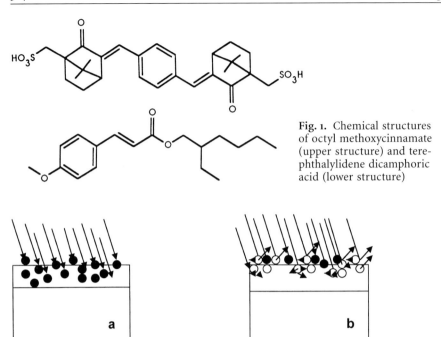

Fig. 1. Chemical structures of octyl methoxycinnamate (upper structure) and terephthalylidene dicamphoric acid (lower structure)

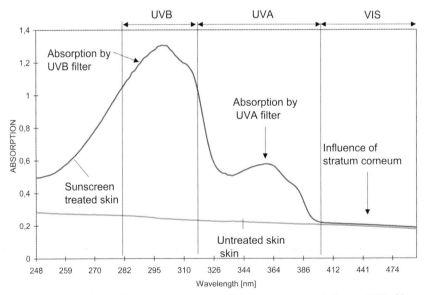

Fig. 2. Mechanisms of (**a**) UV absorbing chemicals and (**b**) physical sunblocking agents

Fig. 3. Combined UV absorption spectrum of a sunscreen containing an UVB filter (4% Eusolex 6300) and UVA filter (1.5% Parsol 1789) as measured on tape-stripped stratum corneum. (Spectrum is courtesy of J. Lademann and H.J. Weigmann)

in the formulated product. Figure 3 shows the combined absorption spectrum of a sunscreen containing an UVB and UVA filter. Physical sunblocking agents such as TiO_2 and ZnO and other particulate agents of organic and inorganic nature protect by reflection, scattering, and absorption of UV radiation (Figure 2b). Broad-spectrum sunscreen products of today contain often both UV absorbing chemicals and physical sunblocking agents.

Sun Protection Factor

The efficacy of a sunscreen preparation is measured by its sun protection factor (SPF). The SPF is defined by the UV energy required to produce a minimal erythema dose (MED) on protected skin divided by the UV energy required to produce an MED on unprotected skin.

SPF = MED (sunscreen-protected skin)/MED (unprotected skin)

There are different methods and norms to determine the SPF of a sunscreen. The most significant parameters of the test methods of the Food and Drug Administration (FDA) in the United States [2], European COLIPA [3], and Australian/New Zealand standard (AS/NZS 2604:1998) are summarized in Table 1. The in vitro absorption or transmission of a sunscreen can be used to estimate its in vivo SPF. In effect, the in vivo SPF is inversely related to the in vitro transmission of a sunscreen as shown in Table 2.

UVA Protection Factor

The FDA has recently recognized that both UVB and UVA radiation are associated with adverse health effects: "The agency is aware that UVA radiation contributes to both acute and chronic skin damage such as erythema, melanogenesis, carcinogenesis, drug-induced photosensitivity, photoaging, and morphological alterations of Langerhans' cells....In addition, the agency is concerned that sunscreens with higher SPF values allow consumers to remain in the sun for long periods of time without burning, thus increasing UVA exposure. Accordingly, protection against UVA radiation is much more important than previously realized. The agency believes that protection against UVA radiation may be as important to consumers' well-being as protection against UVB radiation." Because of UVA testing and labeling issues, the FDA has delayed the implementation of the final monograph on over-the-counter (OTC) sunscreens published in May 1999 until December 2002 [2].

Erythema as endpoint for UVA protection is not suitable for practical SPF testing procedures because high UVA doses are necessary to elicit an erythema response in the skin. When high SPF sunscreens are tested, the necessary UVA irradiation times using standard UVA light sources are, therefore, too long and inappropriate for human volunteers. UVA-induced immediate pigment darkening (IPD) and persistent pigment darkening (PPD) are currently most widely used to determine an in vivo UVA protection factor (Table 3). The IPD response

Table 1. Comparison of the major parameters of the SPF testing procedures published by the FDA, the Australian New Zealand Standards organization, and the European COLIPA

	FDA (1999) [2]	Australian New Zealand Standard (AS/NZS 2604:1998)	COLIPA (1994) [3]
Number of test subjects	20–25	10	10–20
Skin phototypes	I, II, III	I, II, III	I, II, III and subjects with colorimetric ITA°-values>28°
Test area and site	50 cm² (back skin)	30 cm² (back skin)	30 cm² (back skin)
Product quantity and application	2.0 mg/cm²	2.0±0.1 mg/cm²	2.0±0.4 mg/cm²
Product drying time	15 min	15 min	15 min
SPF of sunscreen standards (UV filter)	4.7 (homosalate)	4.0 (homosalate)	P1, low-SPF standard, 4.0–4.4; P2, high-SPF standard, SPF 11.5–13.9 P3: High-SPF standard, 14.0–17.0
UV source and spectrum	Artificial lamp source. Continuous emission spectrum between 290–400 nm, similar to sunlight: sea level, at zenith angel of 10°; UVC (< 290 nm) < 1 %, visible light < 5 %	Artificial lamp source. Spectrum between 290 and 320 nm free from substantial peaks. Continuous spectrum up to 400 nm; UVC < 1°	Artificial lamp source. Output defined by erythemal effectiveness between 290 and 400 nm based on standard sun at 40°N latitude; relative erythema effectiveness below 290 nm < 1 %
Light source filter	WG320/1 mm plus UG5/1 mm or UG11/1 mm	WG320/1 mm plus dichroic or heat absorbing filter	WG 320/1 mm plus UG11/1 mm
Application of light dosages	5 fields of 1.0-cm diameter; dose increments of 1.25	5 fields of 1.0 cm diameter; dose increments of not greater than 1.26	5 fields of 1.0-cm diameter; dose increments of 1.25
Time of MED determination after UV light exposure	22–24 h	16–24 h	20±4 h
Calculation of the SPF	Arithmetic mean of individual SPFs minus correction factor	Arithmetic mean of individual SPFs	Arithmetic mean of individual SPFs

MED, minimal erythema dose; FDA, Food and Drug Administration; COLIPA, Comité de Liaison des Assiociations Européennes de L'Industrie de la Parfumerie, des Produits Cosmetiques et de Toilette.

Table 2. Sun protection factor (SPF) in relation to transmission and absorption of a sunscreen

SPF[a]	Transmission	Absorption %[b]
4	0.250	75
6	0.167	83.3
8	0.125	87.5
10	0.100	90
12	0.083	91.7
15	0.067	93.3
20	0.050	95
25	0.040	96
30	0.033	96.7
40	0.025	97.5
60	0.017	98.3

[a] SPF = 1/transmission.
[b] Absorption % = (1-T)× 100.

is a transient brownish-gray coloration of the skin of subjects with pigmented skin starting within 60 s following UVA irradiation. Whereas the IPD test procedure produces fast results with relatively low dosages of UVA radiation, its results are highly variable and not easy reproducible. The PPD response (determined at 2–24 h after UV exposure) is a longer-lasting tanning response of pigmented subjects after UVA irradiation. The PPD response is stable and its testing results are reproducible. According to the conventional SPF, the UVA protection factor is determined as follows:

PPD (IPD) UVA protection factor = minimal PPD (IPD) dose (sunscreen-protected skin)/minimal PPD (IPD) dose (unprotected skin)

In vitro designation methods (Table 3) to determine an UVA protection factor apply photometric spectral measurements to calculate a theoretical UVA protection factor.

Table 3. Methods for determination and/or designation of the UVA protection factor

In vivo

– Immediate pigment darkening (IPD) immediately after UV
– Persistent pigment darkening (PPD) 2–4 h after UV

In vitro

– Monochromatic protection factor[a]
– English Boots Star Rating System (1–4 stars for UVB/UVA ratio)
– Australian New Zealand Standard (AS/NZS 2604–1998)

[a] According to Diffey [4. 5]

According to Diffey [4] and Cole [5], the following formula can be used to calculate the UVA protection factor.

$$\text{UVA SPF} = \sum(\text{CIE}\lambda \times \text{E}\lambda)/\sum(\text{T}\lambda \times \text{CIE}\lambda \times \text{E}\lambda)$$

where Tλ = sunscreen transmission at wavelength $_\lambda$; CIE = Commission Internationale d'Eclairage (CIE) action spectrum [6] value at wavelength λ; and E = solar simulator irradiance at wavelength λ in the UVA wavelength range from 320 to 400 nm. According to the Australian/New Zealand sunscreen standard (AZ/NZS 2604:1998), a sunscreen can be labeled and promoted as broad spectrum if it reduces UVA in the wavelength range between 320 and 360 nm by at least 90 % using the solution or film method at a sunscreen layer of 8 μm or by at least 99 % using the plate method at a sunscreen layer of 20 μm. The use of differing methods (IPD, PPD, and in vitro measurements) to determine UVA protection does, at present, often not allow us to directly compare the labeled UVA protection factors of commercially available products.

Vehicles of Sunscreens

Sunscreen preparations are available in a variety of forms, including water-in-oil and oil-in-water emulsions, oils, hydrogels, lipogels, alcoholic solutions, and sprays. The basic ingredients of a sunscreen are important for its substantivity, i.e., adhesiveness, which reflects the ability of the vehicle as well as of the active ingredients to remain adherent to the skin and diffuse or penetrate into the stratum corneum when applied in a thin layer. Most sunscreen chemicals are lipophilic in nature, and, thus, they have affinity for oils for solubilization. Water-soluble hydrophilic compounds such para-aminobenzoic (PABA) acid are now less popular to formulate sunscreen preparations because (a) profuse sweating can easily elute or wash off an applied hydrophilic chemical sunscreen product and (b) low humidity and high temperature can cause the product to scale and flak off [1]. Sunscreen formulations can be made more adhesive by incorporating the active ingredients in a water-resistant acrylate polymer base. Liposomes are also used to formulate sunscreen preparations. Liposomes are spheroid particles made of one, two, or several double phospholipid membrane layers, consisting of lecithin, cholesterol, ceramides, and fatty acids. Liposomes exhibit an affinity to the stratum corneum and can penetrate the superficial layers of the skin [7]. They can be loaded in their inner core with hydrophilic substances and in their lipid membranes with lipophilic substances. Liposomal sunscreen preparations have high water resistance and can be used to incorporate and apply classic chemical UV filters or novel photoprotective substances such as DNA repair enzymes to the skin.

Water Resistance of Sunscreens

The labeling of a sunscreen product for water resistance characterizes the substantivity for the resistance to removal of the product by swimming, prolonged

Table 4. Water resistance testing of sunscreens according to FDA protocol [2]

(a) For sunscreen products making the claim of "water resistant" the label SPF shall be the label SPF value determined after 40 min of water immersion using the following procedure for the water-resistance test:
  (1) Apply sunscreen product (followed by the waiting period after application of the sunscreen product indicated on the product labeling)
  (2) 20-min moderate activity in water
  (3) 20-min rest period (do not towel test sites)
  (4) 20-min moderate activity in water
  (5) Conclude water test (air-dry test sites without toweling)
  (6) Begin SPF testing by solar simulator exposure to test-site areas

(b) For sunscreen products making the claim of "very water resistant" the label SPF shall be the label SPF value determined after 80 min of water immersion using the following procedure for the very water resistant test:
  (1) Apply sunscreen product (followed by the waiting period after application of the sunscreen product indicated on the product labeling)
  (2) 20-min moderate activity in water
  (3) 20-min rest period (do not towel test sites)
  (4) 20-min moderate activity in water
  (5) 20-min rest period (do not towel test sites)
  (6) 20-min moderate activity in water
  (7) 20-min rest period (do not towel test sites)
  (8) 20-min moderate activity in water
  (9) Conclude water test (air-dry test sites without toweling)
  (10) Begin SPF testing by solar simulator exposure to test site areas

The standard testing is performed under indoor conditions in a pool, whirlpool, or Jacuzzi with fresh water (of drinking quality) maintained at 23–32 °C.

exercise, or sweating. The FDA has recently standardized the water resistance of a sunscreen into two categories: (a) "water resistant" and (b) "very water resistant." The standard testing is performed under indoor conditions in a pool, whirlpool, or Jacuzzi (Table 4). Importantly however, for practical purposes it needs to be stressed that even if a sunscreen has the label of "water resistant" or "very water resistant," mechanical stress to the skin such as contact to the sand on a beach or towel drying will usually remove most of the applied sunscreen.

UV Filters

In the United States sunscreen preparations are recognized as OTC drugs by the FDA, which has issued in May 1999 a final monograph [2], establishing conditions under which OTC sunscreen products are recognized as safe and effective. An ingredient in sunscreen has been defined as an active ingredient (Table 5) if it absorbs, reflects, or scatters radiation in the UV range at wavelengths from 290 to 400 nm. In the United States a commercial sunscreen product can consist of any of the 16 ingredients listed in Table 5 within the concentration specified for each ingredient, and the finished product must provide a minimum SPF value of not less than 2 as measured by SPF testing. Two or more sunscreen

Table 5. FDA permitted sunscreen ingredients and their maximum concentrations according the Final Sunscreen Monograph of the FDA [2]

Ingredient	Maximum concentration (%)
Aminobenzoic acid (PABA)	15
Avobenzone	3
Cinoxate	3
Dioxybenzone	3
Homosalate	15
Menthyl anthranilate	5
Octocrylene	10
Octyl methoxycinnamate	7.5
Octyl salicylate	5
Oxybenzone	6
Padimate O	8
Phenylbenzimidazole sulfonic acid	4
Sulisobenzone	10
Titanium dioxide	25
Trolamine salicylate	12
Zinc oxide	25

Table 6. UV-absorbing chemicals approved by the FDA listed by groups

Group	Compound	UV Absorbance range (nm)
Aminobenzoates	Para-aminobenzoic acid (PABA)	260–313
	2-ethylhexyl PABA (Padimate O)	264–320
Cinnamates	Octyl methoxycinnamate (Parsol MCX)	280–320
	Cinoxate (2-Ethoxyethyl-4-methoxycinnamate)	280–320
Salicylates	Homosalate	290–320
	Octyl salicylate	280–320
	Trolamine salicylate	260–355
Benzophenones	Dioxybenzone	260–355
	Sulisobenzone	260–360
	Oxybenzone	270–360
Miscellaneous	Avobenzone (butyl-methoxy-dibenzoylmethane)	320–380
	Menthyl anthranilate	300–370
	Octocrylene	290–360
	Phenylbenzimidazole sulfonic acid	290–320
	Titanium dioxide	300–400
	Zinc oxide	300–400

Absorbance ranges of chemicals are from Pathak et al. [1].

active ingredients can be combined with each other in a single product when used in the concentrations established for each ingredient and the concentration of each active ingredient must be sufficient to contribute a minimum SPF of not less than 2 to the finished product. The finished product must have a minimum SPF of not less than the number of sunscreen active ingredients used in the combination multiplied by 2. In Table 6 the UV protecting agents permitted in the United States by the FDA are listed by substance group, i.e., aminobenzoates, cinnamates, salicylates, benzophenones, and miscellaneous, and their effective absorption range is shown. In the European Economic Community (EEC) 19 UV filters are permanently permitted and 3 UV filters are provisionally permitted. The UV filters of the EEC, their absorption ranges, and maximum authorized concentrations are listed in Table 7. In contrast to the United State, in the EEC several permitted UV filters are camphor derivatives (Table 7: No. 2, 7, 9, 18, 19).

Almost all sunscreen products made in the United States, Europe, and Australia contain a mixture of one or more UVB-absorbing chemicals. Broad-spectrum sunscreen products contain, other than UVB filters, at least one highly effective UVA-absorbing filter such as dibenzoyl methane (avobenzone or Parsol 1789), octocrylene, menthyl anthranilate, drometrizole trisiloxane, and tereph-thalylidene dicamphor sulfonic acid, or physical sunblocking agents such as ZnO or TiO_2. Benzophenone derivatives absorbing efficiently both UVB and UVA radiation are often also compounds of broad-spectrum sunscreens.

Photostability

Photochemical reactions due to absorption of UV radiation can change the molecular structure of an UV filter, and as a result lead to the reduction of its UV absorption properties. This process, called photoinstability, is an important issue for the efficacy of UV filters. For instance, para-dimethyl-aminobenzoate (padimate A) was withdrawn by the FDA due to its photoinstability and subsequent photoallergic properties. The UVA filter avobenzone can lose up to 36 % of its activity when subjected to photostability testing [1]. Newly designed UV filters such as drometrizole trisiloxane have improved photostability and do not lose their activity even after long-lasting UV exposure.

Physical Sunblocking Agents

Particulate sunblocking agents of organic or inorganic nature have been used in cosmetic preparations in the past and their use has continued in the topical sunscreen products of today. Physical sunblocking agents include TiO_2 and ZnO as well as other substances such as iron oxide, barium sulfate, gold, talc, kaolin, bentonite, silica, or mica. In contrast to chemical UV filters, physical sunblocking agents reflect, scatter, and also absorb UV radiation (Fig. 2b). At wavelengths above 400 nm, physical sunblocking agents reflect and scatter, but at wavelengths below 400 nm they also absorb UV radiation.

Table 7. Chemical UV filters accepted in the EEC

EEC No.[a]	Substance	INCI[b]	Trade names or other chemical names	Absorption[c]	Maximum authorized concentration (g/100g)
1	4-Aminobenzoic acid	PABA		UVB	5
2	N,N,N-Trimethyl-4-(2-oxoborn-3-ylidene-methyl) anilinium methyl sulfate	Camphor benzalkonium methosulfate		UVB	6
3	Homosalate	Homosalate	Heliopan	UVB	10
4	Oxybenzone	Benzophenone-3	Eusolex 4360 Escalol 567 Uvinul M40 Neo-Heliopan BB	UVB+UVA	10
6	2-Phenylbenzimidazole-5-sulfonic acid and its potassium, sodium and triethanolamine salts	Phenylbenzimidazole sulfonic acid	Eusolex 232 Novantisol Neo-Heliopan-Hydro	UVB	8
7	3,3'-(1–4-Phenylenedimethylene) bis-(7,7-dimethyl-2-oxo-bicyclo-[2,2,1] hept-1-ylmethanesulfonic acid) and its salts	Terephthalylidene dicamphor sulfonic acid	Mexoryl SX	UVA	10
8	1-(4-tert-Butylphenyl)-3-(4-methoxyphenyl) propane-1–3-dione	Butyl methoxydibenzoylmethane	Avobenzone Parsol 1789 Eusolex 920	UVA	5
9	α-(2-Oxoborn-3-ylidene)-toluene-4-sulfonic acid and its salts	Benzylidene camphor sulfonic acid	Mexoryl SL	UVB	6
10	2-Cyano-3,3-diphenyl acrylic acid, 2-ethylhexyl ester	Octocrylene	Uvinul N539	UVB+UVA	10
11	Polymer of N-{(2 and 4)-[(2-oxoborn-3-yliden)-methyl]benzyl} acrylamide		Mexoryl SW	UVB	6
12	Octyl methoxycinnamate	Octyl methoxycinnamate	Parsol MCX Neo Heliopan AV	UVB	10
13	Ethoxylated ethyl-4-aminobenzoate (PEG-25 PABA)			UVB	

Table 7. (Continued)

EEC No.[a]	Substance	INCI[b]	Trade names or other chemical names	Absorption[c]	Maximum authorized concentration (g/100g)
14	Isopentyl-4-methoxycinnamate (Isoamyl-p-Methoxycinnamate)		Neo-Heliopan E1000	UVB	10
15	2,4,6-Trianilino-(p-carbo-2'-ethylhexyl-1'oxi)-1,3,5-triazine (octyl triazone)	Octyl triazone	Uvinul T150	UVB	5
16	Phenol, 2-(2H-Benzotriazol-2yl)-4-methyl-6(2.methyl-3(1,3,3,3-tetra-methyl-1(trimethyl-silyl)oxy)-disilox-anyl)propyl	Drometrizole trisiloxane	Mexoryl XL Silatrizole	UVB+UVA	15
17	Benzoic acid, 4,4-((6-(((1,1-dimethylethyl)aminocarbonyl)phenylamino)1,3,5-triazine-2,4-diyl)diimino)bis-,bis(2-ethylhexyl)ester			UVB	10
18	3-(4'-Methylben-zylidene)-d-1 camphor	4-Methyl-benzylidene camphor	Eusolex 6300	UVB	4
19	3-Benzylidene camphor	3-Benzylidene camphor	Ultren 9 K Mexoryl SD	UVB	2
20	2-Ethylhexyl salicylate	Octyl salicylate		UVB	5
*	2-Ethylhexyl-4-dimethyl-amino-benzoate	Octyl dimethyl PABA	Escalol 507 Eusolex 6007 Padimate O	UVB	8
*	2-Hydroxy-4-methoxybenzo-phenone-5-sulfonic acid and sodium salts	Benzo-phenone-4 Benzo-phenone-5		UVB	5
*	4-Isopropylbenzyl salicylate	Isopropylbenzyl salicylate		UVB	4

* These filters are provisionally permitted until 30 June 2000.
[a] No. 1–20, Chemical UV filters permanently permitted in the EEC according to the EEC Directive 76/768;1999.
[b] INCI, International nomenclature cosmetic ingredient.
[c] Effective absorbance wavelength range.

Macropigments

Cosmetic preparations with high concentrations of pigments of large particle size (> 200 nm) (i.e., macropigments) can grant a total block and broad spectrum protection against UV radiation and visible light. For instance, such preparations contain 20 % ZnO or 20 % TiO_2 with 1 % – 2 % FeO. These sunblocking preparations can be particularly useful in photosensitive disorders such as cutaneous lupus erythematosus to provide broad-spectrum photoprotection (Table 8). They are also used to formulate UV-opaque lipsticks. However, macropigment-based sunblocking preparations are usually not accepted for photoprotection by regular consumers because they need to be applied in a thick creamy layer, which is occlusive, comedogenic, and not always cosmetically pleasant.

Micropigments

A special technology allows the production of TiO_2 and ZnO at a particle size of 1 – 100 nm (i.e., micropigments) [8, 9]. By the reduction of the particle size, these pigments lose capacity to reflect and scatter light in the visible wavelength range and gain absorptive capacity in the UV wavelength range. The marked decrease in whitening of the skin by emulsions containing microparticulate ZnO and TiO_2 has also been aided by adding dimethicone polymer, which changes the spreading coefficients of such physical sun blocking agents. Micropigment-containing sunscreen preparations are more-or-less transparent when applied to the skin; however, they do only protect in the UVB and less efficiently in the UVA but not in the visible waveband range. Micropigments can be ingredients of commercially available sunscreen preparations, particularly in combination with chemical UV filters. Recently, sunscreen preparations solely based on micropigments as active ingredients became commercially available. For instance, a topical preparation containing TiO_2 at a concentration of 5 % can exhibit a SPF of 15 or more. The FDA advisory panel recommends the use of TiO_2 for sun protection particularly in children because, based on long-term experience, TiO_2 is considered very safe and nontoxic.

Biosynthetic Melanin

Certain manufacturers have recently started to incorporate biosynthetic melanin into sunscreen preparations. Similar to natural melanin, biosynthetic melanin can absorb, scatter, and reflect UV radiation [10, 11]. In addition, like natural melanin, biosynthetic melanin can also quench reactive oxygen species. Products containing biosynthetic melanin, but no classic chemical UV filters or physical UV blocking agents, exhibit only low SPF values of up to 6. Biosynthetic melanin added to sunscreens containing common chemical UV filters can slightly increase the SPF. However, the brownish-black color of melanin limits its cosmetically acceptable concentration in a sunscreen.

Non-Classic Sunscreens

Self-Tanning Lotions

Self-tanning lotions or so-called quick tanning lotions contain ingredients [12] that chemically react with proteins (i.e., keratins) in the skin without interaction with UV radiation, and subsequently lead to a change in skin color. Dihydroxyacetone (DHA) is most widely used as the active ingredient in self-tanning lotions [1]. The Maillard browning reaction with skin surface proteins, possibly with histidine and tryptophan, seems to be responsible for the orange-brown to golden brown coloration of the skin after DHA application. The coloration by DHA is completed within 3–10 h after its topical application and protects against radiation in the long UVA wavelength and visible light range [13]. The maximal DHA-induced UVA protection factor lies between 3 and 5. The protective effect of DHA-induced skin coloration fades within 5–7 days due to the physiological desquamation of the superficial keratin layers of the skin. The administration of DHA may be useful for clinical photoprotection in erythropoietic protoporphyria (Table 8) [1].

Tan Inducers

Bergapten (5-methoxypsoralen), which is a constituent of bergamot oil, has been incorporated into suntan preparations. Bergapten-containing preparations lead to UVA-induced photochemical (i.e., PUVA) tanning of the skin. Young and co-workers have experimentally examined the potential photoprotective capacity of bergapten-induced tanning [14]. However, since psoralen and UVA treatment have been shown to be mutagenic and carcinogenic, cosmetic preparations containing significant amounts of bergapten are not any more permitted in most countries, including the United States and the EEC. The results of an epidemiological case-control study from France, Belgium, and Germany indicated that the use of psoralen-containing suntan preparation may have increased the melanoma risk of its consumers by a factor of approximately 2 [15].

Another possible approach of photoprotection by artificial tanning is the use of diacylglycerols, which activate protein kinase D, and thereby increase the activity of skin tyrosinase and synthesis of melanin in the absence of UV radiation [16]. However, there is concern about the safety of such an approach since certain tumor promoters, such as phorbol esters, have protein kinase C-stimulating properties. Recently, the topical treatment with the DNA repair enzyme T4 endonuclease V-containing liposomes was found to increase melanogenesis in human melanocytes in culture [17]. This work was extended by Eller et al. [18] who showed that the topical application of fragmented DNA-repair products such as thymidine dinucleotides (pTpT) also increased melanogenesis in cultured melanocytes in vitro and induced a long-lasting tanning response of at least 60 days in guinea pig skin in vivo.

Antioxidants

Sunscreen products contain, besides UV-absorbing or blocking ingredients, other substances, such as antioxidants, that prevent oxidative damage to UV filters and lipids of the sunscreen vehicle and protect against bacterial colonization. Antioxidants, such as Vitamin C and Vitamin E, do not have intrinsic UV-absorptive capacity, but they have potential photoprotective capacity by neutralizing reactive oxygen species. For instance, a combination of both vitamin E and C added to topical sunscreen preparations containing regular UV filters increased their photoprotective capacity in a swine ex vivo skin model [19].

Topical DNA Repair Enzyme Liposomes

A novel approach in photoprotection is the topical application of DNA repair enzymes to increase DNA repair after UV exposure. In mice, application of liposomes containing the enzyme T4 endonuclease V (T4N5 liposomes) to UV-irradiated skin protected against UV-induced DNA damage (i.e., cyclobutane pyrimidine dimers) and immunological alterations such as suppression of contact allergy and delayed-type hypersensitivity responses to certain antigens [20–22], and reduced the formation of skin cancers [23, 24]. Recently, Wolf and co-workers [7] have demonstrated in human patients with a history of skin cancer that T4N5 liposomes applied topically after UV exposure penetrated human skin and delivered T4 endonuclease into keratinocytes and epidermal Langerhans' cells, and prevented the UV-induced upregulation of the immunosuppressive cytokines interleukin-10 and tumor necrosis factor-α, under circumstances in which the UV-induced erythema response remained unaffected. In another study, Stege et al. [25] showed that the topical application of liposomes containing the DNA repair enzyme photolyase and subsequent exposure to visible light protected human subjects again UVB-induced DNA damage, erythema, sunburn cell formation, and immunological alterations such as suppression of intercellular adhesion molecule-1 (ICAM-1) and nickel hypersensitivity elicitation. DNA repair enzyme containing liposomes are commercially available (Ultrasomes and Photosomes, AGI Dermatics, Freeport, N.Y.) and are formulated by certain manufacturers into sun protection products. DNA repair enzyme-containing liposomes offer new avenues of photoprotection since they are effective even when applied after initiation of a sunburn reaction.

Miscellaneous Topical Photoprotective Agents

Aloe extract has been used for many years in after-sun lotions. Aloe extract in gel form is known for its cooling effect after application, and is used to help in dissolving painful sunburn reactions. Recent work in rodents has shown that aloe (*Aloe barbadensis*) extracts, containing plant oligosaccharides and polysaccharides, had immunoprotective capacity, preventing UV-induced suppression of contact hypersensitivity and delayed type hypersensitivity as well as interleukin-10 production

[26, 27]. An extract from the plant *Polypodium leucotomos*, which is popular in Spain and Central America for the treatment of skin diseases such as atopic dermatitis, vitiligo, and psoriasis [1], has been shown to protect after topical or oral administration human skin in vivo from sunburn, psoralen-induced phototoxic reactions, as well as depletion of Langerhans' cells [28]. *Polypodium* extract may act by its antioxidant and free radical quencher properties [29].

Systemic Photoprotective Agents

Oral beta-carotene ameliorates photosensitivity and prevents phototoxic reactions in patients with erythropoietic protoporphyria [30]. Beta-carotene, which is a natural compound of various vegetables such as carrots, tomatoes, green peppers, and oranges, absorbs radiation in the UVA and visible light range (360–500 nm) with a maximum at 450–475 nm [1]. Beta-carotene is an effective quencher for singlet oxygen produced by photoactivated porphyrins, and this may be the responsible mechanism for its clinical efficacy in erythropoietic protoporphyria. The recommendations for the clinical use of beta-carotene in erythropoietic porphyria are as follows [1]:
Dosage recommendations for beta-carotene:

Children (under 12 years of age):	30–120 mg p.o. daily
Adults:	120–180 mg p.o. daily

The best protective effect of beta-carotene in erythropoietic protoporphyria is usually evident after 6 to 8 weeks of oral administration and target blood levels of 600–800 µg/100 ml are recommended. Beta-carotene is also widely used as an oral sun protective agent in the general population, but studies on its protective effects are sparse. However, a recent study by Stahl et al. [31] revealed that oral administration of beta-carotene alone and beta-carotene in combination with vitamin E given over 12 weeks protected human skin from UV-induced erythema. The efficacy of beta-carotene in photodermatoses such as polymorphic light eruption, hydroa vacciniforme, or chronic actinic dermatitis is questionable and needs to be confirmed by clinical studies [1].

Mathews-Roth and co-workers [32] examined in a double-blind study the sulfur-containing amino acid cysteine as an alternative oral photoprotective agent in patients with erythropoietic protoporphyria and demonstrated its clinical efficacy. Similar to beta-carotene cysteine, which has been shown to act as a radioprotective agent, may act by quenching reactive oxygen species.

Indomethacin, a cyclooxygenase inhibitor, has some efficacy to diminish UVB-induced erythema in human skin [1]. A variety of other substances, including prostaglandin inhibitors such as acetylsalicylic acid (aspirin), and antihistamines failed to provide significant effects in preventing sunburn reactions in human subjects [1].

Green tea, containing unoxidized polyphenolic compounds, may be another candidate for systemic photoprotection. When fed by drinking water to mice, green tea has been shown to delay skin cancer formation induced by UVB and topical chemical tumor promoters [33].

Textiles and Photoprotection

The photoprotection offered by fabrics depends on a number of factors, including the nature of the textile, structure of the fabric, and type of weave [34]. Fabrics exhibit an enormous range in sun protection and their SPF can range from 2 to more than 1,000 [34]. It should be emphasized that clothing generally provides much greater protection against solar UV radiation than topical sunscreen products. However, for maximum photoprotection wool, some human-made fibers, and open weaves such as crepe should be avoided, whereas tightly woven fabrics such as cotton twill or silk, or high-luster polyester materials, should be selected [34]. The clothing industry in the United States in cooperation with the American Society for Testing Materials, and the CEN group of the EEC in Europe are currently standardizing methods for determining SPFs of fabrics.

Adverse Reactions to Topical Photoprotective Agents

The administration of topical sunscreen preparations can occasionally lead to adverse reactions, including contact irritation, phototoxicity, allergic contact sensitization, and photoallergic contact sensitization [1]. Most side effects are irritant reactions due to high concentrations of multiple sun-active ingredients in sunscreen preparations. Allergic contact reactions to sunscreen products can be due to various substances of the vehicle, fragrances, or sun-active ingredients. Phototoxic reactions can occur against sunscreen products containing psoralens, such as bergapten. Photoallergic contact reactions have been reported with sunscreens containing particular chemical UV filters such as para-aminobenzoic acid and its esters. Indeed, the use of PABA, one of the oldest, and since the 1950s, the most widely employed sunscreen agents in both the United States and Europe, strongly declined due to irritant, allergic, and photoallergic reactions [1]. For instance, in the United States amyl-dimethyl PABA (padimate A) was recently withdrawn by the FDA from the approved list of UVB filters. PABA-related allergic cross reactions can occur against other substances containing a primary amino group in the para position, such as para-phenylenediamine, procaine, sulfanilamide, sulfadiazine, and benzocaine. The camphor derivative isopropyl dibenzoylmethane (Eusolex 8200) had to be withdrawn from the products of several European sunscreen manufacturers due to frequent photoallergic reactions. Oxybenzone can also lead to photoallergic reactions; according to EEC regulations, a sunscreen preparation containing this UV filter must have a specific warning on its product label. However, photoallergic reactions can infrequently also be directed against various other UV filters, including Parsol 1789, padimate O, phenylbenzimidazole 5-sulfonic acid and others [1, 12]. Sensitization or photosensitization against UV chemical filters can be assessed by patch and photopatch testing, i.e., topical epicutaneous application of a standard set of potentially photoallergic substances, and subsequent UVA radiation with a standard light dose.

Photoprotection and Skin Cancer

In animal studies chemical sunscreens protected against skin aging [35], tumor initiation [36], and tumor promotion [37]. In a recent molecular biology study [38], sunscreens protected rodents against the formation of p53 mutations, which are an important event in UV skin carcinogenesis.

Sunscreens have been advocated in humans to prevent sunburn in the hope that this will decrease the chance of developing skin cancers, including malignant melanoma. For instance, Stern et al. [39] have estimated that regular use of sunscreen during childhood may reduce the overall lifetime incidence of nonmelanoma skin cancers by 80 %. However, these calculations are of theoretical nature since they do not take into consideration human behavior, by which sunscreen use may lead to extended sun exposures. In a placebo-controlled study from Australia, Thompson et al. [40] found that regular use of a SPF-17 sunscreen containing Parsol MCX and avobenzone reduced the number and prevented the occurrence of new actinic keratoses, which are potential precursors of squamous cell carcinoma. Similar photoprotection against actinic keratoses was reported from a randomized, double-blind trial in Texas, in which an SPF-29 sunscreen was compared to vehicle. In contrast, a prospective epidemiological study by Hunter et al. [41] revealed an increased risk of basal cell carcinoma in women who regularly used sunscreen.

To date, at least 12 epidemiological studies have examined melanoma risk in relation to the use of topical sunscreens [42, 43]. Sunscreen use offered no protection against melanoma in all but two of the studies. Instead, the use of sunscreens was associated with an increased risk of melanoma by a factor of approximately two or three in eight of the studies [42, 43]. Moreover, a recent study by Autier et al. [44] revealed that regular sunscreen use increased in children the number of melanocytic nevi, which are potential melanoma precursors. Roberts and Stanfield [45] recently pointed out that, in some epidemiological studies, potential sampling errors and confounding factors may have been responsible for the observed association of melanoma with the use of sunscreens. They suggested that persons with a history of sunburn are subsequently likely to use sunscreens more frequently and, that ongoing sunscreen use may then appear as a risk factor, while the real cause would be the excessive sun exposure that may have taken place long before. Indeed, in some previous studies, sunscreen use had been positively associated with all types of melanoma due to confounding with fair pigmentary traits and sensitivity of the skin to sunlight [46]. While yet unknown confounding factors cannot be totally excluded from any type of retrospective epidemiological study, the results of the more recent studies on sunscreen use and risk of melanoma were carefully adjusted for multiple parameters, including sun risk awareness, sun behavior, sun sensitivity, tanning response, and host factors, thus making confounding more unlikely [42, 43]. The question remains why sunscreens, which are highly protective against sunburn, may actually not be helpful in preventing melanoma or even lead to an increased risk of melanoma. Although there are no clear answers today, several possibilities may account for it. For example, the exact mechanisms and wavelengths by which sunlight either induces, promotes, or contributes to the development of melanoma have not been determined. Yet there is evidence from experimental studies in the *Xiphophorus* fish model that wavelengths other than UVB radiation may be important in melanoma formation [47, 48]. Indeed, it was reported that in addition to the expected induction of melanoma by UVB, there was appreciable induction in the UVA and even short-wavelength, visible light range, suggesting that wavelengths not absorbed directly by DNA can still induce melanoma. If the action spectra that cause melanomas in humans and fish are similar, the use of common sunscreens that better protect better against UVB than UVA radiation, would have little effect in preventing the induction of melanoma [48]. The hypothesis that UVA radiation is important in the etiology of melanoma is also supported by recent epidemiological observations in which exposure to sunbeds, presumably primarily emitting in the UVA range, was related to an increased risk of melanoma [49, 50]. UV radiation-induced immune suppression seems also to be a significant factor in skin carcinogenesis, including melanoma formation [42]. Studies in animals and humans have yielded conflicting data on the immunoprotective properties of sunscreens. Indeed, depending on the experimental protocol and sunscreen being examined, the use of chemical sunscreen preparations that prevented erythema gave no protection, partial protection, or complete protection against the immunosuppressive effects of UV radiation [21, 22, 51–59]. One study [52] has investigated the effect of three sunscreen preparations containing common chemical UV filters on melanoma growth in a mouse transplantation model, in which the effect on melanoma growth is mediated by the immune system. Whereas all sunscreen preparations completely protected the mice from sunburn and clearly reduced histopathological alterations, they completely failed to protect from UV-induced enhancement of melanoma growth. This study unambiguously indicated that protection from sunburn does not necessarily imply protection from other effects of UV radiation such as immunosuppression. Finally, the increased risk of melanoma observed with the use of sunscreens may be due to human behavior in combination with the use of (partially) inefficient sunscreens: sunscreen protection against sunburn may actually encourage people to prolong sun exposure and thereby increase their risk of melanoma formation when sunscreens are employed that do not or only partially protect against important events in melanoma formation such as tumor initiation or promotion, and immunosuppression [51].

Photoprotection in Photodermatoses and Photosensitive Diseases

The potential clinical efficacy of different photoprotective agents in the most common photodermatoses and photosensitive diseases is summarized in Table 8. Broad-spectrum sunscreen preparations consisting of one or two UVB filters and additional potent UVA filters such as avobenzone (Parsol 1789) or drometrizole trisiloxane as well as physical sunblocking agents such as TiO_2 or ZnO are recommended because UVA or broadband photosensitivity is often present. The exact protective capacity of a sunscreen in a photodermatosis or photosensitive disease is dependent from the action spectrum that describes the triggering

Table 8. Action spectra of common photosensitive diseases and photodermatoses as well as potential efficacy of different sun-protective agents

Photodermatosis/ Photosensitive disease	Action spectrum	Chemical UVB filter	Chemical UVA filter	Macro-pig-ments	Micro-pig-ments	Dihydro-xyace-tone	Beta-caro-tene
Polymorphic light eruption	UVA>UVB	Yes/no	Yes/no	Yes	Yes	Yes/no	–
Actinic prurigo	UVA, UVB	Yes/no	Yes/no	Yes	Yes	Yes/no	–
Hydroa vacciniforme	UVA>UVB	Yes/no	Yes/no	Yes	Yes	Yes/no	–
Urticaria solaris	UVA, UVB, VIS	Yes/no	Yes/no	Yes	Yes/no	Yes/no	–
Chronic actinic dermatitis	UVB>UVA>VIS	Yes/no	Yes/no	Yes	Yes	–	–
Lupus erythematosus	UVB>UVA	Yes/no	Yes/no	Yes	Yes	–	–
Photoallergic/toxic drug eruption	UVA	No	Yes	Yes	Yes	–	–
Erythropoietic protoporphyria	UVA+VIS	No	(Yes)	Yes	(Yes)	Yes	Yes
Xeroderma pigmentosum	UVB>UVA	Yes	Yes	Yes	Yes	–	–

VIS, visible light; Yes, protective dependent on action spectrum; No, not protective; Yes/no, protective or not protective dependent on the action spectrum in the individual patient; (Yes), low protection; –, no scientific evidence for effect.

wavelengths in the individual patient. For instance, in most cases of polymorphic light eruption, photosensitivity is present in the UVA wavelength range but it can also be present in the UVB and both UVA and UVB wavelength ranges [60]. Urticaria solaris often can be provoked by UVB, UVA, and visible wavelengths. When photoprotection is needed in the long-waveband UVA (> 380 nm) or visible light range in diseases such as erythropoietic protoporphyria, the administration of macropigment-containing sunscreen preparations or DHA-induced skin coloration may be helpful.

General Guidelines for Photoprotection

Acute and chronic skin damage can be avoided by protection from sunlight. The available practical approaches for a comprehensive sunlight protection are as follows:
- Reduction of sunlight exposure between 11 A.M. and 2 P.M.[1]
- Use of photoprotective clothing: wearing broad-brimmed hats and caps, use of parasols and umbrellas, wearing sun protective fabrics
- Use of topical sunscreens

---

[1] Between 10 A.M. and 4 P.M. UV intensity is highest

The application of topical sunscreens can help to substantially reduce the effects of sunlight exposure. In the United States, the FDA has established a new product category designation for labeling of sunscreen products [2] to aid in selecting the type of product best suited to an individual's complexion (pigmentation) and desired response to UV radiation. The FDA has set a cap of 30 as the optimal SPF in high-sun protection products [2]. The calculated increase in protection by sunscreen products with SPF of greater than 30 has been considered as limited and negligible, since a product of SPF 30 blocks 96.7 %, and a sunscreen product of SPF 60 blocks 98.3 % of UV radiation (Table 2). Sunscreen products with ultra-high SPFs (SPF>30) may give a false sense of security of protection [1].

1. Minimal sun protection product   SPF of 2 to under 12
2. Moderate sun protection product   SPF of 12 to under 30
3. High sun protection product   SPF of 30 or above (plus 30)

The use of high-SPF sun protection (SPF plus 30) products is recommended for extremely photosensitive subjects with light complexion of skin phototype I and II and non-pretanned individuals of skin type III and IV, particularly when doing outdoor activities in areas with high-UV intensity, such as tropical and subtropical regions, as well as mountains at high altitudes. Sunscreens with SPF value of smaller than 12 may only give partial protection from sunburn and other damaging effects of UV radiation, and thus should not be recommended for use by any normal individual of skin phototype I – III [1]. Manufacturers formulate and sell low-SPF preparations for cosmetic reasons and for users who attempt to achieve a skin tanning response. For children, sunscreen preparations containing physical UV blocking agents are recommended because they are considered as extremely safe and nontoxic.

The amount of sunscreen applied to the skin is important in preventing the acute effects of sunlight [61, 62] and may also be a significant variable in protection against other effect of UV radiation such as immunosuppression [63]. In SPF testing procedures, a sunscreen concentration of 2 mg/cm^2 is applied (Table 1). The use of lower concentrations has been shown to result in a significant loss of photoprotection, at least with regard to sunburn [61]. Sunscreens should be applied 10 – 15 min before beginning of sunlight exposure. This period helps (1) to allow penetration of a sunscreen preparation in the stratum corneum of the skin and subsequently to increase adhesiveness and water resistance and (2) to avoid to be sunburned during product application when being unprotected in the sun. Importantly, sunscreens should be (re)applied every 2 h when being UV exposed outdoors and always be reapplied after swimming because most sunscreen, even when labeled "water resistant" or "very water resistant," is removed by towel drying of the skin.

Finally, it has to be stressed once more: sunscreens are a valid means of photoprotection; however, caution should be taken regarding sunscreens being used to extremely prolong sun exposure because there are no definite data at present that suggest sunscreens protect against the non-sunburn effects of UV radiation, such as immunosuppression and skin carcinogenesis, to the same extent that they protect against sunburn itself [42].

References

1. Pathak MA, Fitzpatrick TB, Nghiem P, Aghassi DS (1999) Sun-protective Agents: formulations, effects, and side effects. In: Freedberg IM, Eisen AZ, Wolff K (eds) Dermatology in general medicine, 5th edn. McGraw-Hill, New York, pp 2742–2763
2. Food and Drug Administration (1999) Sunscreen products for over-the-counter human use. Final monograph FR, federal register, vol 64, no 98, May 21, pp 27666–27693
3. COLIPA Sun Protection Factor Test Method (1994) Published by the European Cosmetic, Toiletry and Perfumery Association (COLIPA), Brussels, Belgium, October 1994
4. Hudson-Peacock MJ, Diffey BL, Farr PM (1994) Photoprotective action of emollients in ultraviolet therapy of psoriasis. Br J Dermatol 130:361–365
5. Cole C (1994) Multicenter evaluation of sunscreen UVA protectiveness with the protection factor test method. J Am Acad Dermatol 30:729–736
6. McKinlay A, Diffey B (1987) A reference spectrum for ultraviolet-induced erythema in human skin. CIE J 6:17–22
7. Wolf P, Maier H, Müllegger RR et al (2000) Topical treatment with liposomes containing T4 endonuclease V protects human skin in vivo from ultraviolet-induced upregulation of interleukin-10 and tumor necrosis factor-α. J Invest Dermatol 114:149–156
8. Robb JL, Simpson LA, Tunstall DF (1994) Scattering & absorption of UV radiation by sunscreens containing fine particle and pigmentary titanium dioxide. Drug Cosmet Ind 154:32–39
9. Woodruff J (1994) Formulating sun care products with micronised oxides. Cosmet Toiletries Manufacture Worldwide 1:179–185
10. Ahene AB, Saxena S, Nacht S (1994) Photoprotection of solubilized and microdispersed melanin particles. In: Zeise L, Chedekel MR, Fitzpatrick TB (eds) Melanin: its role in human photoprotection. Valdenmar, Overland Park, Kansas, pp 255–269
11. Césarini JP, Msika P (1994) Photoprotection from UV-induced pigmentations and melanin introduced in sunscreens. In: Zeise L, Chedekel MR, Fitzpatrick TB (eds) Melanin: its role in human photoprotection. Valdenmar, Overland Park, Kansas, pp 239–244
12. Schauder S, Schrader A, Ippen H (1996) Göttinger Liste 1996. Sonnenschutzkosmetik in Deutschland. Blackwell, Berlin
13. Johnson JA, Fusaro RM (1993) Therapeutic potential of dihydroxyacetone. J Am Acad Dermatol 29:284–285
14. Potten CS, Chadwick CA, Cohen AJ et al (1993) DNA damage in UV-irradiated human skin in vivo: automated direct measurement by image analysis (thymine dimers) compared with indirect measurement (unscheduled DNA synthesis) and protection by 5-methoxypsoralen. Int J Radiat Biol 63:313–324
15. Autier P, Dore JF, Schifflers E et al (1995) Melanoma and use of sunscreens: an EORTC case-control study in Germany, Belgium and France. Int J Cancer 61:749–755
16. Gilchrest BA, Park HY, Eller MS, Yaar M (1996) Mechanisms of ultraviolet light-induced pigmentation. Photochem Photobiol 63:1–10
17. Gilchrest BA, Zhai S, Eller MS, Yarosh DB, Yaar M (1993) Treatment of human melanocytes and S91 melanoma cells with the DNA repair enzyme T4 endonuclease V enhances melanogenesis after ultraviolet radiation. J Invest Dermatol 101:666–672
18. Eller MS, Yaar M, Gilchrest B (1994) DNA damage and melanogenesis. Nature 372:413–414
19. Darr D, Dunston S, Faust H, Pinnel S (1996) Effectiveness of antioxidants (vitamin C and E) with and without sunscreens as topical photoprotectants. Acta Derm Venereol 76:264–268
20. Kripke ML, Cox PA, Alas LG, Yarosh DB (1992) Pyrimidine dimers in DNA initiate systemic immunosuppression in UV-irradiated mice. Proc Natl Acad Sci USA 89:7516–7520

21. Wolf P, Yarosh DB, Kripke ML (1993) Effects of sunscreens and a DNA excision repair enzyme on ultraviolet radiation-induced inflammation, immune suppression, and cyclobutane pyrimidine dimer formation in mice. J Invest Dermatol 101:523–527

22. Wolf P, Cox P, Yarosh DB, Kripke ML (1995) Sunscreens and T4N5 liposomes differ in their ability to protect against UV-induced sunburn cell formation, alterations of dendritic epidermal cells, and local suppression of contact hypersensitivity. J Invest Dermatol 104:287–292

23. Yarosh D, Alas LG, Yee V et al (1992) Pyrimidine dimer removal enhanced by DNA repair liposomes reduces the incidence of UV skin cancer in mice. Cancer Res 52:4227–4231

24. Bito T, Ueda M, Nagano T, Fujii S, Ichihashi M (1995) Reduction of ultraviolet-induced skin cancer in mice by topical application of DNA excision repair enzymes. Photodermatol Photoimmunol Photomed 11:9–13

25. Stege H, Roza L, Vink AA et al (2000) Enzyme plus light therapy to repair DNA damage in ultraviolet-B-irradiated human skin. Proc Natl Acad Sci USA 97:1790–1795

26. Strickland FM, Pelley RP, Kripke ML (1994) Prevention of ultraviolet-induced suppression of contact and delayed type hypersensitivity by Aloa barbadensis gel extract. J Invest Dermatol 102:197–204

27. Strickland FM, Darvill A, Albersheim P, Eberhard S, Pauly M, Pelley RP (1999) Inhibition of UV-induced immune suppression and interleukin-10 production by plant oligosaccharides and polysaccharides. Photochem Photobiol 69:141–147

28. Gonzales S, Pathak MA, Cuevas J, Villarrubia VG, Fitzpatrick TB (1997) Topical or oral administration with an extract of Polypodium leucotomos prevents acute sunburn and psoralen-induced phototoxic reaction as well as depletion of Langerhans cells in human skin. Photodermatol Photoimmunol Photomed 13:50–60

29. Gonzales S, Pathak MA (1996) Inhibition of ultraviolet-induced formation of reactive oxygen species, lipid peroxidation, erythema, and skin photosensitization by Polypodium leucotomos. Photodermatol Photoimmunol Photomed 12:45–56

30. Mathews-Roth MM, Pathak MA, Fitzpatrick TB, Harber LC, Kass EH (1970) Beta-carotene as a photoprotective agent in erythropoietic protoporphyria. N Engl J Med 282:1231–1234

31. Stahl W, Heinrich U, Jungmann H, Sies H, Tronnier H (2000) Carotenoids and carotenoids plus vitamin E protect against ultraviolet light-induced erythema in humans. Am J Clin Nutr 71:795–798

32. Mathews-Roth MM, Rosner B, Benfell K, Roberts JE (1994) A double-blind study of cysteine photoprotection in erythropoietic protoporphyria. Photodermatol Photoimmunol Photomed 10:244–248

33. Agarwal R, Mukhtar H (1996) Chemoprevention of photocarcinogenesis. Photchem Photobiol 63:440–444

34. Robson J, Diffey B (1990) Textiles and sun protection. Photodermatol Photoimmunol Photomed 7:32–34

35. Kligman LH, Akin FJ, Kligman AM (1982) Prevention of ultraviolet damage to the dermis of hairless mice by sunscreens. J Invest Dermatol 78:181–189

36. Kligman LH, Akin FJ, Kligman AM (1980) Sunscreens prevent ultraviolet photocarcinogenesis. J Am Acad Dermatol 3:30–35

37. Synder DS, May M (1975) Ability of PABA to protect mammalian skin from ultraviolet light-induced skin tumors and actinic damage. J Invest Dermatol 65:543–546

38. Ananthaswamy HN, Loughlin SM, Cox P, Evans RL, Ullrich SE, Kripke ML (1997) Sunlight and skin cancer: inhibition of p53 mutations in UV-irradiated mouse skin by sunscreens. Nat Med 3:510–514

39. Stern RS, Weinstein MC, Baker SG (1986) Risk reduction for nonmelanoma skin cancer with childhood sunscreen use. Arch Dermatol 122:537–545

40. Thompson SC, Jolley D, Marks R (1993) Reduction of solar keratoses by regular sunscreen use. N Engl J Med 329:1147–1151

41. Hunter DJ, Colditz GA, Stampfer MJ, Rosner B, Willet WC, Speizer FE (1990) Risk factors for basal cell carcinoma in a prospective cohort of women. Ann Epidemiol Publ Hlth 1:13–23
42. Donawho C, Wolf P (1996) Sunburn, sunscreen, and melanoma. Curr Opin Oncol 8:159–166
43. Wolf P (1999) What can sunscreens do against melanoma? Curr Pract Med 2:27–30
44. Autier P, Dore JF, Cattaruzza MS et al (1999) Sunscreen use, wearing clothes, and number of nevi in 6- to 7-year-old European children. European Organization for Research and Treatment of Cancer Melanoma Cooperative Group. J Natl Cancer Inst 90:1873–1880
45. Roberts LK, Stanfield JW (1995) Suggestion that sunscreen use is a melanoma risk factor is based on inconclusive evidence. Melanoma Res 5:377–378 (letter)
46. Holman CDJ, Armstrong BK, Heenan PJ (1986) Relationship of cutaneous malignant melanoma to individual sunlight-exposure habits. J Natl Cancer Inst 76:403–414
47. Setlow RB, Grist E, Thompson K, Woodhead AD (1993) Wavelengths effective in induction of malignant melanoma. Proc Natl Acad Sci USA 90:6666–6670
48. Setlow RB, Woodhead AD (1994) Temporal changes in the incidence of malignant melanoma: explanation from action spectra. Mutat Res 307:365–374
49. Autier P, Dore JF, Lejeune F et al (1995) Cutaneous malignant melanoma and exposure to sunlamps or sunbeds: an EORTC multicenter case-control study in Belgium, France and Germany. Int J Cancer 58:809–813
50. Westerdahl J, Olsson H, Masback A et al (1995) Use of sunbeds or sunlamps and malignant melanoma in Southern Sweden. Am J Epidemiol 140:691–699
51. Wolf P, Donawho CK, Kripke ML (1993) Analysis of the protective effect of different sunscreens on ultraviolet radiation-induced local and systemic suppression of contact hypersensitivity and inflammatory responses in mice. J Invest Dermatol 100:254–259
52. Wolf P, Donawho CK, Kripke ML (1994) Effect of sunscreens on UV radiation-induced enhancement of melanoma growth in mice. J Natl Cancer Inst 86:99–105
53. Wolf P, Kripke ML (1996) Sunscreens and immunosuppression. J Invest Dermatol 106:1152–1153 (letter)
54. Granstein RD (1995) Evidence that sunscreens prevent UV radiation-induced immunosuppression in humans. Arch Dermatol 131:1201–1204
55. Wolf P, Kripke ML (1997) Immune aspects of sunscreens. In: Gasparro F (ed) Sunscreen photobiology: molecular, cellular and physiological aspects. Springer, Berlin Heidelberg New York, pp 99–126
56. Roberts LK, Beasley DG (1995) Commercial sunscreen lotions prevent ultraviolet-radiation-induced immune suppression of contact hypersensitivity. J Invest Dermatol 105:339–344
57. Bestak R, Barnetson RSC, Nearn MR, Halliday GM (1995) Sunscreen protection of contact hypersensitivity responses from chronic solar-simulated ultraviolet irradiation correlates with the absorption spectrum of the sunscreen. J Invest Dermatol 105:345–351
58. Walker SL, Young AR (1997) Sunscreens offer the same UVB protection factors for inflammation and immunosuppression in the mouse. J Invest Dermatol 108:133–138
59. Whitemore SE, Morison WL (1995) Prevention of UVB-induced immunosuppression in humans by a high sun protection factor sunscreen. Arch Dermatol 131:1128–1133
60. Mastalier U, Kerl H, Wolf P (1998) Clinical, laboratory, phototest and phototherapy findings in polymorphic light eruption: a retrospective study of 133 patients. Eur J Dermatol 8:554–559
61. Stenberg C, Larkö O (1985) Sunscreen application and its importance for the sun protection factor. Arch Dermatol 121:1400–1402

62. Bech-Thomsen N, Wulf HG (1992/1993) Sunbathers' application of sunscreen is prob-
    ably inadequate to obtain the sun protection factor assigned to the preparation. Pho-
    todermatol Photoimmunol Photomed 9:242–244
63. Walker SL, Morris J, Chu AC, Young AR (1994) Relationship between the ability of
    sunscreens containing 2-ethylhexyl-4'-methoxycinnamate to protect against inflam-
    mation, depletion of epidermal Langerhans (Ia$^+$) cells and suppression of alloactivat-
    ing capacity of murine skin in vivo. J Photochem Photobiol B Biol 22:29–36

V Photodiagnostic procedures in daily practice

16 Photodiagnostic Modalities

Norbert J. Neumann, Percy Lehmann

Contents

Introduction

Diagnosis of photodermatoses is based on the patient's history, morphology of the lesions, histopathology, and the results of phototesting. However, generally accepted guidelines for phototesting are still lacking. Laboratory data may help to exclude differential diagnoses, e.g., porphyrias. In most photodermatoses, however, they are of no help. Since skin lesions often subside rapidly after sun exposure, it is desirable to induce the dermatosis in a given test area with appropriate test protocols. This is most important in patients with a vague medical history of sun sensitivity without pertinent skin lesions. Progress has been made to induce a variety of photodermatoses or photoaggravated dermatoses, e.g., polymorphous light eruption, hydroa vacciniforme, chronic actinic dermatitis (including persistent light eruption), solar urticaria, and lupus erythematosus [10–14] in loco.

Material and Methods

At our department of dermatology, all patients with a history of photosensitivity undergo a multistep phototest workup including the following procedures:

I Determination of threshold doses for erythema [24] (minimal erythema dose of ultraviolet radiation B, MED UVB) and pigmentation (immediate pigment darkening, IPD, minimal tanning dose, MTD)

II Reproduction of specific skin lesions by provocative phototesting with standardized irradiation protocols
III Identification of photosensitizers by photopatch test and systemic photochallenge

In the following our experience gained with this workup in a large number of patients with different photosensitivity disorders is described.

UV Sources and Dosimetry

A high-intensity monochromator (Dermolum HI, Müller, Moosinning, Germany) is used for determination of action spectra in solar urticaria. Large doses of polychromatic UVA are applied by a high-pressure metal halide source (UVA-SUN 3000, Mutzhas, Munich, Germany), which has the advantage of a high-irradiance in the UVA band without measurable UVB irradiation [19]. The apparatus is suitable for irradiating large test areas. At a distance of 30 cm, 100 J/cm^2 UVA can be applied within 25 min. The UVASUN proved very useful in experimental reproduction of UVA-sensitive dermatoses. For polychromatic UVB, a bank of ten fluorescent bulbs (Philips TL 20 W/, Hamburg, Germany) is used (UV 800, Waldmann, Villingen-Schwenningen, Germany). The emission spectrum reaches from 285 to 350 nm with a maximum between 310 and 315 nm. At a distance of 30 cm, an average minimal erythema dose (MED UVB) is applied in less than 40 s. Equipped with fluorescent UVA bulbs (Philips TLK 40 W/09 N), the UV 800 serves as the light source for irradiating the photopatch test. The spectral energy distribution reaches from 315 to 395 nm with a peak intensity between 355 and 365 nm. At a distance of 20 cm, 10 J/cm^2 UVA is applied in less than approximately 25 min.

Beside the monochromator, a slice projector with a halogen lamp and cut off filters (Schott, Mainz, Germany) may be used for testing with visible light, e.g., in solar urticaria.

A thermopile attached to a digital wattmeter (Müller, Moosinning, Germany) serves for dosimetry of the monochromator. A UV meter with separate UV detectors for UVA and UVB (Centra, Osram, Munich, Germany) is used to determine the UV irradiance of the UVASUN and UV 800.

Polymorphous Light Eruption

All patients with a history suggestive of polymorphous light eruption (PLE) were tested according to a standard procedure [5, 14]. Best time for testing is early spring before the first intensive sun exposures (Table 1). MED UVB, IPD, and MTD were within the normal range compared with skin-type-matched normal controls. Provocative phototesting was successful in 85 % of the tested patients. In 80 % of these patients, it was induced with UVA alone, in 8 % with UVB alone, and in 12 % both UVA and UVB induced characteristic lesions. Provocative phototesting also enabled us to evaluate the different morphological

Table 1. Test protocol for experimental reproduction of polymorphous light eruption (PLE)

Test site	Area previously exposed
Size of test field	5×8 cm
Light sources	UVA: UVASUN 3000; UVB: UV 800, Philips TL20 W/12
Dose	$3 \times 60 - 100$ J/cm^2 UVA, 3×1.5 MED UVB
Readings	24 – 72 h after irradiation

variants. Most common was the papular type (70 %), followed by the plaque type (16 %). Other variants occurred rarely and included ictus (insect bite)-like type (6 %), erythema multiforme type (3 %), vesiculobullous type (3 %), and hemorrhagic type (2 %).

Erythropoietic Porphyria

UVA and visible light between 400 nm and 600 nm provoke the typical skin lesions of erythropoietic porphyria (EPP) [13]. Unfortunately, in this range of wavelengths, the intensity of irradiation is insufficient in the commonly used irradiation sources. Following our experience, employing 30 – 60 J/cm^2 UVA (UVASUN 3000) is useful to provoke the burning prickling typical for EPP (Table 2) [17]. However, artificially induced skin lesions are often non-specific.

Table 2. Test protocol for experimental reproduction of erythropoietic porphyria (EPP)

Test site	Non-sun-exposed areas
Size of test field	5×8 cm
Light source	UVA: UVASUN 3000 monochromator
Dose	100 J/cm^2 UVA or more, up to eliciting of subjective symptoms 15 J/cm^2 of wavelengths between 380 and 800 nm
Readings	Immediately after and 24 h after irradiation

Hydroa Vacciniforme

Patients with this disease are rare. The induction of skin lesions with UVB as well as UVA has been reported in the literature. It seems likely that the UVA component in sunlight contains the active wavelengths to provoke hydroa vacciniforme in most patients. Our group reported the induction of lesions on the back and arms with repeated doses of 30, 50 and 75 J/cm^2 UVA and even in the oral mucosa with 10 J/cm² UVA [3]. The proposed test protocol is identical to the test protocol for Table 1 despite the differing test site, which in hydroa vacciniforme should be the back or dorsal forearms.

Solar Urticaria

It is usually easy to diagnose solar urticaria (SU) because it can be induced in every SU patient quickly with appropriate testing (Table 3). However, there are various subgroups of patients. Some react only to UVA, others only to visible light, and others to a much broader spectrum. In special settings, inhibition spectra and augmentation can be studied. Injection of preirradiated serum or plasma can also induce lesions. Minimal whealing doses are frequently low; some patients react to doses as low as 0.5 J/cm² UVA or 1.5 J/cm² UVB. Determination of the minimal whealing doses for different wavelengths also is very valuable in order to prove the efficacy of different treatment modalities. In any case, it is advisable to determine the action spectrum [7].

Table 3. Test protocol for experimental reproduction of solar urticaria (SU)

Test site	Non-sun-exposed area (sacral/gluteal area)
Test size	Small (2 × 2 cm)
Light sources	UVA, UVB, UVC, visible light: Monochromator Dermolum HI UVA: UVASUN 3000 (330–460 nm) UVB: UV 800 Philips TL 20 W/12 (285–345 nm) Visible light: Slide projector (> 400 nm) with different absorption filters (Schott, Mainz, Germany)
Dose	Varied with the individual
Readings	Immediately, and up to 1 h after irradiation

Chronic Actinic Dermatitis

Chronic actinic dermatitis (CAD) is defined clinically by chronic dermatitis on skin exposed to the sun, histologically by spongiotic dermatitis, and photobiologically by experimental provocation of spongiotic dermatitis with UVB and often longer wavelengths in the absence of a photoallergen. The traditional names, persistent light eruption, photosensitive eczema, photosensitivity dermatitis, and actinic reticuloid, recently have been considered variants of this condition [18, 21]. Characteristically, the skin of these patients is extremely photosensitive, and one should be able to induce eczematous lesions in every patient via phototesting (Table 4). Additionally, a patch test and photopatch test should be performed, as positive results occur frequently in these patients. Also, in contrast to most other photodermatoses, this is a condition where a lowered threshold dose for the UVB erythema (MED UVB) is a frequent diagnostic sign.

Table 4. Test protocol for experimental reproduction of chronic actinic dermatitis (CAD)

Test site	Uninvolved non-sun-exposed skin
Test size	5×8 cm
Light sources	UVA: UVASUN 3000 UVB: UV 800, Philips TL20 W/12 Visible light: Slide projector with appropriate filters (Schott, Mainz, Germany)
Dose	0.5, 1, 5, 10, 20, 30 J/cm^2 UVA 0.5, 1, 1.5 MED UVB 5, 10, 30 J/cm^2 visible light
Readings	24, 48, 72 h, up to 1 week
Additionally	Patch test, photopatch test

Photoallergy

An outstanding photoallergic example was the epidemic appearance of a photo-allergy due to tetrachlorsalicylanilide (TCSA), which was used as disinfectant in soaps and other toiletries in England 1960–1993. The Austrian, Swiss, and German Photopatch Test Study Group (DAPT) reported that nonsteroidal anti-inflammatory drugs, disinfectants, sunscreens, phenothiazines, and fragrances contemporarily are the most relevant photosensitizers [6, 12, 20, 22].

Photopatch Test

Stephan Epstein emphasized early the eminent role of photopatch testing (PPT) for the identification of photosensitizers [2]. Nevertheless, until the early 1980s the photopatch test procedure was not standardized and varied between countries and dermatological centers with respect to test tray, substance concentrations, vehicles, as well as to the readings and the classification of test reactions [4, 6].

The first standard procedure for photopatch testing was defined by the Scandinavian Photodermatitis Research Group (SPDRG) in 1982 [8]. Guided by the SPDRG, 45 dermatological centers from Austria, Germany, and Switzerland founded the DAPT in 1984 [12]. Their standardized test procedure is summarized in Tables 5–7.

Table 5. Protocol for photopatch testing

Patch test of test materials for 24 h on the upper back by small Finn chambers
After removal of patches, irradiation with 10 J/cm2 UVA (UV 800, Philips TLK 40 W/09, 320–395 nm)
Reading immediately, 24, 48, and 72 h. If necessary, later readings up to 3 weeks
Controls: Patch test without irradiation, irradiation without patch test

Table 6. Photopatch test reaction gradings

0	No reaction
1+	Erythema
2+	Erythema and infiltrate
3+	Erythema and papulovesicles
4+	Erythema, bullae, or erosions

Table 7. Classification of test reactions

Contact reaction	Every positive reaction in the control area other than 1+ immediately after removal of the test tray
Phototoxic Reaction	1+ or 2+, immediate or delayed, as decrescendo reaction
Photoallergic reaction	3+ or 4+, delayed, as crescendo reaction

If the test substance could not penetrate the stratum corneum during the test period, the photopatch test sometimes revealed a false negative result. In such cases, the photoscratch or the photoprick test could be a useful alternative test procedures to detect relevant photoallergens.

Photoscratch and Photoprick Testing

The photoscratch and photoprick tests are modifications of the PPT. In contrast to the PPT, the stratum corneum has to be perforated (e.g., by a lancet) in both test procedures, before the test substance could be applied. Thus, the supposed photosensitizers come in contact with the epidermis without the penetration process through the stratum corneum [1, 23].

Systemic Photochallenge

Systemically applied drugs predominantly revealed false-negative photopatch test results because metabolites are probably the relevant photosensitizers, instead of the topically applied test substances themselves. Therefore, the systemic photochallenge described in Table 8 might be a helpful test procedure [10, 11].

Table 8. Test protocol for systemic photochallenge

Administration of, if feasible, twofold therapeutic dose via the usual mode of application (p. o., s. c. i. m.)
Irradiation (10 J/cm^2 UVA) of different test fields (5 × 5 cm) prior to medication and, according to the pharmacokinetics of the drug, at different times thereafter, usually 1, 2, 4, 8 h
Readings on 3 successive days and up to 3 weeks

Lupus Erythematosus

Sunlight is a well-established factor in induction and exacerbation of all lupus erythematosus (LE) subsets [9, 14–16]. Photosensitivity, although poorly defined, is also one of 11 criteria of the American Rheumatism Association for the diagnosis of systemic LE. In 1993, Kind et al. published [9] a specific standardized protocol for phototesting of LE (Table 9). In our series, skin lesions clinically and histologically compatible with LE were induced in 64 % of patients with subacute cutaneous LE, 42 % of patients with discoid LE, and 25 % of patients with systemic LE. The highest rate of positive test reactions was seen in LE of tumidus type, namely 78 %, a hitherto underestimated feature of this subset. The action spectrum of the induced lesions was within the UVB range in 33 % of patients, in the UVA range in 14 %, and in the UVB and UVA range in 53 %. Characteristically, after provocative testing, LE lesions developed slower than in other photodermatoses. In some patients typical discoid lesions persisted for weeks and even months. Threshold doses for erythema and pigmentation were within the normal range.

Table 9. Test protocol for experimental reproduction of lupus erythematosus (LE)

Test site	Back or upper forearms
Size of test field	5×8 cm
Light sources	UVA: UVASUN 3000 UVB: UV 800, Philips TL20 W/12
Dose	$3 \times 60 - 100$ J/cm^2 UVA 3×1.5 MED UVB
Readings	24–72 h after irradiation, up to 3 weeks after irradiation

Conclusion

It is desirable to induce specific skin lesions of a given photodermatosis, especially when there are no other diagnostic laboratory tests and the patients present no skin lesions when examined in the laboratory. In our laboratory, one of our main efforts over the past few years has been to develop specific standardized test protocols for photosensitivity disorders. Provocative phototesting is the most important diagnostic procedure, and it has established not only a diagnosis with certainty, but also action spectra can be worked out and a objective means of monitoring efficacy of therapeutic measures is provided. Photopatch testing and systemic photochallenge are also instruments of provocative phototesting, which serve to reproduce the dermatosis in loco and, furthermore, to identify the photosensitizing agents. Determination of threshold doses for erythema and pigmentation serves as a screening for high photosensitivity and is a prerequisite for further phototesting. Pathological responses in threshold testing occur mainly in patients with chronic actinic dermatitis (including persistent light reactors). In other photodermatoses, erythemal and pigmentary responses to UV light are within the normal range when compared with normal skin-matched controls.

References

1. Bourrain JL, Paillet C, Woodward C, Beani JC, Amblard P (1997) Diagnosis of photosensitivity to flupenthixol by photoprick testing. Photodermatol Photoimmunol Photomed 14:159–161
2. Epstein S (1964) The photopatch test. Its technique, manifestations, and significance. Ann Allergy 22:1–11
3. Galosi A, Plewig G, Ring J, Meurer M, Schmöckel C, Schurig V, Dorn M (1985) Experimentelle Auslösung von Hauterscheinungen bei Hydroa vacciniformia. Hautarzt 36:449–452
4. Hölzle E, Plewig G, Hofmann C, Braun-Falco O (1985) Photopatch testing. Results of a survey on test procedures and experimental findings. Zentralbl Hautkr 151:361–366
5. Hölzle E, Plewig G, von Kries R, Lehmann P (1987) Polymorphous light eruption. J Invest Dermatol 88:32S–38S
6. Hölzle E, Neumann N, Hausen B, Przybilla B, Schauder S, Hönigsmann H, Bircher A, Plewig G (1991) Photopatch testing: the 5-year experience of the German, Austrian and Swiss photopatch test group. J Am Acad Dermatol 25:59–68
7. Horio T (1987) Solar urticaria-sun, skin and serum. Photodermatology 15:117
8. Jansen CT, Wennersten G, Tystedt 1, Thune P, Brodthagen H (1982) The scandinavian standard photopatch test procedure. Contact Dermatitis 8:155–158
9. Kind P, Lehmann P, Plewig G (1993) Phototesting in Lupus erythematosus. J Invest Dermatol 100:53–57
10. Lehmann P, Hölzle E, Plewig G (1988) Photoallergie auf Neotri mit Kreuzreaktion auf Teneretic Nachweis durch systemische Photoprovokation. Hautarzt 39:38–41
11. Lehmann P, Hölzle E, von Kries R, Plewig G (1986) Übersicht – Neue Konzepte. Lichtdiagnostische Verfahren bei Patienten mit Verdacht auf Photodermatosen. Zentralbl Hautkr 152:667–682
12. Lehmann P (1991) Die deutschsprachige Arbeitsgemeinschaft Photopatch-Test (DAPT). Hautarzt 41:295–297
13. Lehmann P (1994) Photodiagnostische Testverfahren. Aktuel Dermatol 20:41–46
14. Lehmann P (1995) Photodiagnostische Testverfahren bei Lichtdermatosen: Polymorphe Lichtdermatose, Lupus erythematodes und Lichturtikaria. In: Plewig G, Kor ting HC (eds) Fortschritte der praktischen Dermatologie und Venerologie. Springer, Berlin Heidelberg New York, pp 162–167
15. Lehmann P (1996) Photosensitivität des Lupus erythematodes. Aktuel Dermatol 22:47–51
16. Lehmann P, Hölzle E, Kind P, Goerz G, Plewig G (1990) Experimental reproduction of skin lesions in lupus erythernatosus by UVB and UVA radiation. J Am Acad Dermatol 22:181–187
17. Lehmann P, Scharffetter K, Kind P, Goerz G (1991) Erythropoetische Protoporphyrie: Synopsis von 20 Patienten. Hautarzt 42:570–574
18. Milde P, Hölzle E, Neumann N, Lehmann P, Trautvetter U, Plewig G (1991) Chronische aktinische Dermatitis. Hautarzt 42:617–622
19. Mutzhas MF, Hölzle E, Hofmann C, Plewig G (1981) A new apparatus with high radiation energy between 320–460 nm: physical description and dermatological applications. J Invest Dermatol 76:42–47
20. Neumann NJ, Hölzle E, Plewig G, Schwarz T, Panizzon RG, Breit R, Ruzicka T, Lehmann P (2000) Photopatch testing: the 12-year experience of the German, Austrian, and Swiss Photopatch Test Group. J Am Acad Dermatol 42:183–192

21. Norris PG, Hawk JLM (1990) Chronic actinic dermatitis. A unifying concept. Arch Dermatol 126:376–378
22. Rünger TM, Lehmann P, Neumann NJ, Matthies C, Schauder S, Ortel B, Münzberger C Hölzle E (1995) Empfehlung einer Photopatch-Test Standardreihe durch die deutschsprachige Arbeitsgruppe, Photopatch-Test. Hautarzt 46:240–243
23. Schauder S (1990) Der modifizierte intradermale Test im Vergleich zu anderen Verfahren zum Nachweis von phototoxischen und photoallergischen Arzneireaktionen. Z Hautkr 65:247–255
24. Wucherpfennig V (1942) Zur Messung und Bemessung des Ultraviolett. Klin Wochenschr 21:926–930

17 The Photopatch Test

Erhard Hölzle

Contents

Introduction

The photopatch test serves as a tool to diagnose photosensitivity due to photo-toxic or photoallergic substances. Photoallergic reactions require sensitization of the patient before the reaction can be elicited. Phototoxic reactions already occur at first contact with the photosensitizer. Phototoxic reactions are defined as photochemical processes; however, the individual susceptibility varies greatly among patients. The relevance of positive test reactions only can be evaluated concerning the clinical features and history of the patients.

After the introduction of sulfonamides, photoallergic reactions were observed for the first time [1, 2, 3]. Later, phenothiazines gained interest as pho-tosensitizers. To examine such patients, Schulz et al. [21] in 1956 and Epstein and Rowe [4] were the first to devise the method of photopatch testing. In the years between 1962 and 1970 halogenated salicylanilides were identified as the cause of widespread outbreaks of photoallergy [2, 18, 23]. The photosensitivity was traced to the use of deodorant soaps and cosmetics containing halogenated salicylanilides as antimicrobial agents. Workmen manufacturing the soaps were mainly afflicted. In this setting, persistent light reactivity was first described [24].

Photopatch testing is a well-established method to identify phototoxic or photoallergic substances. Until the early 1980s the procedure was, however, not standardized. The first attempt to devise a standard method was initiated by the Scandinavian Photodermatitis Research Group (SPRG) [11, 22]. Following this example in Germany, Austria and Swizerland, the „deutschsprachige Arbeitsge-meinschaft Photopatch-Test" (DAPT, German for photopatch test working group) was founded in 1984 [13] and is still actively working [17]. This group established a standardized protocol for photopatch testing. The procedure described herein is based on this protocol [7, 9, 10].

Indications for the Photopatch Test

The photopatch test is indicated whenever a phototoxic or photoallergic reaction is suspected. Disease entities of the chronic actinic dermatitis spectrum are also indications. Other photodermatoses such as polymorphous light eruption, hydroa vacciniforme, solar urticaria, or porphyrias are diagnosed according to specific criteria of these entities and do not represent an indication for the photopatch test.

For patients who present with unclear photoreactions that cannot be associated with a genuine photodermatosis, photopatch testing should be performed as well. This holds true in particular for patients with eczema in a photodistribution, or those with exacerbated sunburn reactions. Such lesions are suspicious for photoallergic or phototoxic reactions, respectively, and a careful history should evaluate all drugs and topical preparations. Among those, the photosensitizer should be identified in the photopatch test. Following such stringent criteria for photopatch testing, unnecessary test procedures are avoided and positive test reactions obtained are highly relevant for the patients.

Test Substances

Test materials are applied to the back via small aluminum chambers (Finn-Chambers Scanpor, Hermal, Reinbek bei Hamburg) in a duplicate set, one for irradiation, the other as a control. Patches to be irradiated are left on the skin for 24 h; control patches are applied either 24 or 48 h optionally. Non-irradiated patches are used as controls to exclude non-photoinduced, plain contact sensitivity. The procedure of photopatch testing is summarized in Table 1.

Table 1. Photopatch test procedure

Test site	Back
Application of test substances	24 h, small Finn-chambers (Scanpor)
UV source	Fluorescence bulbs (Philips TL-09 N 320–400 nm)
UV dose	5 J/cm^2 UVA<MED UVA
Reading	Immediately, 24, 48, and 72 h after irradiation
Control	Unirradiated patch test

Basically, the prerequisites required for patch testing are also applicable in photopatch testing. The test area must be non-involved clear skin. Topical corticosteroids as well as intense UV exposure have to be avoided 3 weeks prior to testing. Systemic corticosteroids and antihistamines have to be withdrawn 1 week before testing.

Table 2 shows the standard photopatch test substances currently proposed by the photopatch test working group. In addition, tribromsalan, chlorpromazine hydrochloride, thiourea, and olaquindox may be used in special cases. Further drugs or topical preparations used by the patient with a potential of photosensitization also should be tested.

Table 2. Photopatch test substances

Substance	Concentration[a]
Tetrachlorsalicylanilide	0.1 %
5-Brom-4'-chlorsalicylanilide	1 %
Hexachlorophene	1 %
Bithionol	1 %
Sulfanilamide	5 %
Promethazine hydrochloride	0.1 %
Quinidine sulfate	1 %
Musk ambrette	5 %
Fragrance mixture	8 %
4-Aminobenzoic acid	10 %
2-Ethyl-4-dimethyl-aminobenzoate	10 %
1-(4-Isopropylphenyl)-3-phenyl-1,3-propandione	10 %
4-tert-Butyl-4'-methoxy-dibenzoylmethane	10 %
Isoamyl-4-methoxycinnamate	10 %
2-Ethylhexyl-4-methoxycinnamate	10 %
3-(4-Methylbenzyliden)-camphor	10 %
2-Phenyl-5-benzimidazol sulfonic acid	10 %
Oxybenzone	10 %
Sulisobenzone	10 %

[a] All substances in petroleum.

Irradiation and Dosimetry

For irradiation broadband UVA fluorescent tubes are used (Philips TL 09 N 320–400 nm). The UVA dose recommended by the DAPT used to be 10 J/cm^2. In a recent agreement the date can changed to 5 J/cm^2, which is how concordant to most other study groups. In patients with chronic actinic dermatitis highly sensitive against UVA, UVA doses below the minimal erythemal dose UVA have to be used to irradiate the photopatch test.

Reading

Test sites are evaluated before and immediately after irradiation as well as 24, 48, and 72 h later. Control sites are read shortly after removal of the patches as well as 24 and 48 h later. If control patches are applied for only 24 h, a 72-h reading is also done. Evaluation of test reactions is slightly different from the procedure applied to standard patch testing. If erythema only (+) appears in the irradiated patch site, it is read as a relevant reaction and not dismissed, as it were according to the standards of patch testing. Criteria for grading the test reactions are given in Table 3.

In contrast to usual patch testing, grading of photopatch tests is only based on morphological criteria and does not include quantitative aspects. By grading the reactions each day for up to 4 days, reaction patterns can be defined. These

Table 3. Grading photopatch test reactions

Grade	Reaction
+	Erythema
++	Erythema and infiltrate
+++	Erythema, infiltrate, papulovesicles
++++	Erosions, bullae

patterns are helpful in differentiating between phototoxic and photoallergic reactions [16]. Phototoxic reactions are mainly characterized by a maximum in the beginning with a following decrescendo pattern within 24–72 h. Typical are erythema and infiltration, which may exacerbate to bullae. Some phototoxic agents cause an immediate erythema and whealing associated with a burning discomfort ("smarting"). Such reactions occur after testing with coal tar, chlorpromazine, or benoxaprofen. Another reaction pattern presumably caused by phototoxic mechanisms shows a delayed onset 24 h after testing with a plateau-like course consisting only of erythema and infiltration. Examples for such a delayed and prolonged plateau-like pattern are phenothiazine, carprofen, and tiaprofenic acid. Photoallergic reactions are similar to contact allergic reactions and show a delayed onset with a crescendo course. The morphological picture is composed of erythema, infiltration, and papulovesicles. Pruritus is frequent. In cases of doubt, histopathological examination may be helpful to differentiate between photoallergic and phototoxic reactions [12].

Test reactions exceeding erythema (+) in non-irradiated control sites are indicative for plain-contact reactions. In such a case, the reaction on the irradiated site, whatever it may be, is disregarded and the diagnosis is contact sensitization. The simultaneous occurrence of contact and photocontact reactions, as well as the phenomenon of photo-augmentation, is disregarded according to the guidelines of the photopatch test working group.

Relevance of Test Results

Differentiation between phototoxic and photoallergic reactions and judgment of the relevance of a positive test reaction are the most frequent problems in evaluating photopatch test reactions. A positive history of the patient concerning the reacting substance is mandatory in diagnosing relevant photosensitization. Not infrequently, reactions defined as photoallergic by pattern analysis lack a positive history regarding the substance tested. One example is the observation that patients with a contact sensitivity against thiomersal exhibit positive photoallergic reactions against piroxicam [15]. In these cases, it was shown that photoproducts derived from piroxicam upon irradiation exhibit cross-reactivity to thiomersal.

False-negative test results may be observed when systemic drugs are tested. In such cases, modified test procedures are necessary. If lack of penetration of the test substance through the stratum corneum is the problem, tape stripping before applying the test substance or irradiated scratch or prick tests may lead to positive results [19, 20]. If a metabolite of the drug is the true photosensitizer, systemic photoprovocation is the only method to identify the photosensitizing agent [5, 6, 8, 14].

References

1. Burckhardt W (1941) Untersuchungen über die Photoaktivität einiger Sulfanilamide. Dermatologica 83:63–68
2. Calnan CA, Harmann RRM, Wells GC (1961) Photodermatitis from soaps. Br Med J 11:1266
3. Epstein S (1939) Photoallergy and primary photosensitivity to sulfanilamide. J Invest Dermatol 2:43–51
4. Epstein S, Rowe RJ (1957) Photoallergy and photocross-sensitivity to phenergan. J Invest Dermatol 29:319–326
5. Ferguson J, Johnson BE (1993) Clinical and laboratory studies of the photosensitizing potential of norfloxacin, a 4-quinolone broad-spectrum antibiotic. Br J Dermatol 128:185–195
6. Galosi A, Przybilla B, Ring J, Dorn M (1984) Systemische Photoprovokation mit Surgam. Allergologie 7:143–144
7. Hölzle E und die Mitglieder der Deutschsprachigen Arbeitsgemeinschaft Photopatch-Test (1991) Photopatch-Test: Ergebnisse der multizentrischen Studie. Aktuel Dermatol 17:117–123
8. Hölzle E, Neumann N, Hausen B, Przybilla B, Schauder S, Hönigsmann H, Bircher A, Plewig G (1991) Photopatch testing: the 5-year experience of the German, Austrian and Swiss photopatch test group. J Am Acad Dermatol 25:59–68
9. Hölzle E, Plewig G, Lehmann P (1986) Photodermatoses – diagnostic procedures and their interpretation. Photodermatology 4:109–114
10. Hölzle E, Rowold J, Peper S, Plewig G (1989) Die belichtete Epikutantestung. Allergologie 12:13–20
11. Jansen CT, Wennersten G, Tystedt I, Thune P, Brodthagen H (1982) The scandinavian standard photopatch test procedure. Contact Dermatitis 8:155–158
12. Jung EG, Hardmeier T (1967) Zur Histologie der photoallergischen Testreaktion. Dermatologica 135:243–252
13. Lehmann P (1990) Die Deutschsprachige Arbeitsgemeinschaft Photopatch-Test (DAPT). Hautarzt 41:295–297
14. Lehmann P, Hölzle E, von Kries R, Plewig G (1986) Lichtdiagnostische Verfahren bei Patienten mit Lichtdermatosen. Zentralbl Haut 152:667–682
15. Ljunggren B (1989) The piroxicam enigma. Photodermatology 6:151–154
16. Neumann N, Hölzle E, Lehmann P, Benedikter S, Tapernoux B, Plewig G (1994) Pattern analysis of photopatch test reactions. Photodermatol Photoimmunol Photomed 10:65–73
17. Neumann NJ, Hölzle E, Plewig G, Schwarz T, Panizzon RG, Breit R, Ruzicka T, Lehmann P (2000) Photopatch testing: the 12-year experience of the German, Austrian, and Swiss Photopatch Test Group. J Am Acad Dermatol 42:183–192
18. Osmundsen PE (1969) Contact photoallergy to tribromsalicylanilide. Br J Dermatol 81:429–434
19. Przybilla B (1987) Phototestungen bei Lichtdermatosen. Hautarzt 38:23s–28s
20. Schauder S (1990) Der modifizierte intradermale Test im Vergleich zu anderen Verfahren zum Nachweis von phototoxischen und photoallergischen Arzneireaktionen. Z Hautkr 65:247–255

21. Schulz KH, Wiskemann K, Wolf K (1956) Klinische und experimentelle Untersuchungen über die photodynamische Wirksamkeit von Phenothiazinderivaten, insbesondere Megaphen. Arch Klin Exp Dermatol 202:285–298
22. Thune A, Jansen C, Wennersten G, Rystedt I, Brodthagen H, McFadden N (1988) The Scandinavian multicenter photopatch test study 1980–1985: final report. Photodermatology 5:261–269
23. Wilkinson DS (1961) Photodermatitis due to Tetrachlorsalicylanilide. Br J Dermatol 73:213–219
24. Wilkinson DS (1962) Patch test reactions to certain halogenated salicylanilides. Br J Dermatol 74:302–306

18 Fluorescence Diagnosis with δ-Aminolevulinic Acid-Induced Porphyrins in Dermatology

Clemens Fritsch, Kerstin Lang, Klaus-Werner Schulte, Wilfried H.G. Neuse, Thomas Ruzicka, Percy Lehmann

Contents

Introduction and Historical Landmarks

Various examination methods are used in daily dermatological practice to assess the different types of skin diseases. Dermatoscopy is used to evaluate pigmented skin lesions mainly, the ultrasound is applied to reveal the pathology of lymph nodes and to measure the thickness of skin lesions such as sclerodermic or neoplastic ones. However, histopathological examination is the most important diagnostic procedure in dermatology to ensure the clinical diagnosis of any skin disease.

We would like to introduce a new diagnostic procedure, that is mainly used for tumor detection and for guidance of any tumor therapy, the fluorescence diagnosis with δ-aminolevulinic acid-induced porphyrins (FDAP). This diagnostic procedure enables the delineation of neoplastic and inflammatory tissues (e.g., psoriatic skin lesions) from the surrounding normal skin. In FDAP, the diseased skin (e.g., tumor) produces and accumulates high amounts of porphyrins out of the applied porphyrin prodrug δ-aminolevulinic acid (ALA). The porphyrin-enriched tissue then shows a specific red fluorescence when illuminated with a Wood's light [ultraviolet (UV) light].

The predominant uptake of a photosensitizer in the neoplastic tissue and its selective destruction by subsequent irradiation [principle of photodynamic therapy (PDT)] is a fantastic, but not a new, idea. The ability of several dyes (e.g., acridine) to sensitize microorganisms (e.g., paramecium) for their destruction by a following exposure to light was first mentioned in 1900 by Raab [50]. At that time, it was also recognized that the described reaction depends on oxygen, and it was therefore called "photodynamic action" or "photodynamic effect" [61]. In 1903, this photodynamic action was used to treat different skin diseases (i.e., condylomata lata, lupus vulgaris, and skin tumors) for the first time. Other indications tested for photodynamic action were herpes simplex, molluscum contagiosum, pityriasis versicolor, and psoriasis vulgaris [30, 60]. In those early days, eosin was applied as photosensitizer and irradiation was done with white light.

For optimization and standardization of the therapy, different photosensitizing substances, especially porphyrins, were rehearsed in the following years. The first experiments with the photosensitizer hematoporphyrin were done in 1911. Since then, porphyrins have remained the most interesting, effective, and examined substances in PDT.

Concerning the diagnostic potential of porphyrin molecules, the diagnosis of tumors was performed for the first time using hematoporphyrin in 1924 [49]. Hematoporphyrin caused a bright red fluorescence in the tumor tissues when illuminated with UV light. In the 1940s further examinations in experimentally induced sarcomas and mamma carcinomas confirmed the affinity of hematoporphyrin to neoplastic tissues measured by the typical red fluorescence [12]. In the 1950s it was shown that an intravenous application of hematoporphyrin in carcinoma patients led to a preferred accumulation of porphyrins in the tumor tissue. This was again proven by the characteristic red fluorescence during UV illumination [51]. The injection of chemical-purified hematoporphyrin revealed a less selective fluorescence in tumor tissue than injection of unpurified hematoporphyrin [48].

In 1960, Lipson et al. presented the hematoporphyrin derivative (HpD) that consists of a mixture of about ten porphyrin derivatives, dihematoporphyrin esters, and dihematoporphyrin ethers [40]. A preferential enrichment of HpD was found for squamous cell carcinomas and adenocarcinomas [27]. Bladder cancer and pulmonary carcinomas could effectively be detected and treated by intravenous application of HpD and subsequent illumination through a fiber optic device [10, 34]. Until the 1980s, HpD remained the most important photosensitizer in PDT.

Topically applied substances achieved an increasing interest because they avoided the highly generalized photosensitization known from the systematically administered photosensitizers. This disadvantage could be overcome by a "tumor-selective" photosensitization, which was introduced in 1990 by the

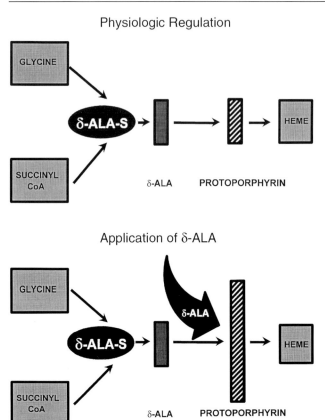

Fig. 1. Scheme of heme biosynthesis. δ-ALA is formed out of succinyl-CoA and glycine. Topical or systemic administration of δ-ALA bypasses the δ-ALA synthase, the limiting step in porphyrin biosynthesis. Consequently, high amounts of porphyrins, in particular protoporphyrin, are synthesized as potent photosensitizers

Canadian researchers around Kennedy [33]: the topical application of the "non-photosensitizing" δ-ALA. This most-important porphyrin precursor leads to an increasing production of porphyrins preferentially in neoplastic and fast proliferating tissues. The exogenous supply of the precursor bypasses the limiting step of the heme biosynthesis, the δ-ALA synthase (Fig. 1).

Over the last 10 years, various research groups confirmed the effectiveness of the topical δ-ALA PDT in the case of superficial skin tumors [8, 13, 17, 18, 20, 21, 57, 63]. Furthermore, there were sporadic reports on the successful use of systemic δ-ALA application in curative or palliative treatment of bronchial carcinomas, tumors of the gastrointestinal tract, and bladder cancer in animal studies as well as in clinical treatments [36, 41, 45, 52]. Finally, the porphyrin fluorescence induced by this new photosensitizer prodrug δ-ALA was used to detect tumors. Usually, the "tumor markers" used in fluorescence detection techniques have been porphyrin-mixtures such as HpD or Photofrin [1, 6, 37]. Although these substances allow a fluorescence description, e.g., in urothelial neoplasm, they have considerable disadvantages, such as a low tumor selectivity. Beyond this, the fluorescence-quantum-profit of the porphyrin mixture in the tissue is quite low and affords expensive techniques of photo-processing for the detection of the tumor fluorescence. Additionally, the systemic application of photosensitizers like Photofrin is always risky as far as phototoxic skin reactions are concerned, even though the substances are only used as a 20 % solution.

The topical use of δ-ALA, in particular in a 20 % mixture with a cream base, for detection of neoplastic tissue has considerable advantages in dermatology: the surrounding healthy skin is barely sensitized and there are no systemic side effects. Over the past few years, the term "photodynamic diagnosis" (PDD) was chosen for the detection of tumors using a photosensitizer and its fluorescence under UV light. Unfortunately, this term is not very suitable, because no reactive species, which would be necessary for a photodynamic reaction, are implicated in this fluorescence-detection technique. For this reason, we decided to introduce the term FDAP.

Fluorescence Diagnosis with δ-ALA-Induced Porphyrins

Physical Background of the Fluorescence in FDAP

The fluorescence detection is the principle basis of FDAP. Therefore, we would like to explain the physical essentials of the fluorescence and its attributes. Fluorescence is a subsiding light emission by atoms or molecules, which are stimulated by absorption of energy.

Absorption of Light. When light runs into a medium, one part of it is reflected, one part is absorbed by the medium and one part penetrates the medium. The absorbed light will be transferred into heat or another form of energy [10].

Semi-Stable Condition of Electrons. In general, material can be stimulated by electricity, light, or radio frequencies and transformed into a higher energy level or a stimulated electron level (semi-stable level). Collision of a molecule with other molecules leads to a quick transfer (approx. 10^{-11} s) of its pulsation energy to the surrounding molecules. The focus of the molecule (being in stimulated electron condition) moves stepwise back to the ground condition. The lifespan of the electron stimulation is sufficient to emit energy as fluorescence spontaneously (approx. 10^{-8} s). By this mechanism, the molecule turns into a higher pulsation level than that of the basic level (Frank-Condon principle). The intensity of the fluorescence Iα is generally proportional to the intensity of the incoming radiation Io and to the concentration of the fluorescing substance C. According to the laws of Lambert-Beer, the intensity ΔIα of the absorbed radiation of a substance is

$$\Delta I\alpha(v) = \alpha(v)\ Io\ (v)\ \Delta x$$

if ΔIα is smaller than Io.

Δx means the thickness, $\alpha(v)$ the absorption coefficient of the substance at the frequency v of the incoming radiation, which is proportional to the concentration C of the substance:

$\alpha(v)=\varepsilon(v)\ C.$

$\varepsilon(v)$ is the molar extinction coefficient of the substance at the light frequency v [7].

Emission. Electromagnetic radiation is released (emission) by the molecule's return to the basic level. All those emission processes are summarized under the generic term luminescence. The radiation or the emission of the molecule can easily be demonstrated if the molecule's concentration in its stimulated condition is very high or if the velocity of the radiationless deactivation is low in relation to the velocity of the radiation. The emission is termed fluorescence if the emission fades quickly (10^{-9}–10^{-3} s) after light absorption depending on the wavelength. In contrast, in the case of phosphorescence, the emission remains longer, characteristically several seconds after absorption.

In most fluids and solutions at room temperature, the radiationless deactivating processes pass so quickly that fluorescence or phosphorescence cannot be observed. However, there are solutions such as the fluorescein solution, which show a clear fluorescence. The part in which the fluorescence emission is a linear function of the concentration is used for the determination of the concentration of the according substances. The following list gives examples for the use of fluorescence in photometry: Determination of riboflavin (vitamin B_6) in cow milk, of thiamin (B_1) in meat and cereals, of polycyclic aromatic compounds in the air, and of porphyrins, enzymes, estrogens, and histidine in blood or urine. Fluorescence can exist in all parts of the electromagnetic spectrum. The fluorescence follows Stock's rule, which states that the emitted radiation cannot be of a shorter wavelength than the exciting light [62].

Previous Indications of FDAP

The professional use of the δ-ALA-induced porphyrin fluorescence in the detection of tumors was first reported in urology. After instillation of a δ-ALA solution into the bladder (1.5 g δ-ALA in 50 ml $NaCO_3$; 0.17 mol/l) fluorescence cystoscopy has been done for the detection of bladder carcinomas. A violet laser light with a wavelength of 406.7 nm is mainly used to visualize the increased biotransformation of δ-ALA into porphyrins in the urothelial tumor tissue [35, 36, 54]. This technique provides a great advantage in tumor detection and post-treatment control of urothelial cancers, because flat mucosa lesions, such as dysplasias or in situ carcinomas, are often not visible by white light endoscopy.

After topical δ-ALA application, the quantitative analysis of the fluorescence intensity revealed a 10-times higher level in the malignant tissue than in the adjacent normal tissue. Fluorescence analysis proved that the accumulation of endogenously built porphyrins, especially protoporphyrin, was tumor selective.

Therefore FDAP seems to be a reliable and easy to perform technique in early detection of urothelial cancer.

The relapse rate and the progression rate depend on the amount of remaining pre-malignant or malignant cells in the mucosa after resection of superficial urinary bladder carcinomas, and therefore an early diagnosis of possible neoplastic tissue is very important for the patient's prognosis.

We biochemically investigated the porphyrin levels in bronchial and colon carcinomas and in the normal tumor-surrounding tissue ex vivo, respectively. Here, as well, we found 1.5- to 2-fold higher porphyrin levels in the neoplastic than in the normal tissues (unpublished data).

FDAP in Dermatology

In the past 10 years δ-ALA PDT was investigated for different dermatological indications, especially for solar keratosis, but also for Bowen's disease, keratoacanthoma, basal cell carcinoma (superficial and solid types), squamous cell carcinoma, mycosis fungoides, and psoriatic lesions [8, 13, 17, 18, 21, 38, 63]. Our own experiences revealed that topical application of δ-ALA and subsequent irradiation with red (570–750 nm) or green light (540–550 nm) can only be curatively used in superficial skin tumors, mainly superficial basal cell carcinomas and initial squamous cell carcinomas, and in cutaneous precanceroses, in particular solar keratosis [18].

We have been treating various tissues with topical δ-ALA and examined the pattern of porphyrin accumulation by irradiation with Wood's light. Thus, we had the opportunity to collect detailed experiences about the fluorescence quantity and quality of skin diseases after topical δ-ALA application [2, 16, 17, 20, 21]. To date, there have been no systematic examinations on the exact distribution of the induced fluorescence in tumor or healthy skin. Strict localization of the porphyrin fluorescence to the tumor tissue would optimize the planning of a surgical treatment or other therapeutic strategies (CO_2-laser, cryosurgery, radiation therapy). To prove this theory, we examined different skin diseases by FDAP, excised the fluorescent skin areas, and examined the tissues histopathologically. An overview of the characteristics and possibilities of this is given in the following section.

Examined Skin Diseases

FDAP was performed in different skin diseases and/or the following situations:
- Clinical and histological diagnosis of precancerosis or skin tumor
- Clinically tumor-suspicious skin changes but not verified by histology
- Precancerosis or skin tumors with the lack of a sharp clinical demarcation
- Tumor relapses
- Other, fast proliferating tissues such as psoriatic lesions

The following skin diseases were investigated with FDAP:
- Skin cancer
    - Basal cell carcinoma (solid and superficial type)
    - Squamous cell carcinoma
    - Malignant melanoma
    - Mycosis fungoides
    - Paget's disease (extramammary type)
    - Kaposi's sarcoma
    - Precanceroses
    - Actinic keratosis
    - Bowen's disease
    - Lentigo maligna
- Other tissues
    - Psoriasis
    - Verrucae vulgares
    - Nevocytic nevi
    - Lupus erythematosus plaques

Furthermore we examined the porphyrin fluorescence in normal healthy skin of various body sites like the trunk, face, capillitium, inguinal and axillary area. In addition, different application times of δ-ALA were chosen.

The aim of the investigation was to find if there were a correlation between the macroscopic fluorescence (intensity) and the microscopic histopathological findings. Furthermore, we wanted to clarify if the tumor fluorescence correlated with the tumor borders histopathologically, and in particular, if clinically unaffected but histopathologically altered skin areas could be detected as pathologically changed by the fluorescence technique.

Implementation of FDAP

For PDT, δ-ALA was applied in a 10 % – 20 % concentration in an ointment. A 10 % mixture was mainly sufficient in the treatment of solar keratosis, whereas a concentration of 20 % was proven best in the treatment of superficial basal or squamous cell carcinomas.

In FDAP, the same δ-ALA concentrations (10 % – 20 %) proved to be effective for the presentation of the typical fluorescence depending on the clinical diagnosis and body location.

We performed the FDAP procedure as described below. Skin was cleansed by disinfecting with Dibromol solution. δ-ALA (Merck, Darmstadt, Germany) was mixed into an ointment (Neribas Salbe, Schering Berlin, Germany) and topically applied on the suspected skin area and, additionally, approximately 1 cm on the surrounding healthy skin. A total amount of approximately 0.2 g of the mixture was applied to a skin area of $1 \, cm^2$ ($20 - 40 \, mg \, δ\text{-}ALA/cm^2$). The treated area was covered by a light-protective bandage (Tegaderm, gazes, aluminum foil, Fixomull) to avoid photobleaching and to maximize substance penetration. After an application-time maximum 6 h (lesser incubation periods can be sufficient depending on the body area and the type of skin disease – see below) the FDAP was carried out with a Wood's lamp (Fluolight; 370–405 nm, Saalmann GmbH, Germany).

The fluorescence intensities in the FDAP were measured in comparison to a fluorescence standard (constantly fluorescing plastic stripes) to allow a semi-quantitative indication: o, no fluorescence; +, slight fluorescence; ++, middle strong fluorescence; +++, strong fluorescence.

It is very difficult to capture the slight differences in the fluorescence quantity photographically. Maintaining adequate stillness for a length of time is an especially difficult task for the older patients. However, it is necessary to achieve optimal conditions for a long exposure time, which is obligatory for the photography of a slight fluorescence picture. We were fortunately able to photographically document the tissue fluorescences in numerous skin diseases. You will find a selection of these photographs in Figs. 2–8. Clinical and fluorescence photos are combined, respectively. The fluorescence patterns allow us to estimate the size and the borders of the lesions and may give information concerning their malignancy.

Character of FDAP Findings

All derived fluorescence intensities are listed in Table 1. Six hours after application of δ-ALA, all epithelial neoplasms, such as basal cell carcinoma (Figs. 2 and 8), squamous cell carcinoma, Bowen's disease (Fig. 3), actinic keratosis (Fig. 4) and extramammary Paget's disease, showed a strong red fluorescence under Wood's light. There was a medium-strong fluorescence in Kaposi's sarcoma, the lesions of lupus erythematosus, and in the plaques of cutaneous T-cell lymphoma (mycosis fungoides) and only a slight or no fluorescence in the pigmented benign and malignant skin changes such as nevocytic nevus, lentigo maligna, and malignant melanoma (Fig. 5). The examined verrucae vulgares (Fig. 6) did not show any fluorescence at all. In psoriatic lesions, there were middle-strong up to strong fluorescence intensities detectable but the fluorescence pattern was often non-homogeneous (Fig. 7).

Histopathological examinations revealed that all middle-strong and strong fluorescent tissues (++ to +++) were found in neoplasms, precanceroses, or fast-proliferating tissues such as psoriasis lesions. The area of the fluorescence correlated with the clinical extension of clinically well-defined tumors as well as with the histopathological borders of clinically ill-defined skin changes. On the face, capillitium, the inguinal and axillary area, the demarcation of tumors and precanceroses by the fluorescence appeared to be more difficult than in other locations. Here, the tumor-specific fluorescence was surrounded and partially covered by a slight but well-seen fluorescence of the normal tissue. This background fluorescence may be partly due to the increased presence of bacteria (e.g., propionibacteria) in these areas. However, the distinguishing of the tumors from the normal skin was nevertheless possible due to the higher fluorescence intensity in tumor tissue compared to normal skin. In addition, the demarcation of tumors in these body areas could improve by diminishing the application time of δ-ALA to 2–4 h.

Table 1. Fluorescence intensities in various cutaneous tissues upon topical application of δ-ALA (20 %)

Skin condition (healthy skin location)	n	Application time (h)	Fluorescence intensity	Borders
BCC – superficial	16	6	+++	Sharp
BCC – solid	12	6	+++	Sharp
SCC	6	6	+++	Sharp
Bowen's disease	6	6	+++	Sharp
Solar keratosis	24	6	++/+++	Sharp
Paget's disease	3	6	+++	Sharp
Mycosis fungoides	4	6	++	Sharp
Kaposi's sarcoma	5	6	+/++	Sharp
Malignant melanoma	8	6	–	Not applicable
Lentigo maligna	4	6	–	Not applicable
Nevus cell nevus	12	6	–	Not applicable
Seborrheic keratoses	8	6	–	Not applicable
Verrucae vulgares	8	6	–	Not applicable
Lupus erythematosus	5	6	++	Sharp
Psoriasis plaques	8	6	++/+++	Sharp
Healthy (trunk)	8	3	–	Not applicable
	8	6	+	Not applicable
	8	12	+	Not applicable
	8	24	+/++	Not applicable
Healthy (face/capillitium)	8	3	+	Not applicable
	8	6	+/++	Not applicable
	8	12	++/+++	Not applicable
	8	24	++	Not applicable
Healthy (inguinal, axillary)	4	3	+	Not applicable
	4	6	+/++	Not applicable
	4	12	++	Not applicable
	4	24	++	Not sharp

–, no; +, little; ++, intermediate; +++, strong fluorescence.

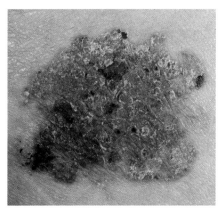 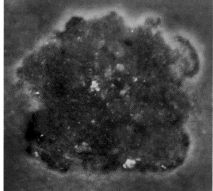

Fig. 2. Bowen's disease (gluteal, m, 72 J). Erythematous plaque, ca. 12 · 10 cm, polycyclic and relative sharply bordered, partly with squama and hemorrhagic crusts. FDAP (δ-ALA 20 %, 6 h): strong reddish fluorescence, sharply limited and correlating with the clinical extension of the lesion

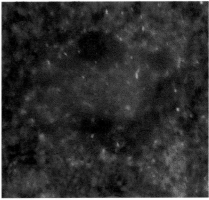

Fig. 3. Superficial basal cell carcinoma (décolleté, w, 48 J). It is impossible to clinically demarcate the borders of the lesion. In FDAP (δ-ALA 20 %, 6 h) the tumor can be very clearly visualized and its borders can be exactly delineated

Discussion

In the recent years, PDT was developed and established as a novel technique for the treatment of superficial skin tumors and precancerous lesions. The application of porphyrins or the porphyrin precursor δ-ALA leads to a preferential enrichment of porphyrins in the tumor tissues. Up to now, there are only a few reports about the effectiveness of the δ-ALA-induced porphyrin fluorescence in the detection and delineation of tumors. There were many studies done on PDT with δ-ALA-induced porphyrins, and the presence of a high fluorescence intensity in neoplasms was often mentioned [8, 13, 18, 20, 38, 63]. In addition, biochemical studies proved that the increased fluorescence intensity correlated with the extracted porphyrin concentrations in the tumor tissues [22, 26, 29, 46]. However, reports on FDAP so far only concern experiences with bladder cancers [35, 54] and intracerebral tumors [56].

In all cutaneous neoplasms examined herein (basal and squamous cell carcinoma, Bowen's disease, actinic keratosis, Paget's disease), we measured an intensive, strong, and sharply bordered red fluorescence under Wood's light 6 h after topical application of δ-ALA. Even in psoriatic lesions, we have been found the typical δ-ALA-induced porphyrin fluorescence strong. However, in the pigmented lesions such as malignant melanomas or nevi, no fluorescence was present. These results illustrate that tumors and psoriasis plaques show an increased porphyrin biosynthesis in comparison to the adjacent "normal" skin. The increased porphyrin biosynthesis seems to be dependent on a damage of the stratum corneum and an increased proliferating rate of the tissue, which is mainly present in neoplastic or inflammatory processes. The δ-ALA-induced porphyrin fluorescence was not visible in verrucae vulgares (Figure 6), seborrheic keratoses (Figure 7), and nevocytic nevi.

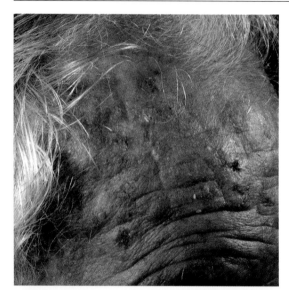

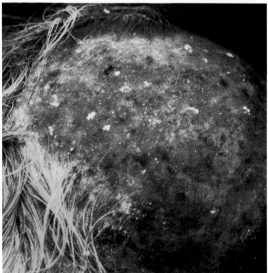

Fig. 4. Solar keratoses (front, m, 73 J). FDAP (δ – ALA 10 %, 6 h): Multiple fluorescing spots indicating solar keratoses. In contrast, clinically, the number of lesions seems to be less

There may be several reasons for the only slight fluorescence intensity in malignant melanomas. On the one hand, it has been well proven by in vitro experiments that melanoma cells can synthesize high levels of porphyrins if δ-ALA is added to the culture medium [5]. However, the generally intact surface of malignant melanomas may limit the penetration of δ-ALA as compared to e.g., basal cell carcinomas with a damaged epidermal surface. Physical factors may also take part in the FDAP behavior of malignant melanomas: the melanin-dependent reduced stimulation or emission of the porphyrin fluorescence.

Fig. 5. Seborrheic keratosis (right temporal area, w, 75 J). FDAP (δ-ALA 20 %, 6 h): In the seborrheic keratosis there is no increased porphyrin fluorescence

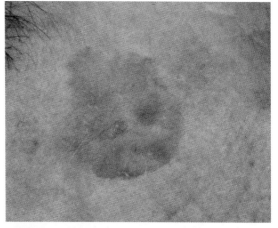

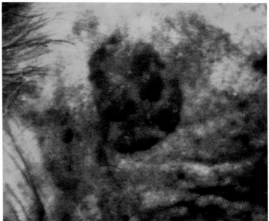

These factors may also be responsible for the relative little fluorescence yield in Kaposi's sarcoma.

Normal skin shows, depending on the body site, different fluorescence kinetics. A stronger intensive fluorescence is proved at the head, in the groin, and in the axillae in comparison with other skin areas. This difference may be based on the fortified colonization of porphyrin producing bacteria (e.g., propionibacteria). After an application time of 24 h, we proved up to middle-strong fluorescence in these locations. Here, the contrast between neoplastic and healthy skin can be improved by reducing the application time of the δ-ALA. Another bacterium, the corynebacterium minutissimum, which is the pathogenic factor in erythrasma, can also form large amounts of protoporphyrin. Therefore, in untreated erythrasma lesions, one can demonstrate a red fluorescence, which is similar to the red fluorescence present in FDAP. In acne patients, there has also been demonstrated a bright follicle-bound fluorescence under a Wood's light [42].

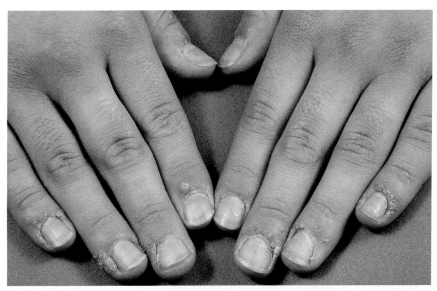

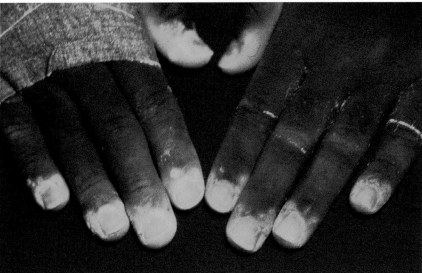

Fig. 6. Verrucae vulgares (w, 12 J). FDAP (δ-ALA 20 %, 6 h): The warts are presenting as whitish spots without any porphyrin fluorescence

Porphyrin Metabolism in Skin

Up to now the porphyrin biosynthesis in human skin has been examined only sporadically [3, 25, 45]. Such examinations were predominantly made to explain the pathomechanism of porphyrias, but nowadays they are increasingly used to measure the effect of PDT with δ-ALA-induced porphyrins.

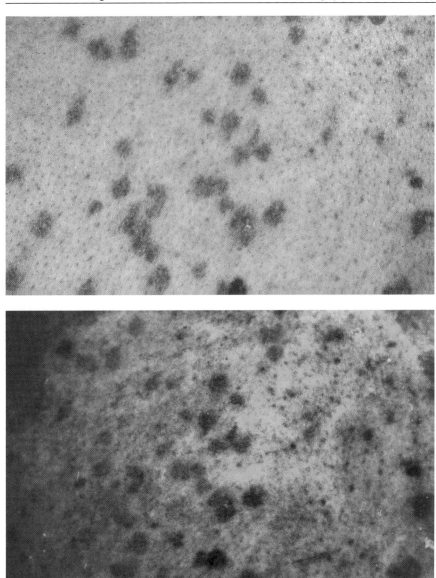

Fig. 7. Psoriasis lesions (back, w, 38 J). Clinic: Multiple erythematous plaques, ca. 2 cm each, sharply bordered, partly confluent, and partly with squamae. FDAP (δ – ALA 20 %, 6 h): The psoriatic lesions are impressing as red fluorescing islands and can be distinguished from the surrounding normal skin

In vitro studies at different cell cultures (K562 leukemia cells, endothelium cells, HaCaT, fibroblasts, Sk-Mel 23, Sk-Mel 28, Bro, HepG2) showed an increased and specific porphyrin synthesis in all cells by application of δ-ALA to the incubation medium. The amount of synthesized porphyrins did not correlate with the "grade of malignancy" of the cell line ([28, 39, 43]; unpublished findings).

In normal human tissues (liver, fatty tissue, skin), the basal porphyrin levels were shown to be low with 0.2–1.2 nmol/g [25]. Basal porphyrin concentrations in human tumors such as bronchial carcinoma and carcinomas of the gastrointestinal tract (unpublished data), or epithelial skin tumors such as basal and squamous cell carcinoma [22], or precancerous lesions such as actinic keratoses [19] were also low with <1 nmol/g. Skin tumors and normal skin samples showed comparable basal porphyrin levels. This finding refuted the theory that tumors may have changed activities of the heme-associated enzymes.

Treatment of cutaneous tissues ex vivo or in vivo with exogenic δ-ALA led to an increased synthesis of porphyrins. In an organic culture model an increased porphyrin biosynthesis with partly tumor-specific porphyrin metabolite patterns (predominantly protoporphyrin or coproporphyrin depending on the tumor) was demonstrated [15]. Topical δ-ALA application in vivo to epithelial skin tumors and psoriatic lesions showed a time-dependent porphyrin synthesis with maximum levels already after 1–4 h for basal cell or squamous cell carcinomas (50–60 nmol/g protein) or 6 h for psoriatic lesions (90 nmol/g protein) [22]. Porphyrin synthesis in normal skin is quite low (at 6 h: 12 nmol/g protein); however, it still increases up to 24 h after δ-ALA application (24 h: 15 nmol/g protein).

Summarizing the available data, we have to proceed on the assumption that in both experimental tumors and different human cutaneous tissues there arises a distinct porphyrin metabolism with variable accumulation of the porphyrin metabolites.

Reception of δ-ALA in Tumors

The δ-ALA concentrations and vehicles used in our department as well as mentioned in the literature show sufficient efficacy in FDAP and PDT. It is still not yet clearly delineated which mechanism makes the δ-ALA penetrate into the skin. The stratum corneum is the main barrier for substances topically applied to the skin. As the keratin layers of superficial skin tumors and precancerosis are pathologically changed, δ-ALA is able to penetrate quickly into those lesions, in contrast to normal skin where the δ-ALA uptake is lower due to an intact surface [32, 47, 58]. The reception of δ-ALA or δ-ALA-induced porphyrins in skin can be fortified by treating the skin with dimethylsulfoxide (DMSO), which leads to a destruction of the skin barrier [47]. This is another hint for the relevance of the stratum corneum in δ-ALA penetration.

The so-far experimental findings will not allow a decision whether the tumor cells in skin accumulate more δ-ALA or show an increased porphyrin biosynthesis in comparison to normal cells. Proceeding on the assumption that δ-ALA is synthesized out of glycine and succinyl-CoA, being a relatively small molecule like amino acids, it could penetrate the cell membrane. Recent examinations showed that there are active as well as passive transport mechanisms taking part in the uptake of δ-ALA into cells and that the δ-ALA uptake can be competitively limited by certain amino acids [44]. Probably, under the aspects of the FDAP and PDT, not only the reception of the amino carbon acid in cells is the limiting and selecting step but also the synthesis and the accumulation of the formed porphyrins preferentially in tumor cells are of extreme relevance.

Porphyrin Metabolism in Tumor Tissues

For many authors, the reason for the preferred accumulation of porphyrins in tumors after δ-ALA application was speculated to be the different activity of the enzymes associated with the porphyrin biosynthesis. The obstacle of the mito-chondrial ferrochelatase, which catalyzes the iron insertion into protoporphyrin, would lead to a reduced heme concentration with a reduced negative feedback. This can justify the accumulation of protoporphyrin in tumor tissue in analogy to fibroblasts [4] or lymphocytes [53] of patients with erythropoietic protopor-phyria (EPP; congenital defect of the ferrochelatase). The relevance of the heme biosynthesis associated enzymes in porphyrin accumulation in skin was indi-cated by testing skin biopsies of patients who suffered from several porphyrias: Patients with acute intermittent porphyria (AIP; defect of the uroporphyrinogen decarboxylase) showed a clear, about 50 % less porphyrin formation in skin, in comparison to healthy persons. Contrary to it, in the skin of patients with por-phyria cutanea tarda (PCT; autosomal dominant defect of the uroporphyrinogen decarboxylase) were found increased amounts of basal porphyrins and a forti-fied porphyrin biosynthesis after application of δ-ALA (in comparison with the skin of healthy people or of AIP patients) [3]. Accordingly, it is conceivable that there is a defect of one or several enzymes of the heme biosynthesis, which leads to an accumulation of the heme precursors (e.g., porphyrins). Other enzymes of the porphyrin biosynthesis, such as δ-ALA dehydratase, which was found to be reduced in tumors (murine mammary carcinoma, human mammary adenocarci-noma) and in liver of tumor-carrying animals, could also contribute to an altered porphyrin production in tumors [9, 45, 59]. Exclusively the δ-ALA synthase is accepted as being the limiting enzyme of the heme biosynthesis [31, 55]. There remains still the question, why do tumor cells receive increased δ-ALA, why do tumor cells predominantly transform and accumulate δ-ALA into porphyrins, and why do they not metabolize porphyrins to heme.

In erythrocytes, there is a limiting in fluence both of the δ-ALA synthase and the ferrochelatase. Erythrocytes offer special circumstances. Here, an X chromo-somal-situated gene regulates the δ-ALA synthase, whereas the chromosome 13-situated gene of a different δ-ALA synthase controls the heme biosynthesis in all other cells [31]. Although erythrocytes and tumor cells are profoundly different, one could assume that in tumor cells or fast-proliferating cells beside the δ-ALA synthase the ferrochelatase is also limiting. This is indicated by fluorescence and biochemical findings, where an accumulation of protoporphyrin arises in tumor models (in vivo, ex vivo) [26, 46, 58]. In addition, at least in particular observations, there was proved a reduced activity of the ferrochelatase.

Further research should focus on the question of why increased porphyrins with partly specific porphyrin metabolite patterns in tumors are formed or accumulated after topical or systemic application of δ-ALA.

Parameter of FDAP

δ-ALA

At present, the δ-ALA is the most appropriate substance for FDAP. Further clinical and biochemical studies have to prove whether other porphyrin precursors, porphyrin products, δ-ALA esters, or even synthesized substances (e.g., porphycenes) for marking neoplastic tissue can be used in the future. Additionally, it has to be clarified, whether the topical δ-ALA application with different vehicles can increase the porphyrin biosynthesis or the penetration ability of δ-ALA. On this occasion, the pretreatment with dimethylsulfoxide seems to improve the effectiveness of FDAP and PDT [47].

Concentration of δ-ALA

The δ-ALA concentrations, which have proved to be effective for the FDAP of skin tumors and precancerosis, come to 10–20% with a total δ-ALA dose of 40 mg/cm^2.

Application Time of the δ-ALA Mixture

In FDAP and PDT, there has been a proven best δ-ALA application time of 6 h in the middle, because at that point the detected porphyrin fluorescence in tumors is marked most severely in comparison with the adjusted normal tissue. The detected porphyrin fluorescence reflects only the accumulation of porphyrins in the superficial, not in the deep-skin, layers. Fluorescence microscopic studies on porphyrin penetration revealed that the porphyrin fluorescence in the deeper dermal layers is only non-homogeneous 6 h after δ-ALA application but becomes visible and partly homogeneous at a later point in time (24–48 h) [47, 58]. The depth of the lesions is not of interest in FDAP. FDAP is performed to evaluate the superficial dimension of a tumor, but FDAP will never give any information on the infiltration depth of a certain lesion. For PDT however, it is important to know if a tumor is entirely sensitized with porphyrins to guarantee a successful treatment; otherwise, the deeply situated parts of the tumor will remain untreated during the light exposure.

Way of δ-ALA Application

FDAP and PDT are mostly performed by topical application of δ-ALA. As already mentioned, sensitization of the tumor tissue with porphyrins is limited to the superficial skin layers. Consequently, only superficial neoplastic tissues can be treated by topical δ-ALA PDT. Depending on the affected area of the body (face, axilla, groin), it may be advantageous to reduce the application time, in order to optimize the contrast between tumor tissue and normal tissue in FDAP.

Interestingly, in the consequence of first reports, the systemic δ-ALA application leads to an even better and more homogeneous sensitizing of the deeper situated tumor parts. To patients with intraoral squamous cell carcinomas, 30 – 60 mg/kg δ-ALA were given periorally [26]. Several biopsies were taken out of the tumors and fluorescence was microscopically evaluated up to 24 h after δ-ALA application. The fluorescence maximum was seated between 4 and 6 h after δ-ALA application, at which a 2 times higher fluorescence was measured in tumor tissue in comparison to the surrounding tissue. The fluorescence was distributed homogeneously in all tumors. The chromatographical analysis of a δ-ALA pretreated tumor specimen revealed protoporphyrin as the predominant porphyrin metabolite. 24 h after the treatment, no porphyrin fluorescence was proved in the biopsies at all. This indicates, in this case, that even the systemic application of relatively high δ-ALA doses does not lead to a long-lasting photosensitivity. Other reports show that patients who took periorally 30 – 60 mg/kg δ-ALA for PDT of tumors of the colon, the rectum, the duodenum, the esophagus, and the bladder suffered side effects such as dizziness, nausea, vomiting, headache, circulatory instability, and both temporary increase of the transaminases and increased photosensitizing ([14, 52], Goetz et al., personal communication). Thus, it is necessary to measure the pharmacokinetics of δ-ALA after its oral and i. v. administration because of the contradictory findings. Further studies should focus on the systemic use of the δ-ALA in the next few years.

Source of Radiation

To get the most effective fluorescence stimulation of the porphyrins, they have to be irradiated in their absorption maximum at 405 nm (Soret-Band). Saalmann's Fluolight (UV-A, 380 – 405 nm) is the light source that leads to a big boost to the δ-ALA-induced porphyrin fluorescence. Although there are many hand lamps emitting Wood's light on the market, in general, their intensity is too low to provoke sufficient porphyrin fluorescence. In addition, many available UV light sources often contain too much visible light, which reduces the profit of the fluorescence because of covering spectrums. As FDAP techniques are increasingly used by dermatological and surgical departments, it is foreseeable, and would be very welcome, that the light industry will cover this shortcoming in the medical light source market.

Unwelcome Side Effects

During the last 7 years we have treated about 1000 patients with topical δ-ALA. Skin irritations, meaning toxic and allergic contact dermatitis were observed rarely (< 2 %). Except for slight tingling, the patients didn't have any complaints during the irradiation with a Wood's light (FDAP). Unlike this, the red-light irradiation (PDT) after δ-ALA application at the PDT has partly led to middle or even strong pains. This pain has been especially strong if the treated lesion was big (such as multiple actinic keratoses on the front or a large basal cell carcinoma) or presented several erosions. Progressing experiments showed that with less δ-ALA (10 %) [20], less-intense irradiation, and with green instead of red light irradiation [23] the painful sensations significantly diminished.

The patients showed no increasing of porphyrins or porphyrin precursors in their blood or urine after topical application of the δ-ALA. This indicates the improbability of a stressed porphyrin metabolism or a systemic photosensitizing after application of these δ-ALA amounts [24]. Consequently, the δ-ALA PDT is a method that can be executed without logistical problems, quickly, without side effects, routinely, and repeatedly.

Conclusion

The basis for the effectiveness of the PDT and FDAP with δ-ALA is the pathogenetically, not clarified, tumor-specific biotransformation of δ-ALA. The methodological foundations of the diagnostic procedure (the FDAP) are already worked out to our content. The FDAP is not a histological examination that defines the malignancy or benignity of tumors or skin changes. The main importance of the FDAP is the specifying of the borders between tumor and normal skin and the better planning of further therapies. It depends on the results of the FDAP to decide whether the respective lesion should be treated by surgical excision, cryosurgery, CO_2-laser therapy, PDT, or radiotherapy. Beyond it, the FDAP can detect post-operatively (or after other tumor therapies) if there are still any tumor residues (Figure 8: FDAP-controlled tumor therapy). The control of a surgical, cryosurgical, or photodynamic treatment with the help of the FDAP is an enrichment for the tumor therapy and tumor aftercare.

Summary

The photodynamic therapy (PDT) is predominantly executed with porphyrin products. In 1990, the porphyrin precursor δ-aminolevulinic acid (δ-ALA) was used in the PDT for the first time and is now used for the treatment of tumors at organ surfaces more and more frequently. The δ-ALA application induces the porphyrin-biosynthesis preferentially in tumor tissue. The tissue that is accumulated with porphyrins can be visible by radiation with a Wood's light due to the emission of a red fluorescence. This principle is called the fluorescence diagnosis with δ-aminolevulinic acid induced porphyrins (FDAP). The indication and efficiency of this novel technique in tumor detection was predominantly mentioned for bladder and intracerebral tumors. In the last few years, the FDAP has become increasingly relevant in dermatology. Ultimate examinations show that the FDAP is a very helpful method for the detection of neoplastic tissue in pre-damaged skin and for delineating clinically ill-defined tumors. The value of the FDAP for the clinical diagnosis of skin tumors, cutaneous precancerosis, inflammatory dermatosis, and pigmented skin lesions was presented and the indications for this method was discussed.

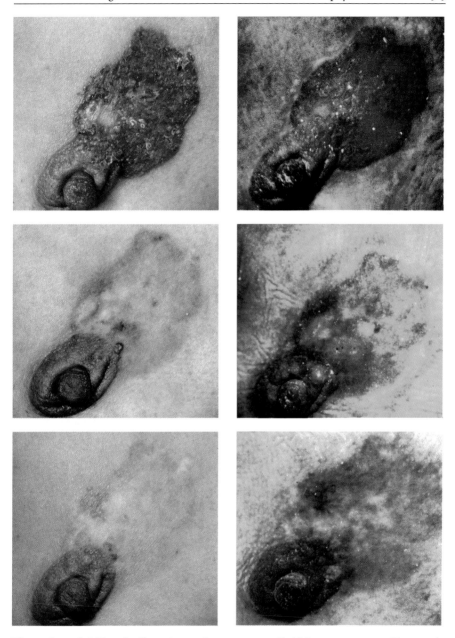

Fig. 8. Superficial basal cell carcinoma (mamma, w, 55 J). This case was treated by repetitive PDT (3 sessions) guided by FDAP. Prior to PDT, on the right mamma an impressing large erythematosquamous plaques with fissures was present. In FDAP the tumor is entirely fluorescing. Five weeks after two PDT sessions (3-week interval; 20 % δ-ALA; 180 J/cm2, 570 – 650 nm) the major part of the tumor is already cured. In FDAP there are still several intensive fluorescing areas indicating remaining tumor tissue. The tumor tissue is

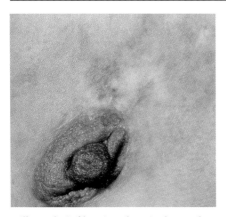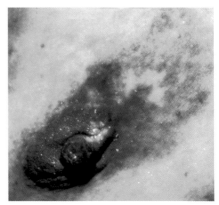

still partly infiltrating the nipple areola complex. Four weeks after the third PDT (not shown), in FDAP, only some little fluorescent spots were present, still infiltrating the nipple areola complex. The fluorescing spots were marked, excised, and the defect was covered by a rotation flap and a reconstructed nipple. Five weeks after repetitive PDT and surgery of the remaining tumor parts, neither clinically nor in FDAP were there any hints of remaining tumor tissue. The patient has now been free of any tumor for 4 years

Acknowledgements. We thank Mrs. Kerstin Kleinert for her help preparing the manuscript.

References

1. Baumgartner R, Fuchs N, Jocham D, Stepp H, Unsöld E (1992) Photokinetics of fluorescent polyporphyrin photofrin II in normal rat tissue and rat bladder tumor. Photochem Photobiol 55:569–574
2. Becker-Wegerich P, Fritsch C, Neuse W, Schulte KW, Ruzicka T, Goerz G (1995) Effektive Kryochirurgie oberflächlicher Hauttumoren unter photodynamischer Diagnostik. H G 70:891–895
3. Bickers DR, Keogh L, Rifkind AB, Harber LC, Kappas A (1977) Studies in porphyria. VI.Biosynthesis of porphyrins in mammilian skin and in the skin of porphyric patients. J Invest Dermatol 68:5–9
4. Bloomer JR, Brenner DA, Mahoney MJ (1977) Study of factors causing excess protoporphyrin accumulation in cultured skin fibroblasts from patients with protoporphyria. J Clin Invest 60:1354–1361
5. Bolsen K, Lang K, Verwholt B, Fritsch C, Goerz G (1996) In vitro incubation of porphyrin biosynthesis in various human cells after incubation with δ-aminolevulinic acid. Arch Dermatol Res 288:320
6. Braichotte DR, Wagnieres GA, Bays R, Monnier P, van den Bergh HE (1995) Clinical pharmacokinetic studies of photofrin by fluorescence spectroscopy in the oral cavity, the esophagus, and the bronchi. Cancer 75:2768–2778
7. Bruls WAG, Slaper H, van der Leun JC, Berrens L (1984) Transmission of human epidermis and stratum corneum as a function of thickness in the ultraviolet and visible wavelengths. Photochem Photobiol 40:485–494
8. Cairnduff F, Stringer MR, Hudson EJ, Ash DV, Brown SB (1994) Superficial photodynamic therapy with topical 5-aminolevulinic acid for superficial primary and secondary skin cancer. Br J Cancer 69:605–608

9. Denk H, Kalt R, Abdelfattah-Gad M, Meyer UA (1981) Effect of griseofulvin on 5-aminolevulinate synthase and on ferrochelatase in mouse liver neoplastic nodules. Cancer Res 41:1535–1538
10. Doiron DR, Profio E, Vincent RG, Dougherty TJ (1979) Fluorescence bronchoscopy for detection of lung cancer. Chest 76:27–32
11. Dougherty TJ (1987) Photosensitizers: therapy and detection of malignant tumors. Photochem Photobiol 45:879–889
12. Figge FHJ, Weiland GS, Manganiello LOJ (1948) Cancer detection and therapy: affinity of neoplastic, embryonic, and traumatized tissues for porphyrins and metalloporphyrins. Proc Soc Exp Biol Med 68:640–641
13. Fijan S, Hönigsmann H, Ortel R (1995) Photodynamic therapy of epithelial skin tumours using delta-aminolevulinic acid and desferrioxamine. Br J Dermatol 133:282–288
14. Fritsch C, Abels C, Goetz AE, Stahl W, Bolsen K, Ruzicka T, Goerz G, Sies H (1997) Porphyrins preferentially accumulate in a melanoma following intravenous injection of 5-aminolevulinic acid. Biol Chem 378:51–57
15. Fritsch C, Batz J, Bolsen K, Schulte KW, Ruzicka T, Goerz G (1994) Exogenous δ-aminolevulinic acid induces the porphyrin biosynthesis in human skin organ cultures with different porphyrin patterns in normal and malignant human tissue. SPIE Proc 2371:215–220
16. Fritsch C, Becker-Wegerich PM, Menke M, Ruzicka T, Goerz G, Olbrisch RR (1997) Successful surgery of multiple recurrent basal cell carcinomas guided by photodynamic diagnosis. Aesthetic Plast Surg 21:437–439
17. Fritsch C, Becker-Wegerich PM, Schulte KW, Neuse W, Lehmann P, Ruzicka T, Goerz G (1996) Photodynamische Therapie und Mamillenplastik eines großflächigen Rumpfhautbasalioms der Mamma. Effektive Kombinationstherapie unter photodynamischer Diagnostik. Hautarzt 47:438–442
18. Fritsch C, Goerz G, Ruzicka T (1998) Photodynamic therapy in dermatology. A review. Arch Dermatol 134:207–214
19. Fritsch C, Homey B, Stahl W, Lehmann P, Ruzicka T, Sies H (1998) Preferential relative porphyrin enrichment in solar keratoses upon topical application of δ-aminolevulinic acid methylester. Photochem Photobiol 68:218–221
20. Fritsch C, Lang K, Neuse W, Ruzicka T, Lehmann P (1998) Photodynamic diagnosis and therapy in dermatology. Skin Pharmacol Appl Skin Physiol 11:358–373
21. Fritsch C, Lehmann P, Bolsen K, Ruzicka T, Goerz G (1994) Photodynamische Diagnostik und Photodynamische Therapie von aktinischen Keratosen. Z Hautkr 69:713–716
22. Fritsch C, Lehmann P, Stahl W, Schulte KW, Blohm E, Lang K, Sies H, Ruzicka T (1999) Optimum porphyrin accumulation in epithelial skin tumours and psoriatic lesions after topical application of δ-aminolaevulinic acid. Br J Cancer 79:1603–1608
23. Fritsch C, Stege S, Saalmann G, Goerz G, Ruzicka T, Krutmann J (1997) Green light is effective and less painful than red light in photodynamic therapy of facial solar keratoses. Photodermatol Photoimmunol Photomed 13:181–185
24. Fritsch C, Verwohlt B, Bolsen K, Ruzicka T, Goerz G (1996) Influence of topical photodynamic therapy with 5-aminolevulinic acid on the porphyrin metabolism. Arch Dermatol Res 288:517–521
25. Goerz G, Link-Mannhardt A, Bolsen K, Zumdick M, Fritsch C, Schürer NY (1995) Porphyrin concentrations in various human tissues. Exp Dermatol 4:218–220
26. Grant EW, Hopper C, MacRobert AJ, Speight PM, Bown SG (1993) Photodynamic therapy of oral cancer: photosensitisation with systemic aminolaevulinic acid. Lancet 324:147–148
27. Gregorie HG Jr, Horger EO, Ward JL (1968) Hematoporphyrin-derivate fluorescence in malignant neoplasms. Ann Surg 167:820–828

28. Hanania J, Malik Z (1992) The effect of EDTA and serum on endogenous porphyrin accumulation and photodynamic sensitization of human K562 leukemic cells. Cancer Lett 65:127–131
29. Hua Z, Gibson SL, Foster TH, Hilf R (1995) Effectiveness of δ-Aminolevulinic acid-induced protoporphyrin as a photosensitizer for photodynamic therapy in vivo. Cancer Res 55:1723–1731
30. Jesionek A, von Tappeiner H (1905) Zur Behandlung von Hautcarcinome mit fluorescierenden Stoffen. Arch Klin Med 82:72–76
31. Kappas A, Sassa S, Galbrath RA, Nordmann Y (1989) The porphyrias. In: Scriver CR, Beaudet AL, Sly WS, Volle D (eds) The metabolic basis of inherited diseases, 6th edn. McGraw-Hill, New York, pp 1305–1365
32. Kennedy JC, Pottier RH (1992) Endogenous protoporphyrin IX, a clinically useful photosensitizer for photodynamic therapy. J Photochem Photobiol 14:275–292
33. Kennedy JC, Pottier RH, Pross DC (1990) Photodynamic therapy with endogenous protoporphyrin IX: basic principles and present clinical experience. J Photochem Photobiol 6:143–148
34. Kinsey JH, Cortese DA, Sanderson DR (1978) Detection of hematoporphyrin fluorescence during fiberoptic bronchoscopy to localize early bronchogenic carcinoma. Mayo Clin Proc 53:594–600
35. Kriegmair M, Baumgartner R, Knuechel R, Ehsan R, Lumper W, Hofstetter A (1994) Fluorescence cystoscopy – a new method in diagnosis of bladder cancer. Urology 44:836–841
36. Kriegmair M, Baumgartner R, Knüchel R, Stepp H, Hofstädter F, Hofstetter A (1996) Detection of early bladder cancer by 5-aminolevulinic acid induced porphyrin fluorescence. J Urol 155:105–109
37. Lam S, Palcic B, McLean D, Hung J, Korbelik M, Profio E (1990) Detection of early lung cancer using low dose Photofrin II. Chest 97:333–337
38. Landthaler M, Rück A, Szeimies RM (1993) Photodynamische Therapie von Tumoren der Haut. Hautarzt 44:69–74
39. Lim HW, Behar S, He D (1994) Effect of porphyrin and irradiation on heme biosynthetic pathway in endothelial cells. Photodermatol Photoimmunol Photomed 10:17–21
40. Lipson RL, Baldes EJ, Olsen AM (1961) The use of a derivate of hematoporphyrin in tumor detection. J Natl Cancer Inst 26:1–4
41. Loh CS, Vernon D, MacRobert AJ, Bedwell J, Bown SG, Brown SB (1992) Endogenous porphyrin distribution induced by 5-aminolaevulinic acid and in the tissue layers of the gastrointestinal tract. J Photochem Photobiol B Biol 20:47–54
42. Lucchina LC, Kollias N, Gillies R, Phillips SB, Muccini JA, Stiller MJ, Tranick RJ, Drake LA (1996) Fluorescence photography in the evaluation of acne. J Am Acad Dermatol 35:58–63
43. Malik Z, Lugaci H (1987) Destruction of erythroleukaemic cells by photoactivation of endogenous porphyrins. Br J Cancer 56:589–595
44. Moan J, Bech O, Gaullier JM, Stokke T, Stehen HB, Ma LW, Berg K (1998) Protoporphyrin IX accumulation in cells treated with 5-aminolevulinic acid: dependence on cell density, cell size and cell cycle. Int J Cancer 75:134–139
45. Navone NM, Frisardi AL, Resnick ER, Del C Battle AM, Polo CF (1988) Porphyrin biosynthesis in human breast cancer. Preliminary mimetic in vitro studies. Med Sci Res 16:61–62
46. Peng Q, Moan J, Warloe T, Rimington C (1992) Distribution and photosensitizing efficiency of porphyrins induced by application of exogenous 5-aminolevulinic in mice bearing mammary carcinoma. Int J Cancer 52:433–443
47. Peng Q, Warloe T, Moan J, Heyerdahl H, Steen HB, Nesland JM, Giercksky KE (1995) Distribution of 5-aminolevulinic acid-induced porphyrins in noduloulcerative basal cell carcinoma. Photochem Photobiol 62:906–913

48. Pimstone NR (1985) Utility of porphyrins and light in the diagnosis and treatment of malignancy (editorial). Hepatology 5:338–340
49. Policard A (1924) Etude sur les aspects offerts par des tumeurs expérimentales examinées à la lumière de Wood. Cr Soc Biol 91:1423–1424
50. Raab O (1900) Über die Wirkung fluorescirender Stoffe auf Infusoriera. Z Biol 39:524
51. Rassmusen-Taxdal DS, Ward GE, Figge FHJ (1955) Fluorescence of human lymphatic and cancer tissues following high doses of hematoporphyrin. Cancer 8:78
52. Regula J, MacRobert AJ, Gorchein A, Buonaccorsi GA, Thorpe SM, Spencer GM, Hatfield ARW, Bown SG (1995) Photosensitisation and photodynamic therapy of oesophageal, duodenal, and colorectal tumours using 5-aminolevulinic acid-induced protoporphyrin IX – a pilot study. Gut 36:67–75
53. Sassa S, Zalar L, Poh-Fitzpatrick MB, Kappas A (1979) Sudies in porphyria IX: detection of the gene defect of erythropoietic protoporphyria in mitogen-stimulated human erythrocytes. Trans Assoc Am Phys 92:268–272
54. Steinbach P, Kriegmair M, Baumgartner R, Hofstädter F, Knüchel R (1994) Intravesical instillation of 5-aminolevulinic acid: the fluorescent metabolite is limited to urothelial cells. Urology 44:676–681
55. Stout AL, Becker FF (1986) Heme enzyme patterns in genetically and chemically induced mouse liver tumors. Cancer Res 46:2756–2759
56. Stummer W, Stocker S, Wagner S, Stepp H, Fritsch C, Goetz C, Goetz AE, Kiefmann R, Reulen HJ (1998) Intraoperative detection of malignant gliomas by 5-aminolevulinic acid-induced porphyrin fluorescence. Neurosurgery 42:518–526
57. Szeimies RM, Abels C, Fritsch C, Karrer S, Steinbach P, Bäumler W, Goerz G, Goetz AE, Landthaler M (1995) Wavelength dependency of photodynamic effects after sensitization with 5-aminolevulinic acid in vitro and in vivo. J Invest Dermatol 105:672–677
58. Szeimies RM, Sassay T, Landthaler M (1994) Penetration potency of topical applied delta aminolevulinic acid for photodynamic therapy of basal cell carcinoma. Photochem Photobiol 59:73–76
61. Tschudy DP, Collins A (1957) Reduction of δ-aminolevulinic acid dehydratase activity in the livers of tumor-bearing animals. Cancer Res 17:976–980
59. von Tappeiner H, Jesionek A (1903) Therapeutische Versuche mit fluoreszierenden Stoffen. MMW 50:2042–2044
60. von Tappeiner H, Jodlbauer A (1904) Ueber die Wirkung der photodynamischen (fluorescierenden) Stoffe auf Protozoen und Enzyme. Arch Klin Med 80:427–487
62. Whitaker M (1994) Fluorescence imaging in living cells. In: Celis JE (ed) Cell biology. A laboratory handbook, vol 2. Academic, San Diego, pp 37–43
63. Wolf P, Rieger E, Kerl H (1993) Topical photodynamic therapy with endogenous porphyrins after application of 5-aminolevulinic acid: an alternative treatment modality for solar keratoses, superficial squamous cell carcinomas, and basal cell carcinomas? J Am Acad Dermatol 28:17–21

VI Appendix

19 Practical Guidelines for Broadband UVB, Narrowband UVB, UVA-1 Phototherapy, and PUVA Photochemotherapy – A Proposal

Herbert Hönigsmann, Jean Krutmann

Contents

This is an overview of the guidelines for phototherapy with ultraviolet (UV) radiation and with psoralen photochemotherapy (PUVA) in the treatment of skin diseases as currently used in the institutions of the authors. There are, of course, other protocols in use that are effective. However, the guidelines presented here have proven safe and successful over many years of phototherapeutic practice and may aim at minimizing potential short-term and long-term side effects by optimizing therapeutic strategies.

UVB therapy and PUVA have well-established places in today's armamentarium of dermatological therapy. In this chapter, we discuss the use of unsensitized UV radiation (phototherapy without exogenous photosensitizers) as well as psoralen photosensitization (PUVA). Treatment regimens will be described primarily with regard to psoriasis, which is the most common indication for both UVB phototherapy and PUVA, while other indications will only be discussed briefly.

Phototherapy Regimens Without Photosensitizers

Phototherapy originally meant the use of artificial broadband UVB irradiations delivered by fluorescent lamps. Today, both broadband UVB and narrowband UVB, as well as combinations of UVA with UVB, are used for phototherapy. The use of narrowband (311–313 nm) phototherapy is superior to conventional broadband UVB with respect to both clearing and remission times in psoriasis. This is due to an improved adjustment of the lamp's emission to the therapeutic spectral requirements. In Europe, narrowband UVB has mostly replaced conventional UVB phototherapy. In the US, the Philips TL01 lamp has only recently come into use, partly due to minor technical incompatibilities. We have been able to show that for psoriasis narrowband phototherapy is nearly as effective as PUVA. Narrowband UVB has also been successfully used in a variety of combination therapies, such as with retinoids, anthralin, and calcipotriol. More recently, UVA-1 radiation (340–400 nm) has been experimentally used for certain inflammatory skin diseases.

Phototherapy with UVB

General Requirements for Safe and Effective Use of UVB Phototherapy

1. Indications: Besides psoriasis there are many other indications for UVB treatment that are discussed in depth in this book.
2. Contraindications: History of skin tumors, photodermatoses and photosensitizing drugs.
3. Informed consent of the patient after information on efficacy, side effects and potential long-term risks of UVB therapy.
4. Knowledge of the kinetics of UVB erythema reaction.
5. Regular exact measurement and documentation of the output of the irradiation source (mW/cm^2) and determination of the dose (J/cm^2; mJ/cm^2).
6. Determination of the individual UVB sensitivity by determining the minimal erythema dose (MED) with the irradiation source used for therapy.
7. Continuous monitoring of the patient during therapy.

Practical Aspects of UVB Phototherapy

Dosimetry

Prior to initiating phototherapy, it is advisable to evaluate the individual UV sensitivity of the patient by phototesting, since skin typing alone does not always reflect the actual sensitivity of an individual. Testing is done by exposing six small template areas (e.g., 1-cm diameter circles) of usually not sun-exposed areas such as the lower back or buttock skin to an incremental series of UVB irradiations. Increases are made by fixed values (e.g., 10 mJ) or by a fraction of the lower dose (e.g., 40 %). An example is given in Table 1. Note that these doses strongly depend on the light meter used.

Table 1. Exposure doses for MED test with broadband and narrowband UVB Sources (mJ/cm²), as measured with an integrated UV meter (Waldmann, Schwenningen, Germany)

Broadband UVB	20	40	60	80	100	120
Narrowband UVB	200	400	600	800	1,000	1,200

Table 2. MED reading

0	No erythema
+	Minimal perceptible erythema with sharp borders (=1 MED)
+	Pink erythema
++	Marked erythema, no edema, no pain
+++	Fiery red erythema, mild edema, mild pain
++++	Violaceus erythema, marked edema, strong pain, partial blistering

The smallest fluence that leads to a minimal detectable erythema reaction 24 h after irradiation is the MED (Table 2). Patients should be instructed to avoid sunbathing or solarium exposure at least 24 h prior to testing. It is of utmost importance to document the type of lamp used for the MED determination since the values obtained with broadband and narrowband sources differ in an order of magnitude.

There is some controversy if a visually assessed MED is the optimal reference value for dosimetry. However, its evaluation is a most practical and easily performed procedure and does not require any apparatus in addition to the phototherapy equipment.

Guidelines for Broadband UVB Therapy

Initial Treatment Phase (Treatment Until Clearing of Disease)
The initial therapeutic UVB dose lies at 70 % of the MED. Treatments are given 2–5 times weekly. As peak UVB erythema appears before 24 h after exposure, increments may be done with each successive treatment. If treatments are given 5 times weekly it is advisable to increase the dose every other treatment. The rate of increase depends on treatment frequency and the effect of the preceding therapeutic exposure. The objective of the dose increments is to maintain a minimally perceptible erythema as a clinical indicator of optimal dosimetry. For example, with thrice weekly treatments, increases of 40 % are given if no erythema was induced, and 20 % with slight erythema. If erythema is mild but persistent, no increment is made. With daily exposures, these rates are no more than 30, 15, and 0 %, respectively. With more intensive or painful erythema, irradiations are withheld until symptoms subside. Treatments are given until complete remission is achieved or no further improvement can be obtained with continued phototherapy (Table 3).

Table 3. Treatment schedule for broadband and narrowband UVB therapy

Step 1	Determination of the minimal erythema dose (MED)	Reading after 24 h	
Step 2	Start of treatment	First therapeutic dose	70 % of MED
Step 3	Treatment continuation thrice weekly (daily)	No erythema	Increase by 40 % (30 %)
		Minimal erythema	Increase by 20 % (15 %) after 2 treatments
		Persistent asymptomatic erythema	No increase
		Painful erythema with or without edema or blistering	No treatment until symptoms subside
Step 4	Resumption of treatment	After resolution of symptoms	Reduction of last dose by 50 %, further increase by 10 %

Maintenance Phase

There is no general agreement whether maintenance treatment is necessary to keep patients in remission for a longer period of time. No precise data exist that would prove the need for maintenance regimens. In cutaneous T-cell lymphoma most therapists use maintenance treatment for several months. For psoriasis, we use a 2-month maintenance phase with twice weekly irradiations for 1 month and once weekly for another month. As a UVB dosage, the last effective dose is given throughout the maintenance phase.

If relapses occur during maintenance treatment, frequency and UVB dose are increased again until clearing.

Guidelines for Narrowband UVB Therapy

Narrowband UVB is much less erythemogenic with regard to physical units (J/cm^2) than broadband UVB. Therefore dosing is different and, as pointed out above, the MED must be determined with these wavelengths. Erythema readings are also performed after 24 h and the initial treatment dose should be not more than 70 %.

Initial treatment phase and eventual maintenance treatment phase are essentially identical to what is recommended for broadband UVB (Table 2).

Switch from Broadband to Narrowband UVB Therapy or Vice Versa

When patients move to another treatment unit it is essential to provide them with detailed treatment data: Type of UVB source, initial MED, last effective dose, and frequency of treatments. If another light source is used for continuation, the current MED has to be determined with the new lamp and treatment is continued with 70 % of this value.

Phototherapy with UVA-1

UVA-1 phototherapy currently represents an investigational treatment form that was originally elaborated and tested for its efficacy for atopic dermatitis. Doses of 130 J/cm^2 are used, but more recently medium- and low-dose regimens are being explored. This area of phototherapy is still developing and further indications may evolve.

General Requirements for Safe and Effective Use of UVA-1 Therapy

1. Indications: Multicenter studies have confirmed the efficacy in severe and acutely exacerbated atopic dermatitis
2. Experimental indications: localized and systemic scleroderma, urticaria pigmentosa, early cutaneous T-cell lymphoma, phototherapy of HIV + patients
3. Contraindications: History of skin tumors, photodermatoses, and photosensitizing drugs. Age less than 18 years, because long-term risks unknown
4. Determination of the individual UVA-1 sensitivity by determining the minimal tanning dose (MTD) with the irradiation source used for therapy
5. Informed consent of the patient after information on efficacy, side effects, and potential long-term risks of UVA-1 therapy
6. Knowledge of the kinetics of UVA-1 pigmentary response
7. Regular exact measurement and documentation of the output of the irradiation source (mW/cm^2) and determination of the dose (J/cm^2)
8. Continuous monitoring of the patient during therapy

Practical Aspects of UVA-1 Phototherapy

Dosimetry

Dosimetry of UVA-1 therapy is adjusted to the individual UVA-1 sensitivity. Before initiating a total-body treatment, it is important to exclude any UVA-1-sensitive photodermatosis that could be provoked during treatment. According to present concepts, irradiation aims at reaching the highest dose of 130 J/cm^2. The test procedure is essentially the same as with UVB sources. Six template areas are irradiated with increasing doses of UVA-1 (Table 4).

Pigmentation readings are performed at 24 h. The smallest fluence that induces a minimal perceptible pigmentation is defined as the MTD (Table 5). In addition, adverse reactions such as erythema, papule, or vesicle formation are documented. The MTD determination does not serve as a parameter for the first therapeutic dose, but is done to obtain information on the individual UVA-1 sensitivity.

Table 4. MTD testing (J/cm^2)

Skin type	UVA-1 test dose					
I–II	10	20	40	60	100	130
III–VI	20	40	60	80	100	130

Table 5. MTD reading

0	No pigmentation
+	Minimal perceptible pigmentation with sharp borders(= 1 MTD)
+	Mild pigmentation
++	Marked pigmentation
+++	Intense pigmentation

Guidelines for High-Dose UVA-1 Therapy: Initial Treatment Phase (Treatment Until Clearing of Disease)

For atopic dermatitis and circumscribed scleroderma, treatments are given daily (with a rest on Saturdays and Sundays) with 130 J/cm^2 without dose increments. The number of treatments for atopic dermatitis is limited to 15, and for scleroderma to 30. For urticaria pigmentosa, treatment is started initially in body quadrants with 60 J/cm^2 and is subsequently increased to 130 J/cm^2. Thereafter patients are switched to total-body treatment with 2–3 irradiations with 60 J/cm^2 and finally 130 J/cm^2 until a total of 15 exposures is reached.

Treatment of Relapses

UVA-1 therapy can be repeated if relapses occur. Yet, because of the uncertainty regarding long-term risks, we have restricted treatment to two cycles per year.

Photochemotherapy (PUVA) Regimens

General Requirements for Safe and Effective Use of PUVA

1. Indications: PUVA is regarded as a treatment for several severe skin diseases, in particular severe psoriasis and cutaneous T-cell lymphoma and other indications that are mentioned in this book.
2. Contraindications: History of skin tumors, photodermatoses, and photosensitizing drugs (other than psoralens).
3. Informed consent of the patient after information on efficacy, side effects, and potential long-term risks of PUVA therapy.
4. Knowledge of the kinetics of the phototoxic PUVA erythema reaction.
5. Knowledge of the pharmacokinetics of psoralens.
6. Regular exact measurement and documentation of the output of the irradiation source (mW/cm^2) and determination of the UVA dose (J/cm^2).
7. Determination of the individual sensitivity by determining the minimal phototoxic dose (MPD).
8. Continuous monitoring of the patient during therapy.

Practical Aspects of PUVA

Two major forms of PUVA are in use, oral PUVA and bath PUVA. More recently, cream PUVA has proven to be ideal for the therapy of limited skin area (hands and feets, head and neck). The general principles of these three types are identical; however, the practical use is different, in particular, regarding dosimetry.

Photosensitizers

Oral PUVA
For oral PUVA 8-methoxypsoralen (8-MOP, Oxsoralen) or 5-methoxypsoralen (5-MOP, Geralen) are used. 5-MOP is currently available in only a few countries in Europe.

Both psoralens are administered according to body weight. 8-MOP is given 1 h, and 5-MOP is given 2 h before irradiation in order to reach the highest tissue level, based on the different kinetics of the two substances.
- 8-MOP (Oxsoralen) 0.6 mg/kg body weight
- 5-MOP (Geralen) 1.2 mg/kg body weight

Bath PUVA
For bath PUVA, 8-MOP and 4,5',8-trimethylpsoralen (TMP) are used. TMP-bath PUVA is currently performed mostly in Scandinavia. TMP induces higher photosensitivity after topical application and is used at lower concentrations than 8-MOP. For practical reasons we will refer here to 8-MOP only. 8-MOP is dissolved in bath water to reach a final concentration of 1.0 mg/l. This is achieved by dilution in bath water (1:5,000) of a stock solution (0.5 % 8-MOP in 96 % ethanol) or, in other words, 20 ml of the stock solution in 100 l bath water. The patients bathe in the tub for 15 – 20 min and are exposed to UVA immediately thereafter. The time interval between bath and irradiation must not be longer than 15 min as photosensitivity declines rapidly and lasts not more than 2 h.

Cream PUVA
For cream PUVA, 8-MOP is used. A 0.0006 %-8-MOP-containing water in oil emulsion (30 % H_2O) has been used for total body treatment. A 2-fold higher concentration is recommended if selected skin areas are being treated. One hour after cream application optimal photosensitivation is achieved.

Dosimetry

Our general recommendations are in accord with the so-called European protocol. This regimen requires initial determination of the individual MPD. MPD testing is done in analogy to MED determination by exposing lower back or buttock skin (after oral ingestion of psoralen or psoralen bath) to a series of graded exposures of UVA. To avoid severe reactions, UVA test doses are given according to skin typing (Tables 6, 7). Since bath PUVA induces a much higher degree of photosensitivity, the test doses must be kept considerably lower (Table 6). As with UVB phototesting, it should be done on previously not sun-exposed skin whenever possible.

Table 6. Exposure doses for MPD test with oral and cream PUVA (J/cm^2)

Skin types I–IV						
UVA dose (8-MOP)	0.5	1	2	3	4	5
UVA dose (5-MOP)	1	2	4	6	8	10

Table 7. Exposure doses for MPD test with bath PUVA (J/cm^2)

Skin types I and II						
UVA dose (8-MOP)	0.25	0.5	1	1.5	2	2.5
Skin types III and IV						
UVA dose (8-MOP)	0.5	1	2	3	4	5

Table 8. MPD reading

0	No erythema
+/–	Minimal perceptible erythema with sharp borders (= 1 MPD)
+	Pink erythema
++	Marked erythema, no edema, no pain
+++	Fiery red erythema, mild edema, mild pain
++++	Violaceus erythema, marked edema, strong pain, partial blistering

The delayed phototoxic erythema reaction is assessed after 72 h (not later than 96 h). The smallest fluence resulting in a minimal perceptible, well-circumscribed erythema represents the MPD (Table 8).

Guidelines for PUVA Therapy

Initial Treatment Phase (Treatment Until Clearing of Disease)
PUVA erythema does not peak before 72 h. Therefore, treatment should never be initiated before the end of the 72-h period after MPD testing. A safe initial therapeutic dose for oral PUVA is 70 % of the MPD (recent studies show that 50 % is often sufficient for effective treatment of psoriasis). For bath PUVA it is advisable to start with only 30 % of the MPD because photosensitivity is up to 10 times higher than with oral PUVA.

	Initial UVA dose
Oral PUVA	50–70 % of the MPD
Bath PUVA	30 % of the MPD
Cream PUVA	50–70 % of the MPD

Irradiations are given up to 4 times weekly. Dose increments are performed not more frequently than twice a week (at least 72 h apart) and never during the first week of treatment in order to avoid an accumulation of delayed cutaneous phototoxicity. However, although not necessary for the therapeutic success, a minimally perceptible erythema is considered a clinical indicator of adequate

Table 9. Treatment schedule for oral and bath PUVA

			Type of PUVA Oral PUVA	Bath PUVA	Cream PUVA
Step 1	Determination of the minimal phototoxic dose (MPD)	Reading after 72 h			
Step 2	Start of treatment	First therapeutic dose	50–70 % of MPD	30 % of MPD	50–70 % of MPD
Step 3	Treatment continuation 2–4 times weekly	No erythema, good response	Increase once weekly by 30 %	Increase once weekly by 30 %	Increase once weekly by 30 %
		No erythema, no response	Increase by 30 %	Increase by 30 %	Increase by 30 %
		Minimal erythema	No increase	No increase	No increase
		Persistent asymptomatic erythema	No increase	No increase	No increase
		Painful erythema with or without edema or blistering	No treatment until symptoms subside	No treatment until symptoms subside	No treatment until symptoms subside
Step 4	Resumption of treatment	After resolution of symptoms	Reduction of last dose by 50 %; if well-tolerated, further increase by 10 %	Reduction of last dose by 50 %; if well-tolerated, further increase by 10 %	Reduction of last dose by 50 %; if well-tolerated, further increase by 10 %

dosimetry. There exists no rigid scheme for dose increments; the major parameter for dose adjustments should be the response of the disease to therapy. It is essential to note that with bath PUVA the MPD can even decrease during the first days after initiation of treatment by up to 50 %, but it increases at later stages. This may be due to persistent psoralen adducts which are converted into crosslinks upon subsequent exposure.

If no erythema is present, in the average case, the UVA dose can be increased safely by 30 % in both, oral PUVA, and bath PUVA (Table 9).

An example for PUVA dosimetry (4 times weekly) is shown below:

Oral PUVA/Cream PUVA
Day	1	2	3	4	5	6	7	8	9	10	11	12	13	14	15	16
J/cm^2	2	2	0	2	2	0	0	2.6	2.6	0	3.4	3.4	0	0	4	4

Bath PUVA
Day	1	2	3	4	5	6	7	8	9	10	11	12	13	14	15	16
J/cm^2	1	1	0	1	1	0	0	1.3	1.3	0	1.3	1.3	0	0	1.7	1.7

Some patients will not need dose adjustments over prolonged periods of time because of erythema formation and/or adequate treatment response.

Maintenance Phase

Maintenance therapy is recommended in the European regimen. It consists of one month of twice-weekly treatments with the last UVA dose used for clearing, followed by another month of once weekly exposures. According to the recommendation of the British Photodermatology Group, maintenance treatment should be considered only if relapses are rapidly following clearance. Although PUVA has been in use now for more than 25 years, the question whether maintenance therapy can prevent early relapses in psoriasis has remained unsolved. For cutaneous T-cell lymphoma, many institutions recommend some type of permanent maintenance therapy. However, due to the lack of prospective studies no valid recommendation can be given. Perhaps a once-monthly treatment would be a feasible compromise.

Mild relapses during the maintenance phase are treated by temporarily increasing the frequency of treatments, in the case of severe relapse the original clearing phase schedule must be resumed until clearing is achieved again.

Suggested Readings

1. Krutmann J (1999) Therapeutic photomedicine: Phototherapy. In: Freedberg IM, Eisen AZ, Wolff K, Austen KF, Goldsmith LA, Katz SI, Fitzpatrick TB (eds) Fitzpatrick's dermatology in general medicine, 5th edn. McGraw-Hill, New York, pp 2870–2879
2. Hönigsmann H, Szeimies R-F, Knobler R, Fitzpatrick TB Pathak MA, Wolff K (l999) Photochemotherapy and Photodynamic Therapy. In: Fitzpatrick TB et al (eds) Dermatology in General Medicine. 5th Edition McGrawHill, New York, pp 2880–2900
3. Morison WL, Fitzpatrick TB: Phototherapy and Photochemotherapy of Skin Disease (1991) 2nd Edition, Raven Press, New York
4. Guidelines of care for phototherapy and photochemotherapy (1994) American Academy of Dermatology Committee on Guidelines of Care. J Am Acad Dermatol 31:643
5. British Photodermatology Group (1994) British Photodermatology Group guidelines for PUVA. Br. J. Dermatol. 130:246–255.

20 Technical Equipment

Helger Stege, Renz Mang

Contents

Introduction

This chapter will provide an overview of irradiation devices that are offered by industry for photo(chemo)therapy in Europe and the United States. An important difference between Europe and the USA is the large number of homecare units that are available in the United States. In Europe, photo(chemo)therapy is almost exclusively being carried out by dermatologists in their offices or in a clinical setting.

The authors would like to point that all the information given in this chapter has been provided by the industry upon contact by the authors. In other words, inclusion or exclusion of a specific company from this chapter might result from ignorance of this company by the authors or from lack of response of the company to the authors' request for information. We have tried to contact every available company and asked them to provide the information that is required for inclusion into this chapter. Despite of these efforts, however, we cannot guarantee completeness. Also, we do not take responsibility for the validity of the information provided by the companies listed here. This applies especially to information on specific emission spectra. These data are the result of measurements conducted by the given company and are not based on measurements performed by us.

Some producers saved registered names or trade names for their products or therapy regimens. Attempts have been made to respect this as much as possible. We do not exclude, however, a wrong or contentious use of single terms, and if trademarks are missing, the reader cannot conclude that this name has not been registered.

Prices given in the tables cannot be guaranteed from the companies due to differences in taxes.

The legal situation concerning the therapeutic use of a given irradiation device system is different in Europe and the United States. As general advice, we would like to recommend that a dermatologist asks for a declaration from the producer or the provider stating that the therapeutic use of a device system of interest is in accordance with the national law.

Abbreviations

I   Intensity
W   Wattage
V   Voltage
IFR   Infrared radiation
pb   Partial body
ms   Modular system
+   Established technique
±   Possible
–   Not possible

Irradiation Device Systems for PUVA Therapy and Broadband UVA Therapy (Tables 1 and 2)

Table 1. Irradiation device systems for PUVA therapy and broadband UVA therapy

Producer	Bulbs/ radiators	Type	Spectrum (in nm)	Technical data	Comment
Cosmedico (Europe, USA)	Fluorescence bulbs	Arimed A Arimed PUVA	350–400 315–400	I: 6–10 mW/cm^2 W: 4,800 W, 220 V/380 V. Panel, cabinet, sunbed, pb irradiation devices, modular system, no special installations necessary Price: 15,000 DM (cabinet)	No integrated dosimetry, dosage via time (single intervals of approx. 20 s possible) Additional UVA dosimeter available Cosmedico offers complete irradiation devices as well as fluorescence bulbs
Dr. Hönle (Europe)	Fluorescence bulbs	Cleo Performance (Philips) dermalight dermalight 3000	320–400	I: 7.3 mW/cm^2; V: 230 V/50 Hz; W: 900–3000 W; cabinet	Integrated dosimetry, opportunity for PC-assisted data and therapy monitoring Combined UVA–UVB irradiation possible
Dr. Hönle (Europe)	Metal halide radiators	Dr. Hönle 400W metal halide radiators dermalight 2005 dermalight 6000	Filter: 1. 320–400 2. 320–400 + IFR-filter	I: 10–20 mW/cm^2 (depending on the filter); W: 2,050 W per column V: 220 V, 50 Hz Filter systems: 1. "Selective UVA-therapy" (SUVA) with blue-filter 2. UVA/PUVA-therapy with h1 filter; columns, cabinets, pb irradiation devices, modular system Price: 9,500–27,500 DM	High-intensity, filter necessary. Caveat: irradiation with wrong spectra possible, if filter missing PC-assisted irradiation with dosage and filter control Standby mode
Narva (Europe)	Fluorescence bulbs	UVA Type 009	320–400	W: 15–160 W V: 220 V, 50 Hz	Only bulbs available, no production of device systems, low UVB contamination, PUVA therapy possible (producer's comment)

Table 1. (Continued)

Producer	Bulbs/radiators	Type	Spectrum (in nm)	Technical data	Comment
National Biological Corporation (USA)	Fluorescence bulbs	FR72T12/BL/HO (UVA); F40/350 BL (UVA); F36T12/BL/HO (UVA); F24T12/BL/HO (UVA); F20T12/BL/HO (UVA); F6T5/BL (UVA); HOUVA II UVA; UVISOL UVA; Panisol UVA	320–400	Different intensities, depending on the type and number of bulbs Price: US $1,695–11,500	Special measuring devices, complete offer of additional equipment
Philips (Europe, USA)	Fluorescence bulbs[a]	Philips TL/08, TL/09 CLEO Performance Cleo Professional	305–400	Detailed technical information via provider or Philips	For medical use: in Europe no direct retail
Photo-TherapeutiX (USA)	Fluorescence bulbs	Model 1600 A (office use) Model 2400 A (office use)	320–400	I: 25 mW/cm^2 V: 30a/240 V/60 Hz Price: US $8,300	Units for UVA phototherapy only for office use, integrated dosimetry
Psoralite (USA)	Fluorescence bulbs	Model 1400 Master UVA Model 1400 Master/Remote UVA Model 2400 UVA	320–400	I: unknown W: unknown V: 110 V Price: US $995–2,750	Dosimetry via time For homecare use
Saalmann (Europe)	Metal halide radiators	Uvapur Uvapur single radiators or ES cabinets	315–380	I: 10–17 mW/cm^2 W: 1,000–2,000 W, 230VAC No installations for cabinets, columns, pb irradiation devices Price: 15,900–30,000 DM	High-intensity, integrated dosimetry, therapy via time or physical units. Stand-by mode. Cabinets for UVA, UVB, PUVA, and combination irradiation

Table 1. (Continued)

Producer	Bulbs/radiators	Type	Spectrum (in nm)	Technical data	Comment
Daavlin (USA)	Fluorescence bulbs	Spectra 350 Spectra 700 (homecare) UV 360 – Home Light Cabinets	320–400	I: 30 mW/cm^2 Price: US \$12,500 US \$1,695–5,495 (homecare units)	All of these units can be manufactured to any desired voltage
Schulze and Böhm (Europe)	Metal halide radiators	450 W UV medisun 6000 medisun 6001L medisun 6311 (ISO) medisun 12000	315–400	I: 15–40 mW/cm^2 W: 5,000–12,000 W, 400 V Sunbeds, automatically change of the filter systems (UVB-UVA), installations necessary Price: 29,500 DM	Computer-assisted irradiation with isodoses, pb irradiation by selection of different bulbs PUVA therapy +, photopatch test possible
Schulze and Böhm	Fluorescence bulbs	medisun 1000 K (Philips TL/10 100 W)	315–400	I: 6–11 mW/cm^2 W: 1,000–3,000 W V: 230 V cabinets, Price: 11,500 DM	Electronic timer, on special request, integrated dosimetry
Sellas (Europe, in USA: Daavlin)	Metal halide radiators	Sellamed System Dr. Sellmeier (2kW-bulbs) Sellamed 12000 Sellamed 18400	320–440 IFR reduced	I: 30–80 mW/cm^2 W: 10–18 kW, 380 V Other voltages possible Sunbeds (horizontal system, irradiation from top), pb units, installation necessary: integrated air condition Price: on inquiry	High-irradiation intensity, integrated dosimetry possible, PUVA: ± Provider in USA: Daavlin

Table 1. (Continued)

Producer	Bulbs/radiators	Type	Spectrum (in nm)	Technical data	Comment
Waldmann (Europe, USA)	Fluorescence bulbs	Waldmann F85/100 W UV6; F86/100 W UV 21 PUVA 1000 L (cabinet) PUVA 3003 (cabinet) PUVA 7001 (horizontal system – irradiation from top)	320–400	I: 3 mW/cm², W: 1,8 (UV3003); 3–5 kW (cabinets), 230/400 V horizontal systems, pb devices, hand/foot box; Installations: pb devices: 220 V, no special installations. Cabinets: 380 V, Installations necessary, modification for different voltages possible. Price: on request	Integrated dosimetry, doses infinitely variable, PUVA therapy +, combinations with UVB-emitting bulbs possible
Wolff (Europe)	Fluorescence bulbs	Wolff System	320–400 (345–365)	Identical to Arimed A (Cosmedico), German market: Cosmedico	Compare: Cosmedico, Switzerland: Wolff

[a] Philips Licht offers also metal halide lamps for UVA-therapy, filters necessary.

Table 2. Partial body irradiation devices for PUVA-, topical PUVA- and for broadband UVA therapy and photodiagnostic procedures (photo-patch, MED, MTD, IPD)

Producer	Bulbs/radiators	Type	Spectrum (in nm)	Technical data	Comment
Cosmedico (Europe, USA)	Fluorescence bulbs	Arimed A (100 W) Cosmedico TK-8	320–400 max.: 340–360	I: 6mW/cm², W: 350 W, 220 V Tripod. Price: ca. 1,300 DM	Pb PUVA +, phototesting +, Dosage via time, portable system configured dosimeter
Daavlin (USA)	Fluorescence bulbs	Spectra Mini I UVA	320–400	I: 30 mW/cm² Price: US $1,350 – 2,300	Dosimetry via time or physical units possible

Table 2. (Continued)

Producer	Bulbs/radiators	Type	Spectrum (in nm)	Technical data	Comment
Dr. Hönle dermalight vario 1; 2 (Europe)	Metal halide radiators	Dr.Hönle metal halide lamps	320–400	I: ca.15–30 mW/cm^2 W: 500–950 W, 220 V. Different filter systems, tripod, top for hand-foot irradiation Price: vario 1: 2,950 DM vario 2: 7,000 DM	Pb PUVA +, phototesting +. High irradiation intensity Dosage via time, no integrated dosimetry. Filter necessary
Dr. Hönle dermalight 180/450 (Europe)	Fluorescence bulbs	PL-S 9 W/10 (Philips)	320–400	I: 12,5 mW/cm^2; V:230, 50 Hz; W: 30–50 W	Pb irradiation, PUVA +
National Biological Corporation (USA)	Fluorescence bulbs	F24T12/BL/HO (UVA) Panisol II UVA Hand/foot II Unit Handisol UVA	320–400	For further information, please contact producer	Company offers also additional equipment, measuring devices, and bulbs
Saalmann (Europe)	Metal halide radiators	Uvapur	315–380	I:10–17 mW/cm^2 W: 0.4–2 kW, 230 V. tripod, Price: 5,000–12,000 DM	Pb PUVA ±, phototesting +, dosage via time, mode for single irradiation areas: pb irradiation
Saalmann (Europe)	Metal halide radiators	Multitester	280–315 315–400	I:up to 50 mW/cm^2 V: 230 V, 00VA, tripod Price: US $9,000	UVA/UVB phototesting unit, integrated light source, system-configured dosimeter
Schulze and Böhm	Fluorescence bulbs	medisun HF-160	315–400	I: 6 mW/cm^2 W: 150–600 W, 230 V tripod, table Price: 1,400–4,000 DM	Electronic timer, dosage via time, portable dosimeter

Table 2. (Continued)

Producer	Bulbs/ radiators	Type	Spectrum (in nm)	Technical data	Comment
Schulze and Böhm	Metal halide radiators	medisun PUVA-HF system 400 W metal halide radiators	315–400	I: 15–30 mW/cm² W: 400–1200 W/230 V Tripod, table Price: 2,900 DM	Electronic timer, dosage via time, portable dosimeter
Sellas (Europe, in USA: Daavlin)	Metal halide radiators	UVA System Dr. Sellmeier 2kW–4 kW Sellamed 2000, 3000, 4000	320–440 IFR reduced	I: 30–150 mW/cm² W: 2.3–4.5 kW, 220 V, other voltages possible, Tripod, Price: on inquiry	Pb PUVA ±, phototesting +, dosage via time
Waldmann (Europe, USA)	Fluorescence bulbs	PL 36 W/09/UV 181AL F8T5 PUVA/UV 200 AL (Mobile support tables) UVA 40 W/UV801AL	315–400 (355)	I: ca. 11–20 mW/cm² V: 230 V, other voltages possible, W: 560 W; Price: on request	Pb PUVA +, phototesting + dosage via time, portable system-configured dosimeter
Waldmann (Europe, USA)	Metal halide radiators	UVA 700 L	330–450	W: 930 W	Phototesting +

UVA-1 Irradiation Devices (Tables 3 and 4)

Table 3. Units for high-dose UVA-1 therapy

Producer[a]	Bulbs/ radiators	Type	Spectrum (in nm)	Technical data	Comment
Dr. Hönle (Europe)	Metal halide radiators	2 kW metal halide radiators Dr. K. Hönle dermalight Ultra 1 24 kW	340–440, IFR reduced	I: 80 mW/cm^2, W: 24 kW, 380 V. Sunbed. Expensive installation for air-conditioning and filters Price: ca. 119,000 DM	Comparable to the dermalight Ultra 1 (12 kW) intensity reduced
Mutzhas (Europe)	Metal halide radiators	UVASUN UVASUN 30000 Biomed	340–400 + visible light	I: 75 mW/cm^2, W: 30 kW, 380 V. Sunbed. Expensive installation for air-conditioning and filters	At this time no production, but spare parts available
Schulze and Böhm (Europe)	Metal halide radiators	medisun 24000 UVA1-high-dosis sunbed 12 × 2000 W radiators	340–410 345–410 IFR reduced	I: 70–120 mW/cm^2 W: 26.5 kW, 400 V. Sunbed. Expensive installation for air-conditioning and filters Price: 89,000 DM	Computer-assisted irradiation with isodoses. UVA-1 irradiation devices for partial-body irradiation available
Sellas (Europe, in USA: Daavlin)	Metal halide radiators	UVA System Dr. Sellmeier Sellamed 24000 A	340–400 + visible light and IFR reduced	I: 50–100 mW/cm^2, W: 26.5 kW, 380 V, other voltages possible. Sunbed (horizontal system, irradiation from top), change of bulbs: after 700 h, expensive installation for filter, air-conditioning and electrics necessary Price: on inquiry	Variation of intensity via distance. Change of filters: depending on measurement of UV-emission by producer (service) Daavlin is exclusive distributor for Sellas in the USA
Cosmedico	Metal halide radiators	12 × 2000 W radiators	340–400 IFR reduced	I: –, W: 24 kW, 400 V. Sunbed	Alarm clock for patients: Software available

[a] On special request Saalmann-Produktionstechnik is able to produce an individually designed UVA-1 unit with an intensity up to 120 mW/cm^2. Technical data by Saalmann.

Table 4. Units for medium- or low-dose UVA-1 therapy

Producer	Bulbs/ radiators	Type	Spectrum (in nm)	Technical data	Comment
Dr. Hönle (Europe)	Metal halide radiators	2 kW-metal halide lamps Dr. K. Hönle dermalight Ultra 1	340–440 IFR reduced	I: 40 mW/cm^2, W: 12 kW, 380 V, further technical data see Table 4: Dr. Hönle dermalight Ultra 1 (24 kW) price: 79,000 DM	Comparable dermalight Ultra 1 (24 kW)
Narva (Europe)	Fluorescence bulbs	Narva UVA1 Type 010 UV	340–400	W: 15–160 W, Length: 43.8–176 cm, Price on inquiry	Only production of bulbs, for pb and wb units. Note the producer's instruction (liability)
Optomed (Europe)	Fluorescence bulbs	OptoDerm radiators (modules) OptoDerm UVA1/ VIS	340–400 Maxima at: 370, 390, 420, 450 IFR reduced	I: 50 mW/cm^2, W: 26,5 kW, 380 V. Sunbed, IFR filter, integrated air-conditioning, expensive installation Price: on inquiry	Narrow-band emission, fluorescence bulbs. Low costs for installations
Philips (Europe, USA)	Fluorescence bulbs	TL 10	340–400		
Saalmann	Metal halide radiators	ESI-Bed (ES I Liege)	340–400	I: 40 mW/cm^2, W: 380 V, horizontal system (irradiation from top) Price on request	System-configured dosimeter
Sellas (in USA: Daavlin)	Metal halide radiators	On request	340–400 visible light IFR reduced	Technical data on request	Sunbed (horizontal system) production of devices for medium-dose UVA-1 possible Details on request Daavlin is exclusive distributor for Sellas in the USA

Table 4. (Continued)

Producer	Bulbs/radiators	Type	Spectrum (in nm)	Technical data	Comment
Cosmedico	Metal halide radiators	12 × 2000 W radiators	340–400 IFR reduced	I: –, W: 24 kW, 400 V. Sunbed	Alarm clock for patients: Software available
Waldmann (Europe, USA)	Fluorescence bulbs	F 85/100 W/TL 10R PUVA 1000L (cabinet) PUVA 3003 (cabinet) PUVA 7001 (horizontal system)	340–400	I: 12–21 mW/cm^2 W: 3–5 kW V: 230/400 V Installation necessary Price: on request Special voltage possible	Cabinets and horizontal therapy systems are available

Irradiation Devices for UVB Therapy (Tables 5–9)

Table 5. Units for conventional broadband UVB therapy

Producer	Bulbs/radiators	Type	Spectrum (in nm)	Technical data	Comment
National Biological Corporation (USA)	Fluorescence bulbs	Light source: FSX72T12/UVB/ HOFS72T12/UVB/ HOFS72T12/UVB/SL; devices: HOUVA II UVB; UVISOL UVB; Panisol UVB; Foldalite	280–320	For further information, please contact the producer	Company also offers additional equipment, measuring devices, etc. Combination with narrow-band UVB possible

Table 5. (Continued)

Producer	Bulbs/ radiators	Type	Spectrum (in nm)	Technical data	Comment
Cosmedico (Europe)	Fluorescence bulbs	Light source: Arimed B Arimed B6 Arimed B 12 devices: GP-24 GP-36 GP-42	300 – 400 290 – 350 285 – 350	I: ca. 0.3 mW/cm^2, W: 4,800 W, 220 V/380 V panel, cabinet, sunbed, pb devices, modular system, price: ca. 18,000 DM (cabinet)	No system-configured dosimeter, dosimetry via time, time intervals a 20 s (for homecare units); pb unit for UVB phototesting usable Office units are equipped with integrated dosimetry
Dr. Hönle (Europe)	Metal halide radiators	Dr. Hönle 400W-radiators dermalight 2005 6000	280 – 400	I: 10 – 20 mW/cm^2, W: 2 – 6 kW, 220 V Columns, cabinets, pb devices, modular system, no requirement for installation for a single column Price: 11,000 – 38,000 DM	Dosimetry via time or physical units possible Advantage: UVB and UVA-therapy by changing of filters possible. Disadvantage: adverse irradiation possible. Compare: Table 1 Dr. Hönle.

Table 6. Units for conventional broadband UVB therapy

Producer	Bulbs/ radiators	Type	Spectrum (in nm)	Technical data	Comment
Metec (Europe)	Fluorescence bulbs	F 85/100 W UV6 Modell: UV 1500 L Arimed 100 W Modell 6100, 1389 Metec UV 1500 L	290 – 340	W: 650 W, 230 V (Modell 6100) W: 2,500 W, 230 V W: 1,000 W, 230 V	Cabinets and sunbeds especially for homecare

Table 6. (Continued)

Producer	Bulbs/radiators	Type	Spectrum (in nm)	Technical data	Comment
Photo TherapeutiX (USA)	Fluorescence bulbs	Model 1600 B (office use), Model 2400 B (office use), Model800B (home unit), Model 1650B (home unit)		I: 3,5–8 mW/cm^2, V: 120/60 Hz, 18 amp; Price: US $6,500–9,400 (office units); Price: US $4,300–5,400 (homecare units)	Cabinets are equipped with a data-control system, and acrylic panels to protect the patient from contact with the bulbs
Schulze and Böhm (Europe)	Metal halide radiators	400 W UV, medisun 6000 K, medisun 12000 K	290–400 peak at 311 nm	I: 1–5 mW/cm^2 (depending on distance); W: 6,500–12,000 W, 400 V; cabinet, columns, sunbeds; Installations necessary; Partial-body systems available; Price: 9,500–39,000 DM	Computer-assisted irradiation with isodoses; pb therapy by selection of radiators; automatic filter change (UVB--UVA), UVA, UVB, and combination therapy UVA/UVB possible
Waldmann (Europe, USA)	Fluorescence bulbs	F 85/100 W UV6; F 85/100 W UV 21; UV 1000 L; UV 7001; UV 3003; partial body: TL20 W/12; UV801BL; F15T8 UVB-UV181BL; F8T5 UVB-UV200BL	280–370, 275–370, 280–370	I: ca. 3 mW/cm^2; Cabinets, horizontal systems: 380 V, installation necessary; pb unit (UV 800): 230 V, no installation; Price: on request (cabinets); partial body-devices: I: 3–6 mW/cm^2; V: 230 V; Price: on request; Special voltages possible for all units	System-configured dosimeter

Table 7. Units for selective UVB therapy

Producer	Bulbs/radiators	Type	Spectrum (in nm)	Technical data	Comment
Dr. Hönle (Europe)	Metal halide lamps	Dr. Hönle 400W-metal halide lamp dermalight 2500 1–3 6000	295–400	I: 10–20 mW/cm^2, W: 2–6 kW, V: 220 V. Filter: h2 (Hönle) Columns, cabinets, pb devices, modular system, low installation costs for single column Price: 11,000–38,000 DM	No integrated dosimetry, dosage via time, high intensity-short irradiation; service-computer; filter change necessary Compare: Table 1 Dr. Hönle.
Saalmann (Europe)	Metal halide radiators	SUP-radiator	290–400 Maximum311 nm	I: 0.5–2 mW/cm^2 cabinets, columns, sunbeds, pb devices W: 0.4–2 kW (cabinet) V: 230 V, Price: 10,000–30,000 DM	System-configured dosimeter Dosimetry via time or physical units possible; short irradiation; service computer, chipcard

Table 8. Units for 311-nm UVB therapy

Producer	Bulbs/radiators	Type	Spectrum (in nm)	Technical data	Comment
Schulze and Böhm (Europe)	Fluorescence bulbs	Philips TL-01 medisun 1000B-311 medisun H-600	311	W: 600–3,000 W, 230 V Cabinets, columns, pb devices Prices: 2,295–29,900 DM	Long-life radiators (approx. 1,000 h), electronic timer PC-assisted irradiation, integrated dosimetry
Cosmedico (Europe, USA)	Fluorescence bulbs	Arimed 311 devices: GH-8/8ST GP-24 GP-36 GP-42	305–315	I: no information W: 9–100 W	Most of the systems can be used with Arimed bulbs

Table 8. Units for selective UVB therapy

Producer	Bulbs/ radiators	Type	Spectrum (in nm)	Technical data	Comment
Photo TherapeutiX (USA)	Fluorescence bulbs	TL-01 Model 1600B (office use) Model 2400B (office use) Model800B (home units) Model 1650B (home units)	311	I: 3.5 cm^2 V: 120 V/60 Hz Price: ca. US $6,500	Cabinets are equipped with a data-control system and acrylic panels to protect the patient from direct contact with the bulbs
National Biological Corporation (USA)	Fluorescence bulbs	TL-01 HOUVA UVBNB UVISOL UVBNB	311	For further information, please contact the producer	Company also offers additional equipment, measuring devices
Metec GmbH (Europe)	Fluorescence bulbs	TL-01 UV 1500 TL	311	W: 1,000 W, 230 V	Special use as homecare units
Waldmann (Europe, USA)	Fluorescence bulbs	Philips TL-01[a] Waldmann F 85/100 W TL-01 UV 1000 L UV 3003 UV 7001 for 311-nm UVB	311	I: 12–13 mW/cm^2 W: 1–5 kW, 230/400 V Price: on request Installation necessary	Emission not only at 311 nm. Low erythematogenicity – high therapeutic safety

[a] Philips TL-01, as well as Cosmedico Arimed 311, or Narva bulbs fit also in irradiation devices of most of the other producers.

Table 9. Units for UVA/UVB combination therapy

Producer	Bulbs/radiators	Name	Spectrum (in nm)	Technical data/comment
Cosmedico (Europe)	Fluorescence bulbs	Arimed B, identical to Photomed Wolff System, Helarium	300–400	Description comp. Table 1 Cosmedico
Waldmann (Europe, USA)	Fluorescence bulbs	Various combination possibilities UVA/UVB	280–400	Description comp. Table 1 Waldmann. Monotherapeutical use for UVB, UVA, PUVA treatment possible
Saalmann (Europe)	Metal halide radiators	Universale	290–400	Partial- and full-body irradiation device systems (sunbeds, cabinets, columns)
Schulze and Böhm (Europe)	Metal halide radiators	medisun 1000AB UV combination cabinet up 26 × 100 W radiators, UVA, UVA1, UVB 311 nm possible	315–400 340–410 311	I: 10–25, 10–25, 6–12 mW/cm^2, W: 1,000–3,000 W, 230 V. Cabinets, spectra selectively usable, Price: minimum 14,000 DM Computer-assisted irradiation with isodoses, electronic timer optional
Schulze and Böhm (Europe)	Metal halide radiators and fluorescence bulbs	medisun 6311 K (ISO)	315–440 311	I: 10–25, 6–12 mW/cm^2, W: 6500 W, 400 V. Cabinets, spectra selectively usable, price: minimum 39,000 DM Computer-assisted irradiation with isodoses optional, pb irradiation possible with different intensities, special kind of cabinets (semi-open)
Schulze and Böhm (Europe)	Metal halide radiators	medisun 4000 K medisun 6000 K medisun 12000 K	290–440 315–440	I: 10–25 mW/cm^2, W: 4500–12000 W, 400 V. Cabinets, spectra selectively usable, Price: minimum 24,900 DM Computer-assisted irradiation with isodoses optional, pb irradiation possible with different intensities, special kind of cabinets (semi-open) Photopatch test function integrated
Photo TherapeutiX (USA)	Fluorescence bulbs	Model 2480 AB		W: 240V-30a. Office units

Photodynamic Therapy and Diagnostics (Table 10)

Table 10. Photodynamic therapy and diagnostic

Producer	Bulbs/radiators	Name	Spectrum	Technical data	Comment
Waldmann (Europe)	Metal halide radiators	PDT 1200 L	600–750 red (other spectra on request)	W: 1200 W -1500 W, 230 V; Price: on request; Special voltages possible	Mobile tripod, relatively large homogeneous irradiation area Integrated dosimetry
Saalmann (Europe)	Metal halide radiators	PDT-Strahler PDD-Strahler	Near 543 (green: PDT), 360–400 (Black: PDD)	W: 150 W, 230 V; Price: 8,500 DM; W: 125 W, 230 V; Price: on inquiry	Portable; Weight, tripod, movable, irradiation area 100 × 100 mm, combination of several units possible (modular system). Different systems for photodynamic diagnostic and therapy
Sellas (Europe, for USA: Daavlin)	Metal halide radiators	Sellamed PDT twin-light	600–750, 500–600, Wood's light	W: 1200 W, 220 V, other voltages possible; Price: 10,000 DM	Device system is equipped with wood-light for additional photodiagnostic procedures
ESC (Europe)	Metal halide radiators	Versa Light	580–720 red, 520–590 green, band at 1250–1600	I: 80-150 mW/cm², W: 1,000 W, 230 V. Price: 60,000 DM	Additional fluorescence at 400–450 nm
Optomed (Europe)	Fluorescence bulbs	OptoDerm	Near 635 red	I: 70 mW/cm²; Price on inquiry	Modular system.
Optomed HD1 (Europe)	Metal halide radiators	Optoderm HD1	600–700	I: 100 mW/cm², W: 1,000 W, 380 V; Price: approx. 9,000 DM	For photodynamic therapy of acne (producer's comment)

Extracorporeal Photopheresis

– Photopheresis UVAR XTS Therakos Inc.

Additional Equipment

Most of the whole-body irradiation devices are equipped with an integrated system for continuous dosimetry. In contrast to whole-body irradiation devices, there is a lack of integrated continuous dosimetry in the use of partial-body irradiation devices. In these cases dosimetry has to be performed using external UV-dosimeters. It is important that the used UV-dosimeter fits to the spectrum emitted by the light source.

– Waldmann: UV dosimeter for UVA und UVB irradiation (UVB: light source UV6 and UV21).
– Dr. Hönle: UVA dosimeter. Because of the constant relation of UVA/UVB radiation in Dr. Hönle metal halide light source (producer's comment) the UVB-dose can be calculated using a given mathematical formula.
– Cosmedico: Cosmolux UVATEST 3000 only for Arimed A light sources.
– Dr. Gröbel UV-Elektronik GmbH: dosimeter for UVA, UVB and spectral radiometer.
– International Light: various UV detectors for scientific and photodermatological use.
– National Biological Corporation: detectors for external dosimetry.
– Polytec: different dosimeter for UV and IFR radiation (scientific, technical, and photomedical use).
– Schulze and Böhm: dosimetry only necessary for calibration.
– Sellas: offers a specific dosimeter for measurement of UVA-1 irradiation, which is adapted to own irradiation devices and filter combinations.
– Solar light: detectors for UVA, UVB, and visible light.
  Adverse effects of UV therapy can be avoided by suberythemal irradiation. The following companies are offering skin-type independent phototest system for determination of the UV-threshold doses (MED, MPD, IPD, or PPD).
– Waldmann: This test system can be used for all irradiation device systems. The irradiation intensity of the device system has to be known. Depending on the different intensities, test areas are automatically covered after irradiation of the skin with predefined UV doses.
– Saalmann: MED test system with integrated light sources, that means determination of UV-threshold doses are only relevant for these or equivalent irradiation device systems.
– Schulze and Böhm: offers a computer-assisted test system.
– Solar Light: offers photodiagnostic units (solar simulators and detectors).

List of Companies or Providers

Devices (Table 11)

Table 11. Device providers

Provider	Address	Telephone/fax	E-mail/Website/telex
Atlas B.V.	Vogelsbergstr. 22 63589 Linsengericht- Altenhaßlau Germany	Tel.: +49-(0)6051 – 7070 Fax: +49-(0)6051 – 707149	
Cosmedico	Kölner Str. 8 70376 Stuttgart Germany	Tel.: +49-(0)711 – 540040 Fax: +49-(0)711 – 54004-55	
ESC-Medizin-technik	Leonhardsweg 2 82008 Unterhaching Germany	Tel.: +49-(0)89 – 66539305 Fax: +49-(0)89 – 6116002	
Dr. Gröbel	UV- Elektronik GmbH Goethestr. 17 76275 Ettlingen Germany		
Gebrüder Haslauer oHG	Kirchenwegstr. 5 83404 Mitterfelden Germany or Moosstr. 131 5020 Salzburg Austria	Tel.: +49-(0)8654 – 488722 Fax: +49-(0)8654 – 488755 Tel.: +43-(0)662 – 830667 Fax: +43-(0)662 – 821740	
Dr. K. Hönle GmbH	Medizintechnik Fraunhoferstraße 5 82152 Planegg Germany	Tel.: +49-(0)89/89922584 Fax: +49-(0) 89/89922580	
Metec GmbH	Medizin-Technische Gesellschaft Buttermelcherstr. 15 80469 München Germany	Tel.: ++ (0)89 – 227221 Fax: ++ (0)89 – 226030	
I. Mutzhas Trading - GmbH	Pilgersheimerstr. 64 81543 München Germany U.S. distribution: National Biological Corporation 1532 Enterprise Parkway Twinsburg OH 44087 USA	Tel.: +49-(0)89 – 668405 Fax: +49-(0)89 – 664809 Phone: +1 – 3300- 425 – 3535 +1 – 0800-338 – 5045 Fax: +1 – 330-425 – 9614	wwWnatbiocorp.com E-mail: nbc@natbiocorp.com

Table 11. (Continued)

Provider	Address	Telephone/fax	E-mail/Website/telex
Narva	Brand-Ebisdorfer Lichtquellen-produktions- u. Vertriebsgesellschaft mbH Erzstr. 22 09618 Brand-Erbisdorf Germany	Tel.: +40-(0)-37322 – 17200/02 Fax: +49-(0)-37322 – 17203	Telex: 322401
Opto-Med GmbH	Rudower Chaussee 5 12489 Berlin Germany	Tel.: +49 – 030-63926540 Fax: +49 – 030-63926544	E-mail: wilkens@optomed.de
Philips Licht	Unternehmens-bereich der Philips GmbH Steindamm 94 20099 Hamburg Germany	Tel.: +49-(0)40 – 28992330 Fax: +49-(0)40 – 28993306	
PhotoThera-peutiX	1260 Palmetto Avenue, Suite C Winter Park FL 32789 USA	Tel.: +1 – 800-290 – 7577 Fax: +1 – 407-628 – 4160	E-mail: rayt@photothrx.com www.photothrx.com or www.homeUVB.com
Photomed Medizin-technik	Robert-Bosch-Str. 5 30989 Gehrden Germany	Tel.: +40-(0)5108 – 4032 +49 – 0172-5113994 Fax: +49-(0)5108 – 7002	
Polytec	Polytec Platz 1 – 7 76337 Waldbronn Germany	Tel: +49-(0)7243 – 6040	
Psoralite			www.psoralite.com
Psori-Med AG	Zürcherstr. 4 8952 Schlieren/ ZH Switzerland or Werner v. Siemens-Str. 62 64711 Erbach Germany	Tel.: +41 – 17322000 Fax: +41 – 17322001 Tel.: +49-(0)6062 – 1081 Fax: +49-(0)6062 – 62304	
Saalmann Lichttechnik	Werrestraße 94 32049 Herford Germany	Tel.: +49-(0)5221 – 2044 Fax: +49-(0)5221 – 27235	
Schulze and Böhm	Kölner Str. 160 50354 Hürth Germany	Tel.: +49-(0)2233 – 933232 Fax: +49-(0)2233 – 933234	E-mail: schulze.boehm@t-online.de www.medisun.de

Table 11. (Continued)

Provider	Address	Telephone/fax	E-mail/Website/telex
Sellas GmbH	Postfach 4029 58272 Gevelsberg Germany	Tel.: +49-(0)2332 – 61225 Fax: +49-(0)2332 – 61031	
Therakos Europe	The Braccans, London Road Bracknell, Berkshire RG 12 2 AT UK In Germany: Therakos Europe Postfach 1364 22803 Norderstedt Germany	Tel.: +44-(0)40 – 52866390 Fax: +44-(0)40 – 52866392	
Trautwein GmbH	Denzlinger Straße 12 79312 Emmendingen Germany	Tel.: +49-(0)7641 – 467730 Fax: +49-(0)7641 – 467770	
Herbert Waldmann GmbH and Co.	Postfach 3720 78026 Villingen-Schwenningen Germany in USA Waldmann Lighting Company 9 West Century Drive 00000 Wheeling, IL 60090 USA	Tel.: +49-(0)7720 – 601-0 Fax: +49-(0)7720/601290 Phone: +1 – 847-5201060 Fax: +1 – 847-5201730	
Wolff System AG	St. Alban-Anlage 29 4020 Basel Switzerland	Tel.: +41 – 61-2741050 Fax: +41 – 61-2741055	

Phototherapeutics

Table 12. Phototherapeutics providers

Provider	Address	Telephone/fax	E-mail/Website/telex
Galderma Laboratorium GmbH (previously: Basotherm)	Munzinger Str. 5 Postfach 600101 79111 Freiburg Germany	Tel.: +49-(0)761 – 45277-0 Fax: +49-(0)761 – 4762215	
Gerot-Pharmazeutika	Arnethgasse 1171 Wien Austria	Tel.: +43 – 1-453505	
Laboratoire Sun-Life	96, Route de Versaille 78460 Chevreuse France		
medac GmbH	Theaterstr. 6 22880 Wedel Germany	Tel.: +49-(0)4103 – 8006442 Fax: +49-(0)4103 – 8006466	www.medac.de
Dusa	181 University Ave. Suite 1208 Toronto, Ontario M5H 3M7 Canada		
Merck KG a.A	64271 Darmstadt Germany	Tel.: +49-(0)6151 – 720 Fax: +49-(0)6151 – 722000	
Phadimed	Industriestr. 40 44628 Herne Germany	Tel.: +49-(0)2323 – 17050 Fax: +49-(0)2323 – 13348	
pro medica	13, Rue Faraday 41260 La Chaussee St. Victor France		

Subject Index